Integrative Chinese Herbal Therapy

The Correspondences of

Dr. Lee Chen-Yu and **Dr. Juno Yang**

Volume III

Roots of Life

Gynecological and Obstetric, Pediatric, Psychological, Musculoskeletal, and Other Conditions

Compiled, Translated, and Authored by
Scott L. Herbster, OMD, LAc

Edited by Marc Wasserman, PhD, LAc

The teacher should never be concerned that a student might surpass him in ability; rather, the teacher should only worry that he doesn't guide the student well enough.

The process of learning is the root of discovery, so don't be hesitant about putting in the extra time and effort; in the end, you will realize it was worth it.

The more complex the pathocondition, the more imperative it is to provide an effective resolution. Though the etiology and pathomechanism may appear opaque at first, you must remain resolute in your efforts to accurately identify the pattern as the basis for administering the optimal treatment. That's the only way to advance the pursuit of scientific discovery and progress—continually striving to improve your fortitude and capacities in the art of medicine.

Dr. Lee Chen-Yu (李政育)

Dr. Lee Chen-Yu (李政育), OMD, LAc, PhD

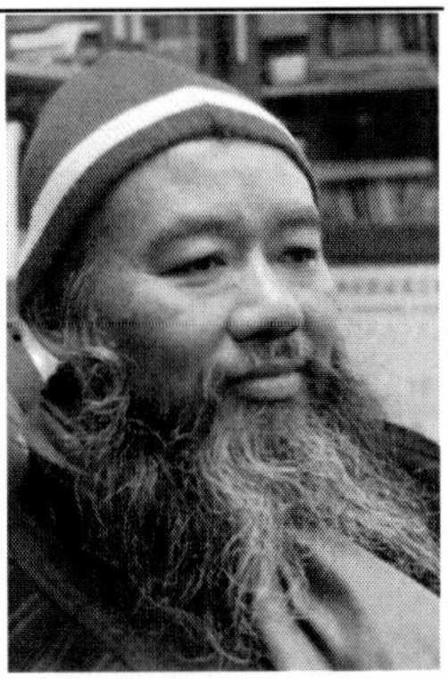

Dr. Lee Chen-Yu is an acclaimed traditional Chinese medicine physician who has practiced and conducted research for over 40 years. Renowned as a pioneering innovator at the forefront of integrative medicine, he is actively engaged in all specializations of clinical medicine. However, he is best known for his seminal research on neurology and oncology, receiving numerous U.S. patents for Chinese medicine formulas that promote nerve tissue regeneration and inhibit cancer cell growth. Dr. Lee is currently the Director of Yu Sheng Chinese Medicine Clinic (founded in 1980), and also serves as the Honorary Chairperson of the Taiwan Chinese-Western Medicine Neurology Association and Honorary PhD Advisor for Liaoning University of Traditional Chinese Medicine. He has authored more than 30 books, coauthored 10 others, written hundreds of professional papers, and been the subject of many masters and PhD dissertations. Dr. Lee has personally mentored hundreds of students from around the world and inspired the pursuit of new vistas in the applications of Chinese medicine.

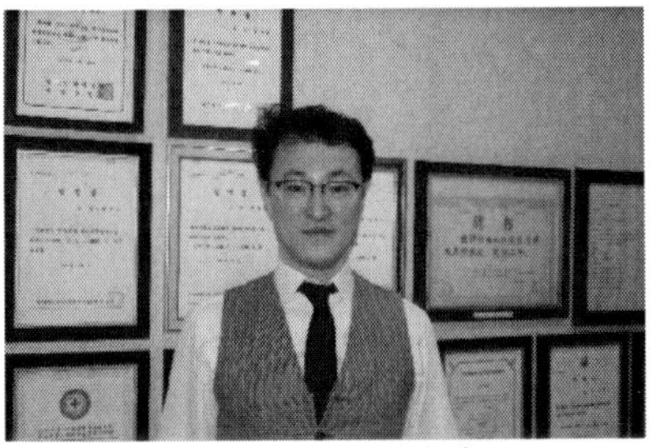

Dr. Juno Yang (梁珠勞), OMD, LAc, PhD

Dr. Juno Yang graduated from the prestigious College of Oriental Medicine at Kyung Hee University in 1998. He later went on to complete his Master of Science in Traditional Korean Medicine Pathology in 2003, and earned a PhD in Radiation Oncology from Ajou University in 2008. After his early years studying with Dr. Lee Chen-Yu, he has been very active writing innumerable professional papers, engaging in experimental research on integrative medicine, and presenting case studies at oriental medicine conferences worldwide. He has also authored three books titled Traditional Korean Medicine Therapies for Miscellaneous Diseases Vol. I (2008), Vol. II (2013), and Vol. III (2017). Dr. Yang is now the director of his own successful medical practice, Kyungheeyedang Oriental Medicine Clinic in Suwon City, near Seoul, South Korea.

ISBN: 978-0-9600303-2-3

TABLE OF CONTENTS

LIST OF CASE STUDIES

I. Gastrointestinal Disorders

Section 1: Liver

Section 2: Gallbladder

V. Neurological Disorders

VI. Hematologic Diseases

VII. Dermatological Disorders

Section 1: Atopic Dermatitis

Section 5: Other Gynecological Disorders

IX. Pediatrics

Section 1: Common Pediatric Disorders

ACKNOWLEDGEMENTS

Immeasurable appreciation and gratitude must be afforded to Dr. Lee Chen-Yu (李政育), whose unwavering guidance and dedication to his student's Dr. Juno Yang (梁珠勞), the compiler, translator, and author and editors of this series, and thousands of other aspiring traditional Chinese medicine (TCM) scholars and practitioners, has made this project possible.

Dr. Lee's nearly 40 years of clinical practice; clinical and laboratory research endeavors in both TCM treatment and integrative TCM and Western medicine; extensive affiliations and cooperation with Western medicine physicians; countless lectures, presentations, and papers; numerous books (both academic and mainstream); and health advocacy radio broadcast programs have reached out to touch the lives of millions of people worldwide. Much gratitude and respect must be given to Dr. Juno Yang, whose quest for knowledge and commitment to the clinical practice and research of TCM has made it possible for us to compile, translate and elucidate this invaluable material.

Further gratitude goes out to these fellow students and preceptees of Dr. Lee's: Frank Delaigue (an accomplished TCM practitioner with over 20 years of clinical experience) and Cyril Oswald (an aspiring TCM educator and practitioner), who together compiled and translated excerpts of this material for a French language book they co-authored titled *Les Hommes de l'Art*, which served as a valuable reference for this book; Dan Altschuler, EAMP, PhD (an acclaimed TCM educator and clinical practitioner with over 25 years of experience and currently a faculty member at the Seattle Institute of Oriental Medicine and Bastyr University), whose *Neuropathy: Traditional Chinese Herbal Treatment in a Modern Medical Environment* (English edition) served as a reference and inspiration for this book; and Chen, Ching-Hui (陳璟徽), OMD, MSc (aka "Big Brother Hui"), who has studied and served as an assistant of Dr. Lee's for nearly 30 years and has been an inexhaustible source of clarifying details about the clinical application of both TCM and integrated TCM and Western medicine.

Finally, a special thanks to Paulo Fonte, a talented physiotherapist and TCM practitioner, now practicing at Estoril Wellness Center in Estoril,

Portugal, whose professionalism and optimism is always a motivating influence on everyone around; and Matthew Stampe, a massage therapist and TCM student at the Virginia University of Oriental Medicine, for providing critical analysis for these books.

FOREWORD

"The teacher should never be concerned that a student might surpass him in ability; rather, the teacher should only worry that he doesn't guide the student well enough." As a pupil of Dr. Lee's, this is something you hear him say often. He doesn't keep secrets and he'll gladly share all of his wisdom with those willing to make a sincere effort.

This three-volume series is an extension of his mission to spread knowledge and healing. Readers will face the same challenges as those traveling thousands of miles to study in his clinic. The knowledge available from the case studies in this collection provides limitless opportunity for gaining clinical experience and opens ongoing opportunities for the practical application of integrated traditional Chinese medicine (TCM) and Western medicine in our modern medical environment.

The familiar nature of the correspondences, the focus on difficult cases, the meticulous translation of source text, and the scrupulous compilation of supplemental material all make for an ideal ongoing learning companion. You'll find it challenging, often getting stuck with questions of your own. This is part of the learning process; it allows for exploration of concepts and growth of new ideas. Anyone who has studied and worked with Dr. Lee has gone through it. Be patient, clarify questions in your mind, and continually search for answers both in this text and beyond.

TCM has always been a system that grows and evolves with each generation. This three-volume series will give you a substantive framework to build upon and find your own ways to innovate. You'll see the way Dr. Lee has updated classical prescription formulas to serve as effective treatments for the severe and intractable diseases of our current times. The balance between classical wisdom and adapting to modern medical trends is his expertise.

If you were to step foot in his clinic, you'd see someone who has mastered his craft. You'd see his ability to diagnose and treat difficult cases. You'd see the comfort and guidance he provides to patients.

And you'd see smiles on the faces of patients and staff. The brightness of his work compared to the gloominess of many medical settings speaks for itself.

I'm excited that this three-volume series makes a small part of the Yu Sheng Chinese Medicine Clinic available for everyone to experience.

Marc Wasserman PhD, LAc
September 2020

PREFACE

TCM Applications and Acceptance

Traditional Chinese medicine (TCM) continues resonating with potential—through a diversity of therapeutic modalities and vast pharmacopoeia, there are few limitations for its efficacy. The starkest limitations are from the institutional confines of academia and modern medicine in step with the pharmaceutical and insurance industries that seem more than often to be holding the reins. Of course, cultural factors also play a role in the acceptance of so-called "alternative" therapies, but based on the perpetual exchange of ideas, adaptation of peoples, and acculturation of societies throughout history, the viability and resounding efficacy of TCM has the persuasive power to overcome.

TCM Education and Status in Societies of Chinese (Han) Cultural Heritage

In societies influenced by Chinese culture (such as China, Taiwan, and South Korea) certified TCM (referred to as traditional Korean medicine (TKM) in South Korea) physicians are required to complete formal TCM medical school programs and pass national licensure examinations authorized by the respective nation's education oversight agency.

In China, 5- and 7-year bachelor's, master's, and doctoral programs are designed for students to receive a doctor of clinical medicine and doctor of integrated medicine, with the option of practicing both Western medicine and TCM and eligibility to take the respective national licensure examinations. In Taiwan, a 5-year post-baccalaureate and an 8-year bachelor's program are designed for students to receive a TCM degree in the former and the option of a dual degree in Western medicine and TCM in the latter, and eligibility to take the respective national licensure examinations. In South Korea, a 4-year post-baccalaureate and a 6-year bachelor's degree program are designed for students to receive a TKM degree and eligibility to take the national licensure examination.

The dual Western medicine and TCM degrees in China and Taiwan require students to fulfill all basic coursework in biomedicine and Western medicine specializations along with clinical internships in both Western medicine and TCM. For TCM (TKM) programs in Taiwan and South Korea, two-thirds of the curriculum focuses on coursework in basic biomedicine and specializations, comparative to the requirements for students in dentistry programs, and one-third on TCM, along with a clerkship in a Western medicine hospital and a clinical internship in the TCM department of a Western medicine hospital.

The relative emphasis on modern biomedicine and Western medicine specializations in the coursework load is balanced out by an intensive TCM curriculum that includes the classics and contemporary texts and their clinical applications. Based on my TCM academic pursuits in Taiwan and relationships with many TCM students, practitioners, and scholars, who have either received TCM educations or are educators themselves in countries such as China, South Korea, the United States, Australia, New Zealand, Israel, France, England, Switzerland, and Canada, I am confident that the depth and breadth of TCM curriculums in East Asian university TCM programs (at least in Taiwan, China, and South Korea) go far beyond that of TCM programs in other countries. To a large extent, this is due to an inherent cultural affinity that accepts this traditional medicine heritage as viable and effective.

There is no question that the institution of modern medicine is synonymous with Western medicine, but despite the enormous amount of funding and energies devoted to research and development, there are still glaring deficiencies. In Taiwan, China, and South Korea, this has opened up the opportunity for TCM to play a role as part of a unified medical system. Just as a major hospital may have dentistry and physiotherapy departments, they also have a TCM department. Indeed, this inclusion within the mainstream institution of modern medicine has in some ways been a boon, ensuring the perpetuation of this form of traditional medicine. However, there has been a price to pay with TCM serving a subservient role—recognized as more of a neoadjuvant, adjuvant, complementary, or palliative therapy—as opposed to primary and secondary care and first-line treatment.

There are still a few TCM physicians with clinical practices outside of the institutional healthcare system, who embrace the powers of integrated TCM and Western medicine, and have been able to achieve success at providing primary and secondary care and first-line treatment beyond the roles of adjuvant, complementary, and palliative therapy. Physicians such as Dr. Lee Chen-Yu (李政育), who have been dedicated to a lifetime of research, clinical practice, and educating, have gained due respect and elevated status within the medical community.

Backed by clinical experience and a thorough understanding of the advantages and disadvantages of Western medicine drugs and procedures, in certain cases Dr. Lee may advise patients to consult with their Western medicine physician about gradually reducing the dose and eventually discontinuing a given drug, or holding off on surgery if the side effects and potential complications outweigh the benefits—particularly if TCM offers a better therapeutic solution. Dr. Lee may also advise patients admitted to the hospital to receive a decocted TCM formula through their nasogastric (NG) tube, which requires both the consent of the patient (and/or family members) and the physician in charge.

Obviously, this type of consent and coordination requires a high degree of trust and communication. This poses significant challenges even in East Asian societies, with the legal ramifications that may arise if something unexpected happens. There is still a lot of work that needs to be done in establishing protocols and fostering universal acceptance. Evidence-based medicine research involving integrated TCM and Western medicine treatment is still sparse. However, based on both the results of evidence-based medicine studies and thousands of years of empirical clinical evidence, there is growing impetus towards recognizing the efficacy of TCM and integrated TCM and Western medicine in the treatment of a broad spectrum of diseases.

Know Your Medicinals and Define Your Paradigm

There is no single TCM medicinal or formula that *must* be administered for a specific symptom, pathocondition, or disease pattern. Classical and contemporary texts and the experience of mentors provide the foundations for the practitioner to clinically apply methodologies, but it is only through experience that dedicated physicians may develop their own paradigm. Medicinals of various properties and chemical constituents are grouped together in pairs and combinations—opposing and complementing, restraining and empowering, accentuating and corresponding—to form a formula composition whose overall action will resolve symptoms and promote the return and/or maintenance of homeostasis. In addition to personal preference based on clinical experience, a variety of factors may influence a TCM physician's selection of medicinals for a formula composition, such as availability, quality, price, storage, legal regulations, and patient preferences (taste, religion, customs, diet, etc.).

Medicinal processing plays an integral role in procuring the intended action, storage life, and mitigation of toxicity. If preparation methods are not tightly monitored and controlled, there could be potentially severe side effects (possibly even fatal). In times of antiquity, it was standard practice for TCM physicians to have their own raw medicinal processing facilities (or a close cooperative relationship with a licensed medicinal dispensary that specialized in preparing and processing medicinals) and dispensaries stocked with decocting pieces of their choice.

Nowadays, even in China, Taiwan, South Korea, and other Asian nations where TCM is a part of mainstream culture, the majority of physicians do *not* have their own processing facilities, and many do *not* even have onsite herbal dispensaries stocked with medicinal decocting pieces. Their medicinal dispensaries are more commonly stocked with medicinal extract powders/granules for the sake of convenience and regulatory oversight. In Taiwan, this is particularly prevalent, in part due to the National Health Insurance program (a single-payer system) that for the most part provides only *nominal* coverage for TCM treatment.

Dr. Lee is among the remaining TCM physicians who carry on the original spirit of the tradition, believing that you have to really "know your medicinals like the back of your hand" in order to fully utilize their best qualities, enhance their weaknesses, temper their volatilities, and harness the extent of their capacity for providing therapeutic efficacy.

Throughout the years, Dr. Lee's relationship with his pharmacopoeia has evolved as he continues to fine-tune his craft, modifying traditional formulas and designing his own to provide the optimal therapeutic regimen for his patients in Taiwan and across the globe. These formulas are referred to throughout the text, either explicitly or implicitly, as "(Yu Sheng)" formulas. Yu Sheng (育生)—literally meaning "the cultivation of life"—simply refers to the name of Dr. Lee's clinic.

Perspectives on the Four Examinations

The four examinations—*inspection*, *listening and smelling*, *inquiry*, and *palpation*—were first recorded in the Warring States period (475–221 BCE) nearly 2,500 years ago. Patient examinations are conducted to determine the correlation of all four examinations and then used to identify the pattern as the basis for determining treatment.

Depending on the type of symptoms, injury, and pathocondition, the four examinations are generally conducted in the following order: *inspection*—including the observation of skin, gait, mannerisms, complexion, color of stool and urine, and the tongue—offers an initial "look" at the patient and is the natural first step; *listening and smelling*—including the sound of speech and breath and the smell of the body, breath, and excretions—provides additional information and is the next natural step; *inquiry*—including patient history, chief complaint, diagnostic images, and lab test results—allows the physician to collect subjective and objective information and data about the patient's condition, which may often be the most valuable; and *palpation*—including touching and feeling the body to determine the presence of heat, tenderness, and accumulations, and also taking the pulse—enables the physician to get a "feel" for the patient's condition and is the last step.

As is often the case with experienced physicians, over the years Dr. Lee has developed a refined application of the four examinations with a keen sense for observing mannerisms, gait, skin manifestations, temperament, disposition, speech, and odor; discerning the nuances of history taking, performing abdominal palpation, and elucidating the significance of pulse.

Early on in Dr. Lee's clinical practice, he would rely on tongue examination much more, but throughout the years this reliance has diminished. He explained that the "natural" variations in size, color, texture, and fur among individuals, and the intake of food and beverages that stain the tongue and alter the appearance of the fur, make tongue examination an unreliable reference. In fact, if one observes Dr. Lee's patient interviews during consultations, you will notice that he rarely examines the tongue except for cases in which patients have pathology of the tongue or mouth proper.

Pulse-taking remains a hallmark of TCM examination and diagnostic protocol, and early on in Dr. Lee's clinical practice he authored a reputable academic book on this topic titled *Illustrated Traditional Chinese Medicine Pulse Reading* (圖解中醫脈學 *Tu Jie Zhong Yi Mai Xue*). Indeed, in its historical context pulse-taking is a vital source that opens up vistas into the discrete inner workings of the human body, revealing information about blood flow, volume, and viscosity; heart rate, cardiac output, and vascular patency; and the organs and physiological systems (endocrine system, autonomic nervous system, and central nervous system) of the entire body.

However, since the advent of modern biomedicine's diagnostic imaging and lab tests, which offer once unimaginable detail in its tangible images and quantitative data, the significance of pulse examination has in many regards been supplanted. This is compounded by the absence of a set, definable and quantifiable standard for interpreting the quality and nature of the pulse, with each individual potentially defining the *feeling* of a pulse differently. Though many well-intended TCM practitioners and devout patients who still cling to the nostalgia may disagree with this assessment, in my opinion pulse-taking is a relatively ambiguous *art* to practice. It is even more difficult to communicate with others, as one pulse-taker's description of a particular pulse may not be the same as another's, even though they may actually be *feeling* the same pulse! However, this doesn't entirely relegate its usefulness for the individual practitioner as a reference for conducting pattern identification, but its subjectivity does limit its function as conveyed to other individuals.

Yet another factor is the widespread administration of Western medicine therapeutic agents for patients with established illnesses and as preventive care. Many of these drugs have a direct affect on the autonomic nervous system and endocrine system, which regulate cardiovascular blood flow and the feedback mechanisms affecting vasoconstriction and vasodilation. The near ubiquitous administration of pharmaceuticals in our modern society makes the "drug pulse" (藥脈 yào mài) phenomenon that much more of a challenge to objectively discern the *feeling* of a pulse.

That said, just as it was applied traditionally, Dr. Lee takes each patient's pulse, records the reading in the patient's medical record, and uses these readings as a baseline for subsequent patient examination. In certain cases where the pulse reading is noticeably inconsistent with the other examination results—presenting signs and symptoms, lab tests, and diagnostic imaging findings—then the pulse may play a vital role in pattern identification (e.g., accurately discerning true and false and complex patterns).

TCM Terminology and Usage

Readers familiar with TCM may know that there are several commonly used terminology systems employed in the translation and explanation of TCM concepts.

I began studying Chinese contemporary and classical texts on subjects such as literature, philosophy, and religion in 1991. Since 2001, I have been focusing energies on studying and practicing TCM. These pursuits have led me through a five-year postbaccalaureate program at a prominent Taiwanese medical teaching college with an affiliated hospital, pursuing studies of classical and contemporary texts in Chinese and English on my own, and also working professionally as a translator of Chinese language TCM texts.

Through these experiences, I have explored the use of the various 'systems,' mixed and matched various 'systems,' and created my own complementary interpretations. At first, this 'trial and error' approach seemed innocuous enough; after all, the objective is simply to get the idea across, right? Well, the more I began to analyze and realize the seamless congruity and irrefutable underlying logic of Prof. Nigel Wiseman's TCM terminology "system," the more I became persuaded to get on board and adopt this lexicon.

Prof. Wiseman's TCM lexicon is the only comprehensive, standardized "system" to date. I find that this system most accurately articulates the original meaning of the source text. Perhaps this particular system appeals to my bilingual sensibilities, providing insight into the underlying historical usage and context of classical terms and expressions used to explain and describe this traditional medical science throughout the millennia.

Naturally, there are limitations in any system, and I admit that some of the usage may seem awkward or unorthodox for those not familiar with the system. But as stated above, the advantages of congruity far outweigh the occasional ambiguity and archaic flavor. It is the comprehensive nature of this system that I believe is the best format to convey and advance the valuable medical insights and scientific methodology of TCM. It may require a bit of getting used to and looking up some terms at first, but in the end, I am confident you will discover the "rhyme to this reason."

INTRODUCTION

This three-volume series comprises the collection of fax and e-mail correspondences between Dr. Lee Chen-Yu (李政育), recognized as one of Taiwan's most accomplished and prominent traditional Chinese medicine (TCM) physicians, and his dedicated student Dr. Juno Yang (梁珠勞) from South Korea. Nearly 40 years of clinical experience and insights are made readily available through these clear and concise interactions, offering practical antidotes for the clinical application of integrated TCM and Western medicine.

In 2000, Dr. Yang came to study under the mentorship of Dr. Lee Chen-Yu at Yu Sheng Chinese Medicine Clinic in Taipei, Taiwan (ROC). Following this period of immersed clinical study, he returned to South Korea where he started his own TCM clinical practice, gradually honing his capacities over the years until becoming confident and competent in treating patients with complex and severe pathoconditions.

At the onset, Dr. Yang lacked experience and thus had a lot of questions about how to accurately diagnose and effectively treat the broad scope of pathoconditions for which patients sought consultation and treatment. Thus, the student would correspond with his mentor by fax or e-mail seeking advice and guidance. Dr. Lee enjoyed sharing the knowledge gained from decades of study, research, and clinical experience. He further imparted the necessity for maintaining "a balance between prudence and confidence" and the importance of "continuing education and developing professional capacities" to make a positive impact on the lives of those who depend on our medical assistance.

This regular correspondence between Dr. Lee (mentor) and Dr. Yang (student) took place from 2001 up until 2008, and consequently these interactions formed the content and outline for the conception of this three-volume series. This material was originally packaged into case study format and published by Yuen Qi Zhai Publishing Co., Ltd. (Taiwan) in 2014 for the Chinese language popular health and wellness book audience under the title *Chinese and Western Integrative Medicine: Chinese Medicine Clinical Applications and Therapeutic Approaches—Volume I,*

II, III (中西結合:中醫臨床治療心法—上中下).

The compiler, translator, and author provides an adaptation of these case studies, devoting extensive efforts to adjust the formatting and presentation and incorporate further details and descriptions—including etiology and pathomechanisms, pattern identification, underlying basis of theoretical concepts and therapeutic approaches, medicinal actions and indications, pharmaceuticals and side effects, lab tests and imaging studies, and invasive and noninvasive procedures. By increasing the depth and breadth of content and making it more informative and authoritative, this three-volume series of case studies now targets the academic and professional audience (TCM students, scholars, and practitioners), as well as those laypersons interested in learning about the potential of Chinese medicine.

These case studies contain troves of information on TCM pattern identification as the basis for determining treatment; the clinical application of TCM medicinals, formulas, and acupuncture regimens; classical TCM pathologic terms and their correlating Western medicine nomenclature; background information on symptoms, diagnostic tests, and therapeutic modalities; and keys to differential diagnosis and prognosis.

The sheer magnitude of this material warranted division into a three-volume series, of which, this is the third and final volume compiled and translated into English. *Volume III Roots of Life* includes chapters on gastrointestinal (liver, gallbladder, spleen, and stomach), genitourinary (kidneys, urinary bladder), diabetes, musculoskeletal (tendonitis, osteomyelitis, fractures), neurological (atrophy, demyelination, neuritis, paresthesia, paralysis), hematologic (anemia), dermatological (atopic dermatitis, lichen, pustules, macules, papules, wheals, dyspigmentation, hyperhidrosis, hair loss), gynecological and obstetric (menstruation, ovaries, uterus, pregnancy, childbirth, postpartum), pediatric (developmental delays, Tourette syndrome, autism, attention deficit hyperactivity disorder), and psychological and psychiatric (psychogenic, psychosomatic, anxiety, depression, insomnia) disorders.

A wide range of other pathological conditions were previously published in *Volume I Beyond the Being* and *Volume II Surfaces in Motion* of this series. The compilation of case studies in this three-volume series covers the gamut of pathologies: oncology, neurology, orthopedics, pulmonology, dermatology, gastroenterology, hepatology, nephrology, endocrinology, cardiology, rheumatology, gynecology and obstetrics, urology, pediatrics, otorhinolaryngology, ophthalmology, hematology, metabolic disorders, proctology, palliative care, infectious diseases, and psychological and psychiatric conditions.

By no means does this series of case studies attempt to present a comprehensive analysis of all the pathological conditions TCM is capable of treating, either independently or through Western medicine integration. Its conception stems from the candid correspondence and guidance between a promising TCM physician (student) and an innovative spirit at the forefront of integrative TCM and Western medicine development (mentor). The scope of the pathological conditions and the descriptions of the cases presented here are simply derived from the questions a dedicated student has asked, seeking guidance from his mentor.

This material will serve as a valuable reference source for practical application—a catalyst that inspires the TCM practitioner to continue applying and integrating the classical traditions within our modern biomedical environment—and an insightful medium for those interested in learning about the vast potential of both the clinical applications of purely TCM and integrative TCM and Western medicine.

UNIT CONVERTER

In this text, the doses of medicinals are given in the traditional Chinese units (fen/qian/liang/jin). This measuring system may be less familiar to the Western reader than the metric system commonly used nowadays. Despite the necessity of an initial learning curve, I have chosen to preserve this element of the text in consideration of honoring the traditional way still practiced in the East. This unified system also provides a simple reading experience and avoids the need for in-text conversions or decimal points.

The gram (g) equivalencies are as follows:

1 fen = 0.375 g
1 qian (10 fen) = 3.75 g
1 liang (10 qian) = 37.5 g
1 jin (16 liang) = 600 g

I. GASTROINTESTINAL DISORDERS

Cases on hepatic diseases, such as hepatitis, cirrhosis, and hepatocellular cancer, were discussed previously in Volume II of this series. However, since these types of pathoconditions affect such a broad portion of the population and manifest in so many different ways, this chapter includes additional hepatobiliary disorders along with other diseases of the digestive tract involving the stomach and spleen.

Section 1: Liver

Case Study #1: Lamivudine Withdrawal Induces "Virologic Rebound"

Q: The first time I ever treated a patient with GPT (ALT) higher than 300 was someone with chronic hepatitis B virus (HBV). He explained that after discontinuing the antiretroviral medication lamivudine his GOT/GPT (AST/ALT), TBil, and DBil levels continued to soar. I prescribed Huang Lian Jie Du Tang (including large doses of The Three Yellows) adding Pu Gong Ying (1 liang each) and Jin Yin Hua (8 qian), but it wasn't effective.

Seeing this type of acute hepatitis case erupt so abruptly, with liver function indices soaring to such high levels, I couldn't sleep at all that night and stayed up researching information about this condition. I even thought about giving up on this case and referring the patient to a hepatologist.

How high can GOT/GPT levels reach before it can be considered dangerous? Will levels fall back down after the initial rise? Or will levels fluctuate in surges? What are the signs and/or symptoms that indicate TCM treatment has been effective? Please offer your advice and guidance.

A: These are what I call therapeutic drug withdrawal symptoms or "virologic rebounds." Lamivudine is a commonly administered drug for the treatment of HIV and hepatitis B (HBV). Regular administration effectively reduces GOT/GPT levels, resolves symptoms, and prevents exacerbations that could lead to more severe, life-threatening conditions (e.g., fulminant hepatitis, hepatomegaly). However, the downside of lamivudine is that once it has been completely discontinued, and no other adjuvant or remedial treatment is administered (e.g., TCM medicinals), then withdrawal symptoms may manifest with an abrupt "virologic rebound."

Based on my clinical experience, after complete withdrawal the majority of patients will incur withdrawal symptoms that may manifest abruptly within 1 week or appear up to 6 months (or only very rarely up to 3 years) later, with symptoms including severe hepatitis, hepatomegaly, *reversible* liver failure (aka acute liver failure

(ALF)/fulminant hepatitis), or even *irreversible* liver failure. At that time, the liver function indices may have returned to normal and it would appear the patient was well on the way to recovery, thus causing you (and other physicians) to fail to accurately identify the pattern and misinterpret the condition.

Remember! You can't simply rely on GOT/GPT levels to determine the presence and/or severity of liver disease. Typically, GOT/GPT fluctuate along with TBil and DBil levels, and in severe cases result in hepatorenal syndrome (HRS). If the serum BUN and Cr increase, then the patient may develop uremia; and if ammonia levels increase, then the patient could develop hepatic encephalopathy (HE) that may result in death. The best way to prevent the manifestation of these exacerbations ("rebounds") is to continue administering TCM medicinals, treating the underlying condition and regulating the constitution so the patient is able to safely ride through the storms of "virologic rebound."

In response to your question of how high GOT (normal range 0–40 u/L) and GPT levels (normal range 1–30 u/L) can reach before it is considered critical, there really is no exact number, but I have personally had a case where the GPT reached 3,000, and recently one patient reached 1,680. Each case is different for how high "rebound" (flare-up) levels reach, the tendency for recurrence and fluctuations, and the rate of progression back down to normal levels.

I once had an unusual "virologic rebound" case where the patient initially presented with GPT 1,000. After administering TCM medicinal treatment, levels dropped back down to normal, then suddenly, GPT levels spiked back up again to 800. As before, administration of TCM medicinals dropped levels back down, and then GTP levels jumped back up again to over 500. This sequence of events continued through 5 consecutive "rebounds" (flare-ups), up until the patient's condition finally stabilized and has remained that way for over 1 year now.

Typically, during the acute (flare-up) stage, the TCM formula composition must be modified accordingly up until GOT and GPT levels return to normal. And then, you must continue administering this formula for 1 to 2 months afterwards, evaluating lab test results to ensure that the condition has stabilized. Once the condition has stabilized, then you can begin reducing the dosage from 1 packet of decocting pieces per day (approx. 600 cc of decoction) to 1 packet over 2 days; and then gradually with time, 1 packet over 3 days, 4 days and so on. Evaluate lab test results after 2 months, and if they remain normal, then gradually discontinue administration.

Remember! Once the condition has stabilized and medicinals have been discontinued, you must advise the patient to avoid staying up late, get 8–10 hours of sleep each night, do *not* engage in strenuous overexerting exercise, do *not* drink alcohol or take any drugs (e.g., over-the-counter medications, folk remedies) without a physician's consent, and eat a healthy, well-rounded diet (i.e., grains, legumes, fruits, vegetables, meat, fish, seafood, eggs, and dairy products).

Case Study #2: Hepatitis During Pregnancy – Elevated GOT and GPT

Q1: This 33 y/o female chronic hepatitis B virus (HBV) patient is a mother of two children. She explained that 2 months after discontinuing administration of lamivudine her liver function tests (GOT and GPT) had increased. Her gastroenterologist then switched her over to adefovir, which resulted in an initial decrease and then an increase in GOT/GPT. Subsequently, she was referred to a hepatologist who prescribed pegylated interferon alpha 2a (PEG-IFN alpha-2a).

To everyone's surprise, her GOT and GPT levels gradually increased, and upon further examination, they discovered that she was already 5 months pregnant! The patient was concerned about the potential of adverse effects and also the high cost of the interferon drug, so she decided to seek TCM treatment. I prescribed the following formula regimen:

Week 1: Sheng Yu Tang adding Huang Qin (6 qian)

Week 2: Changed to Xiang Sha Liu Jun Zi Tang adding Huang Qin (8 qian), Ma Huang (1.5 qian), and Lian Qiao (8 qian)

Week 3: Changed to Huang Lian Jie Du Tang (including Huang Qin, Huang Lian, and Huang Bo (8 qian each) and Zhi Zi (5 qian)).

The strange thing is that after taking TCM medicinals her condition worsened. Over this period of administration her GOT/GPT levels gradually rose from 110/214, 118/184, 170/180, and 212/251. I am perplexed! Why would a chronic HBV patient's condition worsen during pregnancy? I have searched through pathophysiological texts and medical information online, but have found no logical connections.

I am wondering if the reason for these poor results is because I was overly cautious about the patient being pregnant, and either failed to include high enough dosages or chose the wrong medicinals. How would you proceed with this case? Please offer your advice and guidance.

A: Chronic HBV patients who have been prescribed lamivudine for long periods of time and happen to become pregnant, and then abruptly discontinue taking this drug due to concerns of adverse effects on the fetus will typically experience a "virologic rebound" within 1 week up to 6 months after withdrawal. In severe cases, the condition may develop into fulminant hepatitis (aka acute liver failure (ALF)). This type of antiretroviral medication really only offers short-term efficacy, while long-term administration in large doses can even lead to liver failure. In fact, long-term administration of most -dine and -vir classification of drugs will have an adverse effect on the fetus and may lead to liver cirrhosis and failure in the patient.

Interferon and adefovir offer about the same results. Based on statistical data, regardless of whether interferon and adefovir are administered independently or combined, this treatment only offers short-term efficacy. Efficacy following 6 months of administration is 30%, 1 year only 15%, and after 1 year the percentage dips below 10%.

That being the case, then by all means, the patient's pregnancy offers an opportune moment for TCM medicinal intervention to gradually discontinue and replace the Western medicine drugs. Naturally, complete discontinuation of these drugs may lead to a "virologic rebound," with markedly elevated liver enzyme levels that may be high enough to cause concern of developing into fulminant hepatitis. However, under the care of an experienced TCM physician, with accurate pattern identification as the basis of treatment, GOT and GPT levels will gradually fall and return to normal.

At the initial stage of "virologic rebound" resulting from withdrawal of hepatoprotective agents, I would prescribe a fire-draining toxin-resolving formula such as Huang Lian Jie Du Tang (including large doses of The Three Yellows (1 liang each)) adding Ma Huang, Lian Qiao, and Pu Gong Ying.

If this formula does *not* effectively lower GOT and GPT, then bleed the well points of the liver, spleen, and stomach channels—Yin Bai (SP1), Li Dui (ST45), and Da Dun (LV1)—and the corresponding back transport points (背俞穴 bèi shù xué) of the urinary bladder channel on the back—Gan Shu (UB18), Pi Shu (UB20), and Wei Shu (UB21). This should expedite the process and provide effective results.

If jaundice presents, then include large doses of Zhi Zi; and if loose stools present, add Bai Zhu, Fu Ling, and Ze Xie. If liver function levels initially decrease, but fail to continue progressing back down to normal levels, then you can consider changing the formula to Blood Desiccation Formula adding Wu Wei Zi, Huang Qin, and Shan Zha. Plus, you can also perform acupuncture (warm needle) on the following acupoints: Tai Chong (LV3), Zhong Feng (LV4), Tai Bai (SP3), Gong Sun (SP4), and San Yin Jiao (SP6).

Remember! The TCM medicinals that you prescribe for treating this condition are all non-toxic and mild in nature. There is *no* need to worry about any adverse effects on pregnancy and the fetus.

Q2: Thanks for your advice! I prescribed Huang Lian Jie Du Tang (including large doses of The Three Yellows (8 qian each) and Zhi Zi (5 qian)) adding Da Huang (0.5 qian) for this pregnant patient with lamivudine withdrawal "virologic rebound." GOT and GPT levels have already fallen back down to 220 and 250 respectively. I have regained some confidence!

A: I am also thrilled and proud of you! Remember! This serves as a good reminder: Virtually all types of Western medicine drugs administered over long periods of time will result in dependence and adverse effects, including the seemingly most innocuous of them, such as antacids and Compound Glycyrrhiza Mixture (a commonly prescribed expectorant and cough suppressant that also contains opium). Once medication is discontinued these patients are susceptible to withdrawal "rebound," which often manifests with even worse symptoms.

There are Western medicine drugs designed to limit the potential for "rebound," but most of these are classified as second- or third-line drugs and do *not* offer the efficacy of the first-line drugs. Conversely, TCM formulas and medicinal combinations offer flexibility to "customize" formulas for each patient's specific condition and pattern presentation at any given interval throughout the period of treatment.

However, this requires the care of a competent physician with ample knowledge of both TCM and Western medicine (e.g., anatomy, physiology, pathology, pharmacology) and ample clinical experience in the practice of integrative TCM and Western medicine. That is the only way to ensure that the patient will receive the best treatment possible.

Q3: As you advised, I prescribed Huang Lian Jie Du Tang (including The Three Yellows (1 liang each) and Zhi Zi (6 qian)) adding Pu Gong Ying (1 liang). After taking this formula the patient's GOT and GPT dropped down to 120 and 150, respectively, and platelet count (PLT) decreased from 108,000 to 92,000. She should be ready to give birth anytime now. Should I consider adding Gan Jiang and Rou Gui (or possibly Xi Lu Rong and Han Lian Cao)?

A: Withdrawal "rebound" following discontinuation of lamivudine can be identified as heat pattern, thus you should *not* add those great heat yang-supplementing medicinals (i.e., Gan Jiang, Fu Zi, Rou Gui, and Xi Lu Rong). When I first started my clinical practice about 30 years ago, I would prescribe Han Lian Cao, but later on the quality of this medicinal on the market here in Taiwan declined (stringy twigs and woolly leaves!), making me apprehensive about its efficacy. Thus I have *not* used it since. I *can* guarantee that The Three Yellows, Zhi Mu, Long Dan Cao, Lian Qiao, Jin Yin Hua, and Pu Gong Ying are effective. Just make sure to prescribe large doses!

These TCM medicinals are all mild and will *not* have any adverse effects on the pregnant mother or her fetus. During the postpartum period you may want to consider adding Sheng Du Zhong. If PLT continues to decline, simply add Xu Duan, Gu Sui Bu, and Niu Xi and the count will rise. Remember! You do *not* need to add Xi Lu Rong or Zhu Jie Qi*.

*Note: Zhu Jie Qi (竹節七/*Tupistra ensifolia* Wang et Tang/aka Zhu Qi) appears in *Selected Medicinal Plants of Yunnan* (雲南中草藥選 *Yunnan Zhong Cao Yao Xuan*). It has a bitter and slightly sweet flavor and cold nature, and heat-clearing toxin-resolving, blood-quickening pain-relieving, water-disinhibiting swelling-dispersing, and platelet count-increasing actions.

Q4: It's been 2 months postpartum now and the most recent lab test results for this patient are as follows: GOT/GPT 60/40 and PLT

113,000. Do you have any advice on what to look out for in the future?

A: You will always get good results through accurate pattern identification and prescribing adequate doses of the right medicinals. Remember! After discontinuing medication, such as lamivudine, adefovir, and interferon, a withdrawal "virologic rebound" may occur up to 3 to 5 times, manifesting as abrupt spikes in GOT and GPT levels. Administering TCM treatment right at the onset of the first "rebound" will rapidly stabilize the condition and also function as a preemptive measure that minimizes the severity of and potential for future "rebounds."

The TCM treatment regimen for these acute "rebounds" (or flare-ups) is as follows:

1) Bleed the well points of the liver, spleen, and stomach channels—Yin Bai (SP1), Li Dui (ST45), and Da Dun (LV1);
2) Perform acupuncture on Tai Chong (LV3), Zhong Feng (LV4), Nei Guan (P6), and Zu San Li (ST36);
3) Prescribe a fire-draining toxin-resolving formula such as Huang Lian Jie Du Tang (including large doses of The Three Yellows) adding Shan Zha and Gu Sui Bu; and
4) In cases of extremely high liver function tests, you can also bleed the corresponding back transport points (背俞穴 bèi shù xué) of the urinary bladder channel on the back—Gan Shu (UB18), Pi Shu (UB20), and Wei Shu (UB21).

Case Study #3: Ectopic Pregnancy Treatment Induces Hepatitis Flare-Up

Q1: A 35 y/o female patient with a history of chronic HBV had been administered lamivudine and adefovir without effective results. At the time she was 6 months pregnant and the liver function tests (GOT and GPT) were still 200 and 280, respectively, and PLT 90,000. She worried that the medication would have adverse effects on childbirth, so she decided to visit me for TCM treatment.

My first formula was Huang Lian Jie Du Tang variant, which effectively improved her condition, bringing liver function indices (GOT and GPT), PLT, and IgM antibody levels back to normal. Both of us were very happy about the positive results. Unfortunately, two years later GPT levels unexpectedly increased from 60, 104, 129, to 172, and following thorough testing and examination, ectopic pregnancy located in the left fallopian tube was discovered. Since T-Bil was only 1.4, her doctors decided against performing surgery and instead tried to treat the patient with medication (i.e., methotrexate (MTX).

My approach was the same as before, I prescribed Huang Lian Jie Du Tang variant, which resulted in bringing GPT back down to 75, but T-Bil increased to 1.94, 1.98, and 2.89. However, as I continued administering this formula, GPT gradually increased back up to previous highs (approx. 170), while T-Bil dropped back down (approx. 1.5).

Do you think this is a case of chronic hepatitis or cirrhosis? Could administration of methotrexate (MTX) induce idiopathic hepatitis or reactivate chronic hepatitis? What's the best approach for treating this patient? Please offer your advice and guidance.

A: From your description, it is difficult to definitively determine whether this is a case of idiopathic (drug-induced) hepatitis (e.g., acute hepatitis, hepatoxicity) or whether it is a reactivation of chronic hepatitis. Considering HBV had remained stable for 2 years and it has been so long since withdrawal from lamivudine and adefovir administration, I do *not* think this case involves reactivation of chronic hepatitis induced by lamivudine and adefovir withdrawal. It is common for a "rebound" (flare-up) in GPT levels to occur up to 6 months after withdrawal, but extremely rare for it to occur 1 to 2 years later, unless of course the patient has been reinfected.

Since it wasn't until *after* the patient presented with ectopic pregnancy and subsequently received treatment with MTX that GOT and GPT levels began gradually increasing, this strongly suggests idiopathic (drug-induced) hepatitis. Hepatic tumors may also cause a rise in liver function test levels, so you should advise your patient to have an ultrasound performed to rule out this possibility. Methotrexate (MTX) is a chemotherapeutic agent and immune system suppressant that can damage the liver. Almost all chemotherapeutic agents carry the risk of hepatic and renal toxicity, with adverse effects varying from dosage and each patient's unique condition and constitution.

Remember! Even though TCM medicinals are mild in nature compared to the adverse effects posed by Western medicine pharmaceutical agents, administered in excessive doses TCM medicinals may also have damaging effects on liver function. Thus, your formula composition must be well balanced, with the appropriate doses of medicinals possessing both mutually complementary and counteractive actions.

I recommend closely observing this patient for a period of time, having blood samples taken every 1–2 weeks to monitor GOT and GPT. The best approach for treatment during this stage is as follows:

1) Bleed the well points of the liver, spleen, and stomach channels—Yin Bai (SP1), Li Dui (ST45), and Da Dun (LV1)—and the corresponding back transport points (背俞穴 bèi shù xué) of the urinary bladder channel on the back—Gan Shu (UB18), Pi Shu (UB20), and Wei Shu (UB21);
2) Needle Tai Chong (LV3), Zhong Feng (LV4), and Nei Guan (P6); and
3) Prescribe a fire-draining toxin-resolving formula such as Huang Lian Jie Du Tang adding Shan Zha, Gu Sui Bu, Dan Shen, Chi Shao, and The Four Lings (Fu Ling, Cang Zhu, Zhu Ling, and Ze Xie). These additions will clear away the metabolic waste resulting from the break down of inflammatory factors that would otherwise encapsulate the inflamed hepatocytes and prevent the medicinals from promoting further therapeutic actions.

This well-balanced three-step therapeutic approach functions like a "radar" that allows the medicinals to detect, zoom in on, target, and destroy the enemy! The pharmacodynamics involved in the clinical effectiveness of TCM medicinals in the treatment of this pathocondition are as follows:

- Heat-clearing toxin-resolving medicinals function as an anti-inflammatory and also inhibit the viability of mutant cells;
- Blood-quickening and stasis-transforming medicinals inhibit the enemy's vascular endothelial growth factor (VEGF) involved in angiogenesis and a host of other related enzymes; and
- Dampness-disinhibiting by bland percolation medicinals promote the dehydration of mutant cells, thus reducing their viability, and open up pathways for the TCM formula to attack the DNA of these mutant cells, thus eradicating them.

Q2: I have another question about this chronic HBV patient whom incurred a sudden spike in GPT levels after receiving treatment with methotrexate (MTX) for ectopic pregnancy (tubal pregnancy in the left fallopian tube). After following through on your advice by administering Huang Lian Jie Du Tang (including large doses of The Three Yellows) adding Pu Gong Ying and Lian Qiao, initially GOT and GPT decreased, but then rose back up again.

Subsequently, the patient underwent further examination at a hospital which revealed mild hepatic cirrhosis, and afterwards I decided to modify my original Huang Lian Jie Du Tang formula by including larger doses of The Three Yellows (8 qian each) and adding Shan Zha, Gu Sui Bu, Fu Ling, Ze Xie, Chi Shao, and Dan Shen.

Why is methotrexate (MTX) prescribed for the treatment of ectopic pregnancy (aka tubal pregnancy)? Is its action directed at opening up the occlusion in the fallopian tube?

A: This sounds like a case where the chronic HBV was rendered inactive, but the administration of MTX for the treatment of ectopic pregnancy induced a flare-up causing reactivation of chronic hepatitis (i.e., drug-induced hepatitis). In this situation, you must administer a three-step therapeutic approach—bleeding, needling, and prescribing medicinals. Once the flare-up peaks, the inflammation will gradually resolve.

Mild cirrhosis may indicate a certain degree of fibrosis, but the condition has *not* evolved into full-blown cirrhosis. Many heat-clearing with cold and bitterness medicinals will effectively treat hepatitis, including the formula you prescribed above. Just remember! Long-term administration of Zhi Zi may cause transient blue-gray or bronze skin dyspigmentation. You should advise the patient about the potential for this cosmetically unappealing adverse effect, and if you notice any signs of skin discoloration, then immediately subtract this medicinal from your formula composition.

MTX was originally used as a chemotherapeutic agent (e.g., breast, skin, lung cancer) and immune suppressant (e.g., rheumatoid arthritis, psoriasis) and is now also administered for the treatment of ectopic pregnancy, hydatidiform mole (aka molar pregnancy), endometriosis, and increased follicle-stimulating hormone (FSH) and □-hCG concentrations. MTX treats ectopic (tubal) pregnancy by inhibiting nucleic acid synthesis, thus effectively killing the rapidly dividing ectopic trophoblast. However, liver disease is one the main contraindications of MTX and there is a significant possibility for this drug to have adverse effects on a patient such as yours.

Tubal occlusion (with or without ectopic (tubal) pregnancy) can be classified as:

1) Phlegm-heat pattern—Administer a Shao Yang depressed heat-clearing and phlegm turbidity harassing the inner body-dispelling formula such as Wen Dan Tang adding Ge Gen, Mai Men Dong, and Lai Fu Zi; or
2) Static blood pattern—Administer either a blood-nourishing blood-quickening, stasis-dispelling pain-relieving, and network vessel-freeing channel-regulating formula, such as Ru Mo Si Wu Tang; or a blood-breaking, channel-freeing, pain-relieving, and liver- and kidney-supplementing formula, such as Tong Jing Fang. This approach will provide effective treatment for this pathocondition.

Case Study #4: Hepatitis During Pregnancy – Fortify the Spleen, Resolve the Exterior, and Clear Heat

Q: I have another patient (32 y/o) who has hepatitis and is now pregnant. Her most recent liver function tests are as follows: GOT 168, GPT 200, and PLT 104,000 (down from 110,000 about 1 month ago).

I prescribed Sheng Yu Tang adding Huang Qin (6 qian), but liver enzyme levels did not decrease. Do you think I should change the formula to Ma Huang Lian Qiao Chi Xiao Dou Tang? What dose of Lian Qiao would you recommend?

A: For patients with hepatitis and low PLT count during pregnancy, prescribing Sheng Yu Tang (supplements blood and qi, dispels stasis, and nourishes yin) does *not* sound like a good idea. The yang jaundice with exterior pattern formula Ma Huang Lian Qiao Chi Xiao Dou Tang (resolves the exterior and promotes sweating and clears heat and disinhibits dampness) is more in the right direction for sure!

If the patient has a poor appetite and poor digestion, I would consider prescribing a qi-boosting spleen-fortifying and qi-moving phlegm-transforming formula such as Xiang Sha Liu Jun Zi Tang adding Huang Qin, and Ma Huang and Lian Qiao (the respective sovereign and minister medicinals in Ma Huang Lian Qiao Chi Xiao Dou Tang).

In fact, if the patient has a good appetite and healthy digestion, I would even consider prescribing a fire-draining toxin-resolving formula such as Huang Lian Jie Du Tang adding Ma Huang and Lian Qiao, which is directly aimed at treating the root (治本 zhì b□n)—liver inflammation. In a cold climate like South Korea, it is common for patients to tolerate a relatively large dose of Ma Huang (3 qian); and for Lian Qiao, I would consider initially prescribing up to 3–5 qian, but it really depends on the patient's constitution and condition.

Recently, I have been treating a patient with buccal carcinoma. On the patient's initial visit, the tumor had already ulcerated, with multiple nodules producing exudation and pus. As my treatment regimen progressed it was necessary to prescribe Lian Qiao (4 liang) and Wan Ling Dan (20 pills/3x/day) in order to make headway in attempting to get the condition under control. This is an example of what I mean by my mantra: "Design your formula composition based on each patient's unique constitution, presentation of signs and symptoms, the stage of the pathocondition progression, and identification of the resulting pattern that manifests."

Case Study #5: Hormone Replacement Therapy – Induces Spike in GOT and GPT

Q1: A 51 y/o female patient having a history of chronic hepatitis B infection (HBV) presented with liver depression and blood stasis pattern. I prescribed Ru Mo Si Wu Tang adding Gan Jiang, Fu Zi, Rou Gui, Chuan Qi, Huang Qin, Ma Huang, and Di Long. To my dismay, after only taking several days of this formula GOT and GPT soared up to 200.

This unexpected spike made the patient lose some confidence in my capacity to provide effective treatment and wedged some awkwardness into her follow-up visit. Actually, I thought that my prescription was very conservative and prudent, with only small dose of Ma Huang (1 qian) and Fu Zi (3 qian) plus a bit of Huang Qin (3 qian). Do you think it is conceivable this could have caused a flare-up in a patient with preexisting chronic hepatitis? What's the best way to approach this type of patient?

A: This suggests that your patient has preexisting chronic *active* hepatitis. It is *possible* that your original blood-nourishing blood-quickening, stasis-dispelling pain-relieving, and network vessel-freeing channel-regulating formula adding The Three Great Yang-Supplementers (Gan Jiang, Fu Zi, and Rou Gui) could have induced this sudden spike!

If you want to continue prescribing Ru Mo Si Wu Tang, then you need to subtract The Three Great Yang-Supplementers and add large doses of The Three Yellows—Huang Qin (8 qian–1 liang), Huang Lian (5 qian), and Huang Bo (5 qian). Or, you could simply change the formula to a fire-draining toxin-resolving formula such as Huang Lian Jie Du Tang combining Ru Mo Si Wu Tang adding Niu Xi, Sheng Du Zhong, Ma Huang, and Di Long. These approaches should prove effective in improving symptoms and ensuring that the chronic hepatitis does *not* reactivate and cause irreversible damage to the liver.

Typically, the treatment objective for chronic active hepatitis is to reduce inflammation and lower GOT (0–40 u/L) and GPT (1–30 u/L) levels. Once the enzyme levels drop back to normal, you should still continue administering this formula for 3–5 more weeks. After that, you can change back to your original blood-nourishing blood-quickening, stasis-dispelling pain-relieving, and network vessel-freeing channel-regulating formula.

Q2: Whew!...after undergoing follow-up examination and further investigation, Western medicine doctors determined that the cause of this patient's spike in liver enzyme levels was due to administration of female hormones (i.e., hormone replacement therapy (HRT)) for menopause and not a flare-up of chronic hepatitis.

A: Now that you know HRT is the cause of elevated liver enzyme levels, naturally, you should advise the patient to gradually discontinue this treatment and administer TCM medicinals instead. I would consider prescribing your original formula Ru Mo Si Wu Tang subtracting The Three Great Yang-Supplementers and adding large doses of The Three Yellows.

If menopausal symptoms of tidal heat, palpitations, dizziness, and insomnia present, then consider adding combinations of Qing Hao,

Zhi Mu, and Di Gu Pi; Sheng Long Gu and Sheng Mu Li; Gan Cao and Long Yang Rou; Tian Ma; Zi He Che (powder); and Yu Sheng Wan.

This approach will effectively reduce and maintain normal GOT and GPT levels and resolve the menopausal transition symptoms.

Case Study #6: Steep in Rice Wine and a Bit of Vinegar

Q: I have a 53 y/o female patient with a history of chronic active HBV. She is the same patient that I administered TCM treatment to over a period of time about 2 years ago, successfully resolving symptoms and reestablishing healthy liver function. Recently, she came back for a visit, with lab tests once again indicating elevated GPT levels.

I prescribed Huang Lian Jie Du Tang (subtracting Zhi Zi) adding Da Qing Ye, Ban Lan Gen, Dan Shen, and Chi Shao (formula composition first steeped in wine and then decocted) at a dosage of 3 packets of decocting pieces per week*. After 2 weeks of treatment, GPT levels have already dropped down from 330 to 108 (normal range 1–30 u/L). Do you think I should continue prescribing this same formula?

A: Huang Lian Jie Du Tang variant for the treatment of a chronic hepatitis flare-up will offer excellent efficacy, especially if you first steep the medicinals in rice wine before decocting. Now, it is evident that you really have a firm grasp of my therapeutic concepts and methodology! Steeping the decocting pieces in rice wine prior to decoction enables the procurement of higher levels of the bioactive constituents in The Three Yellows and enhances the blood-supplementing actions of Dan Shen and Chi Shao.

If a flare-up occurs after liver enzyme levels had dropped back down to normal, then I would also add 2–3 tablespoons of distilled white vinegar (liver channel conductor medicinal) during decoction. Once levels return to normal, then you can return to decocting as normal. Distilled white vinegar also enhances the blood-quickening stasis-dissipating and qi-moving actions of Dan Shen and Chi Shao and promotes the body's absorption of the bioactive constituents in these medicinals, which may be necessary if the gastrointestinal tract or accessory organs involved in digestion are compromised.

This just goes to show you that in addition to understanding each medicinals' nature, flavor, qi, and channel entry, you must also know their distribution, varieties, harvest season, preparation and decoction methods, and how the individual actions of each medicinal combine in opposing or complementary relationships to form the overall formula composition!

*Note: Typically, 1 packet of decocting pieces is boiled in approximately 1,200 cc (depending on the types and amount of medicinals) of water down to approximately 600 cc of decoction and administered as a standard 1-day dosage (200 cc/3x/day).

Case Study #7: "Hematologic" Fibrotic Change – Prescribe Xiang Sha Liu Jun Zi Tang Variant

Q: A 40 y/o female patient explained that she first tested positive for hepatitis B virus (HBV) about 20 years ago, and has tried all types of medication, but nothing has proven effective.

Recently, a computed tomography (CT) scan showed that her spleen had enlarged by 6 cm (10 yrs ago it was 15 cm and now it is 21 cm). GOT, GPT, and AFP (alpha-fetoprotein) tumor marker index were all normal; T-Bil was elevated at 1.60 (0.2–1.2 mg/dL); PLT was very low at 58,000 (150,000–400,000 μL); and she has had sloppy stools with poor appetite.

I prescribed Xiang Sha Liu Jun Zi Tang adding The Three Great Yang-Supplementers (Gan Jiang, Fu Zi, and Rou Gui), Fu Ling, Huang Qin, Zhi Zi, Ren Shen, and Chuan Qi. Do you think this is a good approach? Please offer your advice and guidance.

A: Normal levels of GOT, GPT, and AFP in this patient with chronic active HBV and splenomegaly indicates rapid hepatocyte damage, lysis, or fibrotic change, and suggests the presence of "hematologic" liver fibrosis. You should closely monitor T-Pro, A/G (albumin/globulin) ratio, and BUN and creatinine levels to ensure you can make the optimal formula modifications necessary to prevent the onset of hepatorenal syndrome (HRS) and edema. The cause of the splenomegaly is likely due to hematological abnormalities (e.g., congenital, genetic, immune-mediated blood cell, or myeloproliferative disorders).

For these types of patients, I typically prescribe Xiang Sha Liu Jun Zi Tang, gradually increasing the dose of Da Huang up until the patient maintains 2–3 stools/day. Considering your patient's low PLT count, I would subtract Chuan Qi and Ren Shen from your original formula and add Xi Lu Rong (invigorates kidney yang, boosts essence-blood, regulates the thoroughfare and controlling vessels, and promotes homatopoeisis) and wine-steeped Zhu Jie Qi (clears heat and resolves toxin, quickens the blood and relieves pain, disinhibits water and disperses swelling, and increases platelet count) instead. You could also consider changing your formula to Sheng Yu Tang adding The Three Great Yang-Supplementers, Ren Shen, Huang Qin, Bai Zhu, Fu Ling, Ze Xie, Xi Lu Rong, Zhu Jie Qi, Shan Zha, and Ji Nei Jin. Either approach should provide effective results.

Case Study #8: Benign Hepatic Cyst – Typically Does *Not* Require Treatment

Q: A benign hepatic cyst was found incidentally following a routine physical examination of this 48 y/o male patient. Aside from slight fatigue and mild tenderness along the right hypochondriac region, he has *no* other signs or symptoms. Do you think this patient needs treatment?

A: Benign hepatic cysts are typically asymptomatic so it would seem unlikely that it is causing fatigue and tenderness. With that in mind, I think this may be a psychosomatic disorder or chronic fatigue syndrome (CFS) (both of which are pathoconditions that commonly affect urban dwellers!), or possibly intercostal neuralgia.

Frankly, considering it is a relatively asymptomatic benign hepatic cyst, you really do *not* need to initiate treatment. However, many Asians, especially older people, feel like the physician is "neglecting" them or that they are somehow being "diminished" if treatment is *not* administered (even though they may really *not* even need it!).

If this is the case with your patient, then you can consider prescribing either a spleen- and stomach-supplementing, phlegm-damp-transforming, and blood-nourishing wind-stabilizing formula such as Ban Xia Tian Ma Bai Zhu San adding Gan Cao, Long Yan Rou, Yan Hu Suo and Mu Xiang (quicken the blood, move qi, and relieve pain), and Yu Sheng Wan; a heat-clearing and phlegm-damp-transforming water-disinhibiting formula such as Chai Ling Tang adding Ren Shen (powder) and Yu Sheng Wan; or an exterior-interior resolution and concurrent elimination of cold formula such as Chai Hu Gui Zhi Tang adding Ru Xiang, Mo Yao, and Chuan Qi, and if necessary, San Leng, E Zhu, Yan Hu Suo, and Bin Lang (break blood and move qi and disperse accumulations and relieve pain).

Remember! You should advise the patient to have an ultrasound performed every 3–6 months to follow-up on any changes or complications.

Case Study #9: Automobile Accident – Hepatomegaly, Jaundice, and Dark Stool

Q: A 42 y/o male with a history of duodenal ulcer got into an automobile accident 2 weeks ago injuring his lower back and was admitted into the hospital for 1 week of treatment and follow-up examination. After being released from the hospital, he has suffered from right hypochondriac distention and pain, glomus below the heart (心下痞 x□n xià pi), jaundice (T-Bil 6.6), and dark stool. How would you treat this patient?

A: For this patient who incurred a traumatic injury from an automobile accident 2 weeks ago, I would prescribe a blood-nourishing blood-quickening, stasis-dispelling pain-relieving, and network vessel-freeing channel-regulating formula such as Ru Mo Si Wu Tang adding Huang Qin, Chuan Qi, Mu Dan Pi, and Zhi Zi.

Remember! Hepatomegaly alters normal blood flow in the abdominal region and may result in congestive disorders involving the GI tract and heart, which makes the patient susceptible to hemorrhage. So be sure to inform the patient of these potential complications and encourage him to continue following up with lab tests and imaging studies.

Case Study #10: TCM Medicinals Inhibit RNA Synthesis and Formulas Offer Antiviral Effects

Q: There was an article in the June 2003 issue of the *Journal of Integrative Chinese-Western Medicine Neurological Association* that presented the results of experimental research on 20 heat-clearing toxin-resolving medicinals, including Long Dan Cao, Shan Dou Gen, Huang Qin, Zhi Zi, and Ku Shen. I was surprised to read that despite having the action of inhibiting RNA synthesis, these medicinals do *not* contain antiviral properties.

This seems strange to me, because in clinical practice these types of heat-clearing toxin-resolving medicinals irrefutably offer antiviral effects. Why would the results of this experiment indicate otherwise? Please offer your advice and guidance.

A: In my humble opinion, I think it *may* be possible for single medicinals to inhibit viral hepatitis (e.g., HCV, HBV), but only with *limited* efficacy. I have cooperated with other university professors and Western medicine physicians on conducting both animal and human experiments and the results have always shown that a major or compound formula far exceeds the efficacy of administering a single medicinal. Of course, it's also possible that there are discrepancies between the cell line and virus strain tested in the experiment compared with how viruses manifest in the human body.

As for pharmacodynamics, the heat-clearing toxin-resolving medicinals used in this study likely "slow down" the cycle of viral proliferation by disrupting the RNA synthesis of the virus after it has entered the host cell, thus inhibiting the capacity of the viral nucleic acid to redirect ("hijack") the metabolism of the host cell. "Slowing down" the cycle of viral proliferation effectively "buys time" for the TCM medicinal formula (composition containing multiple medicinals) to initiate therapeutic actions and for the body's immune system to "gather forces" to directly fight the virus.

But remember! Worm-killing medicinals, such as Xiong Huang and Liu Huang, *do* indeed contain properties that directly kill microbes (bacteria, virus, and fungi). However, due to the risk of adverse effects caused by their toxic nature, if prescribed for oral administration, they can only be prescribed in miniscully small doses within a well-balanced formula composition, or applied sparingly for external application (e.g., topical application of Xiong Huang for the treatment of herpes zoster skin rash).

Depending on the specific case, a well-rounded formula composition may also include medicinals that function to boost the immune system (e.g., spleen-, qi-, kidney yang-supplementing medicinals), which heightens the body's capacity to fight the invaders (e.g., microbes, cancer cells). I encourage you to continue exploring and discovering the wonders of TCM. Let's go!

Case Study #11: Acute HVA Infection – Stay Vigilant for Rapid Fluctuations

Q: A 25 y/o male was diagnosed with hepatitis A (HAV) infection (confirmed through blood tests), and at the onset presented with generalized jaundice. Liver function tests were performed regularly to monitor the condition, with the results as follows: GOT/GPT (0–40 u/L)/(1–30 u/L) was initially 2,650/4,076, and decreased to 900/2,289 and then 77/128; and T-Bil (0.2–1.2 mg/dL) was initially 8.5, and increased to 13.1 and then 21.

I prescribed Huang Lian Jie Du Tang (including Huang Qin (8 qian)) adding Da Huang (1 qian), Da Qing Ye, and Ban Lan Gen. Subsequently, liver function tests showed GOT/GPT 80/73 and no data for T-Bil. After taking my formula, the color of the patient's urine lightened (it had been dark) and the patient maintains 2–3 stools/day. How would you proceed from here?

A: In cases where the acute stage of HAV infection resolves with GOT/GPT levels coming back down, but total bilirubin (T-Bil) continues to rise (hyperbilirubinemia), you must be vigilant of the possibility for acute liver failure (ALF) developing.

If a fire-draining toxin-resolving formula, such as Huang Lian Jie Du Tang adding large doses of Zhi Zi, is *still* unable to bring down bilirubin levels, then you should consider adding Mu Dan Pi and Di Gu Pi (cool and quicken the blood) and Chuan Qi (quickens the blood and transforms stasis). If T-Bil levels *still* do not come back down, then consider adding The Three Great Yang-Supplementers, or change to a liver channel blood-supplementing formula such as Sheng

Yu Tang, Xue Ku Fang, or Qi Bao Mei Ran Dan adding Zhi Zi, Wu Wei Zi, Gan Jiang and Fu Zi (starting out at small doses and incrementally adding if necessary), and Huang Qin (counterbalances the heat). Also, advise the patient to have liver function tests performed every 2–3 days in order to closely monitor the condition.

Remember! Administration of TCM medicinals for patients presenting with acute liver failure (ALF) may initially reduce bilirubin levels, but then abruptly spike back up again. Thus, you must closely monitor the condition and be prepared for all potential outcomes. It may even be necessary to ask the patient's family members to have blood cross-matching tests performed just in case the patient does need a liver transplant at some point.

You must continually modify your formula composition in response to changes in liver function tests and complete blood count (CBC). In the event that hepatorenal syndrome (HRS) or hepatic encephalopathy (HE) arises, your first line of treatment should be (Yu Sheng) Wu Ling San (Nephritis Formula) variant.

Case Study #12: Allergic Purpura – Hepatorenal Syndrome

Q: A 15 y/o female diagnosed with Henoch-Schönlein purpura (HSP) (aka anaphylactoid purpura, IgA vasculitis, or purpura rheumatica) recently visited me. Her father explained that when the patient was 10 y/o she caught what at the time they thought was simply a common cold, but later developed into nephritis (proteinuria), and eventually she was diagnosed with HSP.

She presented with non-palpable purpura (reddish-purple spots that look like bruises (petechiae and ecchymoses) on the back of both lower legs and palpable purpura (vasculitis) on the front of both lower legs. She has tried the gamut of Western medicine treatments (i.e., steroids, anti-inflammatories, analgesics) as well as TCM treatment, saying that the TCM treatment effectively relieved symptoms for a period of time, but the symptoms eventually came back strong again. How would you treat this patient? Please offer your advice and guidance.

A: Patients with progressive Henoch-Schönlein purpura (HSP) that fails to resolve are susceptible to developing severe kidney disease (e.g., nephritis, nephrotic syndrome, kidney failure), and in some patients liver involvement may occur, resulting in hepatorenal syndrome (HRS) that could lead to hepatic cirrhosis, fulminant hepatitis, and liver cancer.

In these types of patients, depending on the presenting signs and symptoms (e.g., extent of low serum albumin levels, edema, nutritional status) and pattern, I would consider prescribing either Wu Ling San (Nephritis Formula) (including large doses of Fu Ling and Ze Xie) adding Ren Shen/Chuan Qi Powder and Xi Lu Rong; or Chai Ling Tang (including large doses of Fu Ling and Ze Xie) adding Gan Jiang, Fu Zi, Huang Qi, and possibly Si Shen Tang. And if GOT/GPT remain high then make sure to add large doses of The Three Yellows.

Remember! You must also be aware that patients who discontinue long-term administration of corticosteroids may incur a "withdrawal rebound" with exacerbations in symptoms, requiring you to modify your formula to provide effective relief and expedite the recovery process. Once the patient's condition stabilizes, then you can gradually discontinue administration of TCM medicinals.

Section 2: Gallbladder

Case Study #1: Small Gallbladder Polyps and Peptic Ulcer – Surgery *Not* Necessary, Just Treat the Ulcer

Q: A 40 y/o female visited me with a chief complaint of poor appetite and indigestion. Suspecting gastrointestinal tract etiology, I advised her to have an ultrasound performed with the results showing two small polyps and also a gastric ulcer. I prescribed Xiao Chai Hu Tang adding a large dose of Dang Gui (8 qian), Chuan Qi, Da Huang, and Hai Piao Xiao. Do you think this is a good approach?

A: For cases of small (≤ 1 cm) benign cysts or solitary gallbladder polyps in the *absence* of symptoms such as fever, pain and distention in the abdominal and/or hypochondriac region, abdominal glomus and hardness, nausea, and vomiting, it's *not* necessary to initiate aggressive intervention, or any type of treatment for that matter. These small polypoid growths are simply abnormal accumulations of mucous membrane tissue that may remain in the body without any symptoms or complications.

Any type of surgery, whether it be minimally invasive (e.g., laparoscopic) or open, runs the risk of infection. So, unless the patient has other notable risk factors (e.g., primary sclerosing cholangitis, cystic duct obstruction) that may preclude a potential for malignancy, either a *non-invasive* therapeutic approach or *none at all* would suffice.

Modern medicine abounds with all sorts of high tech instruments, devices, and pharmaceuticals. There seems to be a tendency, at least here in Taiwan anyways, for physicians to send patients to the operating table or take potent drugs even though a particular pathocondition really doesn't warrant such invasive, extreme treatment. This not only is a waste of resources, but may result in unnecessary adverse effects that are much more detrimental to the patient's health than the completely benign condition it attempts to treat. It seems somewhat ironic to me that I always remember one of the mantras of Western medicine being "the best treatment is observation." Oftentimes, though not always, as long as the lesion has *not* yet formed or there is uncertainty as to whether or not it will eventually form at all, these treatments are completely unnecessary.

Of course, if the patient presented with symptoms of fullness and pain in the stomach duct and abdomen, hard glomus below the heart (epigastric region), and/or vomiting, which strongly suggest peptic ulcer, then I would treat the peptic ulcer accordingly and *not* worry about the benign gallbladder polyp(s). On the other hand, if the patient visited me with results of an endoscopy revealing a gastric ulcer in the *absence* of any signs (other than macroscopic appearance) or symptoms whatsoever, then I would likely *not* even administer treatment at all.

If the patient presents with symptoms of clamoring stomach (嘈雜 cáo zá), including pain on an empty stomach, dull pain that at times is imperceptible and at times gnawing, and a feeling of hunger but no desire to eat, then I would prescribe a fire-draining toxin-resolving formula such as Huang Lian Jie Du Tang or one of the Xie Xin Tang (Heart-Draining Decoction) variants. If the patient presents with symptoms of "heartburn," then I would prescribe a Shao Yang-harmonizing and -resolving formula such as Xiao Chai Hu Tang variant as you have done here, but make sure to add Lai Fu Zi (disperses food and eliminates distention and downbears qi and transforms phlegm) along with the other medicinals.

So many people in today's world are stressed out and full of anxiety (e.g., liver depression and qi stagnation). This psychological stress alters the metabolism and the gut microbiota, creating a caustically acidic environment which can lead to ulcerations in the gastric mucosa and intestinal epithelium. I've had a lot of success with Xiao Chai Hu Tang variant for these types of patients.

Case Study #2: Intrahepatic Cholangitis and Autoimmune Hepatitis

Q: A friend of mine with hepatitis visited me for consultation and treatment. Liver function tests were GOT 69 (0–40 u/L), GPT 95 (1–30 u/L), and T-Bil 2.89 (0.2–1.2 mg/dL). I prescribed Huang Lian Jie Du Tang (including large doses of The Three Yellows (6 qian each)), and after only 3 days GOT and GPT had decreased to 49 and 77, respectively, and T-Bil to 1.60, but he is still HBsAb (-). If these results were to drop back down to normal, what would be the best approach moving forward?

A: Based on your description of this patient with hepatitis and increased T-Bil, it sounds to me like the patient may have intrahepatic cholangitis. In this case, I would continue prescribing Huang Lian Jie Du Tang (drains fire and resolves toxin) up until liver function tests return to normal and then switch to a medicinal extract powder for 3–5 more weeks. Naturally, you should advise the patient to follow-up with periodic examinations. The presence of HBsAb (-) really doesn't impact your therapeutic approach, plus other serologic test results would be needed to more accurately interpret any potential significance.

For cases of autoimmune hepatitis, I would prescribe either (Yu Sheng) Hyperactive Immune Formula (clears heat and resolves toxin, enriches yin and drains fire, cools the blood and eliminates steam, and clears vacuity heat) or Huang Lian Jie Du Tang (including large doses of The Three Yellows) adding Qing Hao, Zhi Zi, and Di Gu Pi. In the acute stage, it is critical to add Qing Hao, Zhi Mu, and Di Gu Pi, Lian Qiao, and Ma Huang. And for cases of bacterial or viral hepatitis, in the acute stage, I would prescribe Ma Huang Lian Qiao Chi Xiao Dou Tang variant.

These formulas offer exceptional therapeutic efficacy. Honestly, I am at a loss as to why these types of therapeutic approaches, rooted in the foundations of classical theory and practice, are *not* embraced by more of today's TCM physicians.

Case Study #3: Elevated Total Bilirubin Levels – Biliary Obstruction

Q: A 32 y/o male patient presented with elevated T-Bil 10.3 mg/l, normal GOT/GPT and stool and urine, and poor food intake (reduced appetite), indigestion, and glomus and oppression in the abdominal and epigastric region.

I diagnosed the patient with cholecystitis and prescribed Xiao Chai Hu Tang adding Dang Gui, Zhi Zi, and Da Huang. However, after taking this formula for 2 weeks, there was no significant improvement. Please offer your advice and suggestions.

A: Elevated T-Bil with normal liver enzyme lab test results suggests either biliary stricture (e.g., trauma, iatrogenic) or biliary blockage (e.g., choledocholithiasis (aka gallbladder stones)), which could lead to cholangitis. You may want to advise your patient to have imaging studies performed, which will provide a more definitive diagnosis.

As for treatment, I would consider prescribing a classical heat-clearing dampness-disinhibiting and jaundice-dispersing and -abating formula such as Yin Chen Hao Tang or Zhi Zi Bo Pi Tang adding Da Huang, Huang Lian, and Huang Bo. Of course, you could prescribe Xiao Chai Hu Tang variant, but it really does *not* address the Shao Yang internal damp-heat pattern as directly as the classical remedies (經方 j□ ng f□ ng).

Section 3: Spleen and Stomach

Case Study #1: Ruptured Spleen – Ru Mo Si Wu Tang Prevents Bleeding

Q: A relative of mine accidentally fell off his 12th floor balcony and was sent to the emergency room where examination revealed a ruptured spleen. Apparently, an awning below his apartment served as a "life net" so that he was lucky enough to avoid brain trauma and paralysis or death. His chief complaint is the ruptured spleen. Can TCM provide effective adjuvant treatment for this pathocondition?

A: TCM medicinals can prevent chronic bleeding caused by abdominal visceral injury and supplement the center and boost qi so the body is able to more quickly recover.

At the onset, to prevent chronic bleeding caused by abdominal visceral injury I would prescribe Ru Mo Si Wu Tang adding Huang Qin, Fu Ling, Ze Xie, Bai Zhu, Tian Ma, Chuan Qi, Du Zhong, Di Long, and a small dose of Da Huang.

Then, in the post-acute stage, after the condition has stabilized with no signs of bleeding, clotting, or infection, I would change to a center-supplementing qi-boosting formula such as Bu Zhong Yi Qi Tang adding Yan Hu Suo, Mu Xiang, Huang Qin, Du Zhong, Tian Ma, and Chuan Qi.

For the final phase of the therapeutic regimen, I would continue prescribing Bu Zhong Yi Qi Tang adding The Three Great Yang-Supplementers (Gan Jiang, Fu Zi, and Rou Gui).

Case Study #2: Perforated Peptic Ulcer – Postoperative TCM Treatment

Q: Last night my father had a sudden attack of severe abdominal pain. After being rushed to the hospital, examination revealed a perforated peptic ulcer (PPU), with emergency laparotomy and closure of the perforation performed. He seems to be doing ok now. After being discharged from the hospital, what's the best approach for helping him recover and regulate the constitution?

A: Laparoscopic repair is being used increasingly more for the management of perforated peptic ulcer (PPU), so just to make sure, you may want to verify if it was laparotomy (open surgery) or the less invasive laparoscopic repair, which tends to result in less postoperative pain.

Regardless of the type of surgery performed, if there is postoperative pain, then you can perform acupuncture on the distal acupoints Nei Guan (P6), He Gu (LI4), Zu San Li (ST36), and Tai Chong (LV3); or local acupoints along the stomach and controlling vessel channels.

As for postoperative TCM medicinal treatment, during the initial wound healing stage (i.e., hemostasis and inflammatory phase) right after surgery, I would start out by prescribing a fire-draining toxin-resolving formula such as Huang Lian Jie Du Tang adding Yan Hu Suo and Mu Xiang (quicken the blood, move qi, and relieve pain). This approach will resolve inflammation, minimize the potential for sepsis, and relieve pain. If there is only mild heat pattern (e.g., possible inflammation and mild bleeding), then I would prescribe a dual exterior- and interior-resolving and heat-clearing formula such as Ge Gen Qin Lian Tang adding Ban Xia, Fu Ling, Lai Fu Zi, Chuan Qi, and Hai Piao Xiao (or Bei Mu (powder)). This formula will provide the necessary heat-clearing toxin-resolving (anti-inflammatory), acid-controlling (antacid), blood-stanching, and sore-closing (wound healing) actions. If pain is severe, you can also add medicinals such as Ru Xiang, Mo Yao, Lai Fu Zi, Chuan Wu, Cao Wu, and Yu Sheng Wan to your formula.

After administering this formula throughout the initial wound healing phase (i.e., hemostasis and inflammatory phase) and there are *no* longer any signs or symptoms of pronounced heat or complications (e.g., postoperative leak, surgical site infection, pneumonia, wound dehiscence, peritonitis) that arise, then you can change to a spleen-fortifying qi-supplementing formula such as Bu Zhong Yi Qi Tang adding Huang Qin, Ban Xia, Lai Fu Zi, Chuan Qi, and Hai Piao Xiao (or Bei Mu (powder)).

Once the wound has progressed through the proliferative and into the remodeling phase of healing, then you can change to a simple formula for long-term regulation of the constitution up until the wound (i.e., ulceration) has completely healed—*no* presenting signs or symptoms and verification from imaging studies. For long-term regulation of the constitution, I would consider prescribing a dampness-drying phlegm-harmonizing and qi-normalizing center-harmonizing formula, such as Er Chen Tang, or a qi-boosting spleen-fortifying and qi-moving phlegm-transforming formula, such as Xiang Sha Liu Jun Zi Tang. Just make sure to include Lai Fu Zi, Huang Qin, and Hai Piao Xiao (powder). Or, even simpler, you could prescribe Ban Xia, Lai Fu Zi, Huang Qin, and Hai Piao Xiao (powder).

Naturally, throughout the treatment process, if the patient incurs symptoms such as pain, distention, fullness, or indigestion, then you can perform acupuncture on points such as Nei Guan (P6), Tai Chong (LV3), Zu San Li (ST36), Wei Shu (UB21), and Pi Shu (UB20) as well.

Remember! When you administer formula decoctions for the treatment of peptic ulcers (or in this case postoperative treatment), you must instruct patients to take the decoction at either room temperature or chilled, first retaining it in the mouth after drinking and then slowly swallowing, allowing a steady, gradual stream of liquid to coat and seep into the wound. In fact, you should advise these patients to ingest or drink all foods and beverages either at room temperature or chilled, and it is best to avoid spicy foods, such as chili or raw garlic (cooked garlic should be ok though), at least up until the lesion has completely healed.

Case Study #3: "Belching" – Differential Diagnosis and Treatment

Q: A 60 y/o male patient explained that he had a 30-year history of excessive belching and glomus and oppression below the heart (epigastric region). While conducting a physical examination, I happened to press lightly on Shang Wan (CV13) acupoint, which elicited an immediate response of repetitive belching, with the patient saying that he felt like there was "something suspended and hanging from" the middle of his chest (Jiu Wei (CV15) acupoint). His stool and urine are normal and he gets at least 8 hours of sleep a night, does *not* eat spicy foods, and has *no* other physical or neurological symptoms.

Originally, I was thinking about prescribing Xiao Chai Hu Tang, but then I considered how long these symptoms have persisted, so I decided to administer Ban Xia Tian Ma Bai Zhu San variant instead. The problem is that this formula has *not* been effective. Please offer your advice and guidance.

A: First, you must clearly distinguish the type of sound produced (e.g., belching (aka burping, eructation), hiccups, or sigh) in order to determine the etiology and accurately identify the pattern. There are many nuances to the various sounds and accompanying presentation of signs and symptoms that go along with "belching." In my clinical practice, I conduct differential diagnosis for this type of condition based on the following distinctions:*

- Belching (噎 y□) refers to either a narrowing or obstruction of the esophagus that leads to the inability to get food down and immediate vomiting of ingested food.
- Belching (嗝 gé) refers to either duodenal or high jejunal narrowing or obstruction.
- Belching (噎嗝 y□ gé) refers to a feeling of blockage or obstruction upon ingestion, and then exhalation and belching.
- Belching (噫氣 y□ qì) refers to a big exhalation or sighing, which is emotionally or psychologically derived and thus is a type of psychosomatic disorder.
- Belching (噯氣 ai qì) typically refers to belching and acid swallowing (acid regurgitation), dry belching with food malodor, or belching of sour putrid qi, and occurs after overeating or ingesting foods that are not fresh, resulting in belching or exhalation of this sour, putrid odor.
- Belching (打嗝 da gé) refers to spasm of the diaphragm that induces paroxysmal retching.
- Belching from satiation (飽嗝 da bao gé) (may also manifest as hiccups (呃逆 è nì)) results from bloating or dyspepsia following satiation (overeating), which stimulates the diaphragm, causing spasms that resolve upon the release of gas (stomach qi ascending counterflow (胃氣上逆 wèi qì shàng nì)) and prevents vomiting.

  Another example of belching from satiation is when you burp infants after ingesting milk by gently patting her on the back to release the qi occlusion (e.g., a form of dysphagia-occlusion (噎嗝 y□ gé)), producing an ascending counterflow of qi and undigested milk. When an infant is hungry and aggressively grasps for milk she may swallow too much air in the process and this air will naturally be released through burping. If the baby isn't burped, this may result in spitting up or regurgitating milk.

- Sour belching (噯酸 ai su□n) occurs in patients with acid reflux (gastroesophageal reflux disease (GERD)) whose esophageal sphincter relaxes abnormally or has weakened, thus allowing upward counterflow of backwash (i.e., stomach acid (possibly bile as well) and sometimes fermented stomach content) and causing the stereotypical "heartburn" sensation.
- Air belching (打氣嗝 da qì gé) is another type of belching that may present in some patients with Tourette syndrome, a neuropsychiatric disorder marked by uncontrollable motor and vocal tics.

  Also, some people with physically inactive sedentary lifestyles may go long periods of time without stretching the chest wall muscles, resulting in depressed qi in the chest; and once the torso is stretched an ejection of depressed qi (吐鬱氣 tu yù qì) is emitted.

  There are also cases of running piglet (奔豚氣 b□ n tún qì) that may present with this type of air belching.

The repetitive belching you described this patient as having suggests belching (打嗝 da gé) caused by spasm of the diaphragm, stomach, or esophagus, and *not* belching (噫氣 y□ qì) derived from psychosomatic origins. For this type of patient with *long-standing* belching (打嗝 da gé), I would consider prescribing a center-warming counterflow-downbearing formula, such as Ding Xiang San adding Ban Xia, or the composition Ban Xia (5 qian), Gan Jiang (5 qian), Gan Cao (3 qian), Huang Qin (1.5 qian), and Shi Di (8 qian).

However, if the patient's symptoms were of *recent onset*, then I would consider prescribing a stomach-harmonizing counterflow-downbearing and phlegm-dispersing rheum-eliminating formula such as Xiao Ban Xia Tang (simply composed of the medicinal pair Ban Xia and Sheng Jiang) adding Shi Di and Fu Ling. And in cases where heat pattern presents, I would prescribe either Wen Dan Tang adding Shi Di or Ju Pi Zhu Ru Tang adding Shi Di.

For patients with belching (噫氣 y□ qì) and ejection of depressed qi (吐鬱氣 tu yù qì), you can prescribe a liver-repressing and -coursing and depressed heat in the liver- and gallbladder-clearing formula such as Yi Gan San, Wen Dan Tang, Si Ni San, Wu Ling San, Xiao Chai Hu Tang, Xiao Yao San, and Yue Ju Wan. And you should also emphasize the importance of getting regular exercise and keep in good spirits.

If ascendant hyperactivity of liver yang pattern belching (噫 y□) and ejection of depressed qi (吐鬱氣 tu yù qì) presents, you can consider prescribing a Shao Yang-harmonizing and fright-settling spirit-quieting or liver-settling wind-extinguishing and yin-enriching yang-subduing formula such as Chai Hu Long Gu Mu Li Tang, Jian Ling Tang, Zhi Bo Di Huang Tang adding Long Gu Mu Li Tang, Huang Lian Jie Du Tang adding Long Gu and Mu Li, Chai Hu Qing Gan Tang, or Si Ni San.

In cases of qi, blood, phlegm, spleen, and stomach cold or vacuity pattern belching (噯氣 ai qì) and ejection of depressed qi (吐鬱氣 tu yù qì), I would consider prescribing a spleen- and stomach-supplementing and phlegm-damp-transforming or a qi-, blood-, and kidney yang-supplementing formula such as Ban Xia Tian Ma Bai Zhu San, Xiang Sha Liu Jun Zi Tang, Shi Quan Da Bu Tang, Bu Zhong Yi Qi Tang, You Gui Wan, or Shen Qi Wan.

If these symptoms are of *recent onset*, then you can needle (draining method) acupoints such as Nei Guan (P6), Zu San Li (ST36), Tai Chong (LV3), and He Gu (LI4); in the *post-acute* stage you can consider adding Pi Shu (UB20), Wei Shu (UB21), and Ge Shu (UB17); and for *long-standing*, chronic conditions, warm needle Nei Guan (P6), Zu San Li (ST36), Tai Chong (LV3), Pi Shu (UB20), Wei Shu (UB21), and Ge Shu (UB17).

*Note: A variety of TCM medical diagnostics terms have accumulated over the millennia to describe the different types of sounds and accompanying symptoms that manifest under an umbrella term commonly known as "belching" (aka burp or eructation).

Many of these terms overlap and some have specific connotations. However, there is a significant degree of ambiguity among these terms due to the limitations of the written language and subjectivity involved in describing a *sound*. In the same way that pulse-taking is very much an individual, subjective interpretation of a *tactile* sensation, so is determining and defining the nuances of the *sound* of "belching."

Case Study #4: Gastric Polyps – Stomach Channel Damp-Heat with Static Blood

Q: A 43 y/o male patient with a 20-year history of glomus below the heart (epigastric region) complained that recently symptoms have been more pronounced. Sometimes it is even difficult to swallow food, and when he forces himself to eat, he often gets dyspepsia (bloating, indigestion, and pain in the epigastric region).

A thorough medical examination, endoscopy, and biopsy revealed a gastric polyp that was histopathologically identified as a hyperplastic polyp. His gastroenterologist recommended that he undergo surgical excision, but the patient doesn't want to have surgery and that's why he wants to try TCM instead.

The patient's stool and urine are normal, but he has thick white tongue fur with a purplish-red tongue body. Can TCM treat this pathocondition? Or do you think I should advise the patient to go ahead with preventive surgery? Please offer your advice and guidance.

A: Gastric polyps can be identified as stomach channel damp-heat with static blood pattern. For now, I would advise the patient to *hold off* on surgical excision and take TCM medicinals instead. There are many approaches you could take based on accurate pattern identification.

For instance, you could prescribe a stomach-clearing fire-draining and blood-cooling formula, such as Qing Wei San adding Mu Dan Pi, Zhi Zi, and Long Dan Cao (or possibly Chuan Qi, Niu Xi, and Liu Ji Nu), or a blood-nourishing blood-quickening and stasis-dispelling pain-relieving formula, such as Ru Mo Si Wu Tang adding Huang Qin, Huang Lian, Zhi Zi, and Pu Huang. Of course, with this type of aberrant growth I would also prescribe Wan Ling Dan (resolves toxin and disperses welling-abscesses, dispels wind and relieves pain, and has anticancer actions).

Remember! Just to be on the safe side, advise the patient to have periodic follow-up endoscopy performed to rule out the possibility of dysplasia.

Case Study #5: Sour Belching – Gastrointestinal Esophageal Reflux Disease (GERD)

Q: South Korea has been in a period of economic recession for a while now and this seems to have increased the incidence of stress-induced disorders. In particular, I have had many patients coming in complaining of fullness and pain below the heart and gripping pain in the epigastric region, which some patients explain can be almost unbearable at times.

Based on the stereotypical presentation of dyspepsia and heartburn, I have diagnosed most of these patients with gastrointestinal esophageal reflux disease (GERD). Accordingly, I have tried administering a number of different formulas with Chai Hu and Ban Xia as the sovereign medicinals, but have not had very much success. How would you treat these types of patients?

A: Gastrointestinal esophageal reflux disease (GERD) correlates with sour belching (嗳酸 ai su□n) described in TCM classical texts, and typically results from transient lower esophageal sphincter relaxations and sphincter pressure abnormalities. In principle, I would prescribe formulas based on the Xie Xin Tang (Heart-Draining Decoction) variants such as Ban Xia Xie Xin Tang, Sheng Jiang Xie Xin Tang, or Gan Cao Xie Xin Tang.

Depending on the specific presentation of signs and symptoms and pattern identification, at the onset I might prescribe a phlegm-dispelling water-moving and qi-dissipating glomus-dispersing formula such as Xiao Ban Xia Jia Fu Ling Tang adding Lai Fu Zi and Hai Piao Xiao (controls acid). Some patients with pronounced heat bind and qi stagnation may require formula variants such as Zhi Zi Shi Tang, Zhi Zi Hou Po Tang, or Xiao Ban Xia Jia Fu Ling Tang adding Zhi Zi and Huang Qin.

For patients presenting with only minor symptoms that do *not* present serious discomfort or complications, you can consider simply advising the patient to cut fresh Chinese white radish (*Raphanus sativus* var. *longipinnatus*) or fresh ginger (pre-cut slices of processed ginseng will work as well) into thin slices and suck on them like a "lozenge" throughout the day. Do *not* bite or chew on these lozenges, just keep a slice in between the teeth and cheek and swallow the saliva until the lozenges naturally become saturated, soften and begin dissolving. At that point, spit the lozenge out and replace it with another piece.

Remember! Prevention of sour belching is the best way for treating any disease, so advise your GERD patients to be mindful of the Three *Don'ts*: *Don't* overeat, *Don't* lie down immediately after eating, and *Don't* eat food two hours prior to going to bed. These helpful precautions will effectively reduce the severity of GERD symptoms.

Case Study #6: Antireflux Surgery Complication

Q: A 47 y/o female underwent laparoscopic antireflux surgery (Nissen fundoplication) for persistent and unmanageable reflux esophagitis. Following surgery the patient suffered from reduced stomach motility, bile reflux, was unable to eat rich, oily foods, and could only tolerate small amounts of food at one meal setting.

For the past 2 years now, she has been taking an antacid and a gastroprokinetic agent (enhances stomach motility) prescribed by her gastroenterologist, but the symptoms have not improved. The patient told me she thinks her vagus nerve may have been severed during surgery. If this really is a case of idiopathic vagus nerve damage (i.e., compression or severed), do you think she has any chance of recovery?

A: Laparoscopic surgery (a minimally invasive technique) is most commonly performed as the first choice for surgery. Although laparoscopy reduces the risk of postsurgical complications (e.g., infections, hiatus hernia, nerve damage) compared to an open procedure, these complications still do occur in some cases, especially bloating and difficulty swallowing (dysphagia), which may resolve once the swelling from surgery resolves.

In your patient's case, the swelling from surgery which could have caused temporary compression should have gone down a long time ago. It is possible that the vagus nerve has either been severed (or partially severed) or is being physically compressed somewhere along its pathway as a result of surgery.

As for treatment, I would focus on prescribing TCM formulas that treat the symptoms and pattern. Based on the description of your patient, I would consider prescribing Ban Xia Tian Ma Bai Zhu San adding Da Huang (small dose), Di Long, Ma Huang, Ren Shen, and Chuan Qi. If the patient's condition does *not* improve, then increase the dose of Huang Qi and add Chuan Xiong, Chi Shao, Yin Xing Ye, and Yu Sheng Wan. This therapeutic approach, along with the appropriate lifestyle modifications, should successfully resolve these symptoms.

Case Study #7: Epigastric and Back Pain in the Middle of the

Night

Q: A 24 y/o female explained that she has had back pain in the middle of the night since she was in junior high school (13 years old). Throughout her life people around her always said, "Oh, it's nothing serious, once you get married and have kids it will be fine!" Well, after she grew up, got married and had a child, to her dismay, these symptoms got even worse. She told me, "I can't believe I fell for that old wives' tale!"

Every night at around 1 a.m., she has symptoms of glomus below the heart and epigastric region and back pain (extending from Shen Dao (GV11) to Ji Zhong (GV6)). She said that when these episodes occur the pain is so unbearable that she "curls up like a prawn." The strange thing is that these symptoms resolve spontaneously every time at around 5–6 a.m. She has no symptoms in the daytime and her stool and urine are normal. These intensified symptoms have been occurring for the past 3–4 years now. What do you think this could be?

A: Mmh!...Glomus below the heart and epigastric region and back pain when the patient is lying down in the middle of the night. It sounds to me like a case of gastrointestinal esophageal reflux disease (GERD), with the gastric acid "burning" the gastroesophageal sphincter and/or esophagus and thus causing unbearable pain.

I would try prescribing a phlegm-dispelling water-moving and qi-dissipating glomus-dispersing formula such as Xiao Ban Xia Jia Fu Ling Tang adding Lai Fu Zi and Hai Piao Xiao (3 qian), and if the "burning" pain is severe, also add Huang Qin. Administer this formula decoction at a dosage of 600 cc (200 cc/3x/day) and advise the patient to take the decoction by sipping the liquid slowly like a beverage (don't just gulp it down!). You can also consider advising the patient to suck on fresh ginseng slices like a lozenge during waking hours and swallow the juice; and if convenient, she can even sleep with the ginseng slice between her cheek and teeth at night.

Naturally, you should recommend that she have a thorough gastrointestinal examination and workup performed. This will enable you to verify for sure if she has GERD and also give your patient the peace of mind that you are on the right track.

And one last thing! Always remember to rule out the possibility of psychosomatic disorder, especially for this type of patient with "enduring pain" that spontaneously resolves.

Case Study #8: Gastrectomy – Sloppy Stool Following Surgery

Q: A 31 y/o male patient underwent a total gastrectomy as a part of the treatment regimen for stomach cancer. Since then, every time he eats any type of food at all he has sloppy stool, and right now he's very thin and his hands tremble slightly. What's the best way to treat this patient?

A: Sloppy stool (便溏 biàn tang) (diarrhea or loose stool) is a common malady for patients whom have undergone gastrectomy. For this type of patient, I would prescribe a dampness-drying spleen-fortifying and qi-moving stomach-harmonizing formula such as Ping Wei San (including large doses of Cang Zhu). This is one of the few situations in which I would prefer administering powdered medicinals (either extract powder or decocting pieces pulverized into powder) over a decoction, because the powder is easier to digest.

There are troublesome post-gastrectomy complications that the patient may incur (e.g., dumping syndrome (malabsorption), intestinal blockage), but the key factor in alleviating, and/or resolving these complications if they do arise, is to promote digestion. Your patient's gastroenterologist should have already advised him about diet, such as eating small meals spread throughout the day and sticking to a high protein, low fat and low sugar diet. TCM medicinals will aide in the process of promoting digestion and absorbing the nutrients he puts in his body.

Once the condition has stabilized, you can either administer the digestant Ji Nei Jin (disperses food (promotes digestion) and fortifies the stomach) yourself for decoction or simply advise the patient to take Ji Nei Jin as a tonic on his own to regulate the constitution in the long-term.

Case Study #9: NSAIDs – Look Out for Gastric Ulcer!

Q: A 43 y/o female presented with palpable swelling (Du Bi (ST35) and Xi Yan (EX-LE5)) and pain (more pronounced when walking and going upstairs) in both knees, but *no* heat. She said that she has been taking non-steroidal anti-inflammatory drugs (NSAIDs) for about 2 years now in attempts to resolve the discomfort in her knees.

Recently, every time after taking these pills she feels a sharp, aching pain below the heart (epigastric region) and occasionally after eating. Stool and urine are normal. I am wondering if the patient might have a peptic ulcer. What do you think about this case? Please offer your advice and guidance.

A: Yes, NSAID-induced gastric ulcer is definitely a possibility in this case. You may want to advise your patient to undergo a thorough medical examination, including gastrointestinal endoscopy, if you think it is necessary to definitively verify your diagnosis. The fact that the patient still has persistent swelling (in the depressions along the joint line) and pain despite taking the NSAIDs suggests the possibility of anterior cruciate ligament (ACL) injury and swelling from the collection of synovial fluid.

A good therapeutic approach that will effectively address both the knee swelling and pain and peptic ulcer is Huang Lian Jie Du Tang (including Huang Bo (5–8 qian)) adding Bai Zhu, Fu Ling, Ze Xie, Lai Fu Zi, and Niu Xi. Lai Fu Zi is very effective for the "heartburn" of gastrointestinal pathoconditions. Don't forget to bleed locally at the site of swelling and pain on the knees and needle the two acupoints where the vastus lateralis and vastus medialis muscles taper into tendons approximately diagonal from the upper edges of the patella, Yin Ling Quan (SP9), Yang Ling Quan (GB34), He Ding (EX-LE2), Xi Yang Guan (GB33), Nei Guan (P6), and Tai Chong (LV3).

Case Study #10: Huang Lian Jie Du Tang – Sloppy Stools?

Q: Recently, I have noticed that when prescribing Huang Lian Jie Du Tang that includes relatively large doses of each medicinal (6 qian or more) many patients will incur as many as 5–6 sloppy (loose) stools per day. Has this been your experience with prescribing large doses of these fire-draining toxin-resolving type medicinals? Is this a normal reaction? How do you resolve this problem?

A: Yes, it *is* possible for some people to have sloppy (loose) stools after taking large doses of fire-draining toxin-resolving medicinals such as the The Three Yellows—Huang Qin, Huang Lian, and Huang Bo. This goes for large doses of other types of medicinals as well (e.g., yin-nourishing blood-supplementing, blood-quickening stasis-transforming, yin-enriching yang-subduing).

It may take a period of time for some people's digestive systems (including the gut microbiome!) to adjust and be able to absorb larger doses of these decocted medicinals. Most people only incur mild episodes of sloppy (loose) stool before their bodies' spontaneously adjust after only a short period of administration. But if the symptoms are more severe and the patient does *not* seem to be adjusting on their own, you can consider reducing the doses and/or adding Cang Zhu, Ze Xie, and Fu Ling. Both of these methods have been successful for me.

On a related note, I have even seen a few patients who have developed an "indigo" blue-green pigment discoloration on the face after taking Da Qing Ye (dried leaves), Lan Ban Gen (root), and Qing Dai (process dried powder of the leaves and stems), which all come from the same indigo plant (*Isatis indigotica* Fort.). Don't worry! The "indigo" tint fades back to normal after adjusting the formula accordingly and the patient has completely metabolized the medicinals.

II. GENITOURINARY DISORDERS

Section 1: Kidneys

Case Study #1: Fetal Renal Asymmetry

Q: My wife went for a routine prenatal ultrasound recently and results showed that the kidneys of the fetus (male) are not the same size. The larger kidney measured 10 x 7 mm and the smaller was 9.5 x 6 mm.

I am thinking about prescribing Zhi Bo Di Huang Tang variant for my wife. Do you think this will help promote growth of the smaller kidney and balance out the sizes?

A: The size of your son's kidneys is well within the normal range and the discrepancy is statistically insignificant at less than 1 cm. If it's anything at all, there is a possibility of mild hydronephrosis. That means you really don't have anything to worry about and you don't need to administer Zhi Bo Di Huang Tang variant. The best approach to ensure a healthy pregnancy is the natural way without any medication at all. Typically, any size discrepancy and/or hydronephrosis will resolve spontaneously either during the fetal stage or after birth. If your child really does end up being born with an abnormality, you can treat it at that time.

For instance, if hydronephrosis (the obstruction of urine output usually caused by either narrowing of the ureter, blockage in the kidney or bladder, or vesicouretal reflux) presents, with *no* other underlying renal damage or infection, then you can simply prescribe a kidney yang-warming qi transformation-promoting and water-disinhibiting dampness-percolating formula such as Wu Ling San (Nephritis Formula).

If hard bind (fibrosis) (硬結 yìng jié) of the kidney presents, then prescribe a blood-breaking, channel-freeing pain-relieving, and liver- and kidney-supplementing formula such as Tong Jing Fang. And in the case of a congenital deficiency, you can prescribe a kidney-supplementing yang-assisting formula such as Shen Qi Wan variant.

Remember! Right now the most important thing is to make sure your wife gets enough sleep, eats healthy, and stays in good spirits!

Case Study #2: Hypertension, Hematuria, and Proteinuria – Chronic Glomerulonephritis

Q: A 24 y/o overweight (height: 180 cm, weight: 110 kg) male patient explained that he has had intermittent hematuria (light brown urine) ever since high school, which is more pronounced when he is really tired or has had a lot of exercise. Worried that he may have a problem with his kidneys, he went in for a thorough examination upon which urinalysis revealed 24-hour total protein at 500 mg (normal level <150 mg within a 24-hour period).

The patient is currently taking antihypertension drugs for high blood pressure. What's the best approach for treating this patient?

A: Hematuria, proteinuria, and hypertension suggest chronic glomerulonephritis. How about your patient's BUN and CR levels? Is your patient simply overweight or does he have edema as well? You need to further clarify the patient's condition (i.e., signs, symptoms, lab workup) in order to conduct accurate pattern identification as the basis for your prescription.

Assuming the patient does have chronic glomerulonephritis, Western medicine really doesn't have any specific therapeutic regimen other than dietary restrictions, controlling blood pressure, and diuretics (if there is edema).

As for TCM treatment, I would first find out whether the patient has received long-term administration of immunosuppressants, such as corticosteroids or Imuran.

If *not*, then I would consider prescribing a formula variant such as Zhi Bo Di Huang Tang (enriches yin and downbears fire), Zhi Zi Bo Pi Tang (clears heat and drains fire), Wu Ling San (warms kidney yang and promotes qi transformation and disinhibits water and percolates dampness), or Ba Zheng San (clears heat and drains fire and disinhits water and frees strangury).

If *yes*, then I would prescribe a formula variant such as Xiang Sha Liu Jun Zi Tang (boosts qi and fortifies the spleen and moves qi and transforms phlegm), Bu Zhong Yi Qi Tang (fortifies the spleen and supplements qi and upbears yang), or You Gui Yin (warms and supplements kidney yang, quickens the blood and dissipates stasis, and eliminates dampness and relieves pain). Regardless of which formula you choose, start out by adding small doses of The Three Great Yang-Supplementers and Huang Bo (gradually increasing the doses of each), Huang Qi (gradually increasing the dose up to 2 liang), Shan Yao, Tu Si Zi, and blood-stanching and astringing medicinals such as Chuan Qi, Ce Bo Ye, Ou Jie, and Bai Guo.

You should administer this formula up until the hematuria (microscopic and macroscopic) resolves and then continue regulating the constitution with TCM medicinals for 3–6 more months to ensure the condition has been completely cured. During the therapeutic regimen, it is *possible* that some patients may develop canker sores (aphthous ulcers) in the mouth as a result of the great heat medicinals. If this occurs, you can simply add Huang Liang and Huang Qin (to counterbalance the heat and heal the sores) and/or consider reducing the dose of Gan Jiang and Fu Zi. After a 1–2 weeks the sores will resolve and you can gradually reduce the amount of Huang Qin and Huang Lian and begin increasing the doses of The Three Great Yang-Supplementers.

Case Study #3: Purplish-Red Macules on Lower Legs

Q: A 47 y/o female patient explained that 3 years ago a routine health examination revealed proteinuria (+), and she has been taking medication (unspecified) to treat this condition since then.

Recently, she had a bout of enteritis, prompting her to visit a doctor whom ordered blood tests that indicated the patient was anemic. Her doctor recommended that she receive erythropoietin (EPO) infusions (3 infusions spaced 10 days apart) at the hospital to treat the anemia, but the patient thought it was a hassle to take time off from work, so she decided to see what TCM could do for her.

During her initial visit I noticed that she had purplish-red macules

(紫紅斑 zi hóng b□n) (ecchymosis) on her lower legs, and the patient said that they were "a little itchy" when they first appeared, but now they don't itch and "seem to be fading away." I'm not sure where to start with this patient. Can you give me any advice?

A: You just mentioned proteinuria (+), a sign that something may be wrong with the patient, but you did not indicate whether further lab workup (e.g., urinalysis (RBC casts) and blood tests (BUN and creatinine)) or imaging tests were performed, or if there was a definitive diagnosis given by a nephrologist.

Based on the patient's history and the fact that she was prescribed EPO, it sounds like she may have glomerulonephritis and possibly be either uremic and/or extremely undernourished. The bruising (ecchymoses) on her lower legs is likely due to low platelet (PLT) count. I would consider prescribing either You Gui Yin or Shen Qi Wan adding Rou Gui, Gan Jiang, Huang Bo, Ren Shen, Xi Lu Rong, Shan Zha, and Zhu Jie Qi. This therapeutic approach will help remedy the patient's anemia and glomerulonephritis.

Section 2: Urinary Bladder

Case Study #1: Neurogenic Bladder

Q1: One year ago, a 65 y/o female received a spinal injection (unspecified agent) near the acupoints Ming Men (GV4) and Yao Yang Guan (GV3) for the treatment of lingering lumbar pain. Following the injection, she experienced an episode of *transient* palsy in both lower legs (which spontaneously subsided about 1 month later) and *continues* to suffer from urinary incontinence (she has to void about every 10–15 minutes as a precautionary measure otherwise she would need to wear adult diapers). This is very difficult for her to deal with because it dramatically affects her quality of life. How would you treat this patient?

A: She still has some functional capacity and control over urination. In this case, I would consider prescribing a qi-, blood-, and kidney yang-supplementing formula such as Bu Zhong Yi Qi Tang, Gui Qi Jian Zhong Tang, Bu Yang Huan Wu Tang, or Paralysis Formula #3 (You Gui Yin Variant) (subtracting Da Huang). Just make sure to include Huang Qi (large doses), Ma Huang, Di Long, Bai Guo, and Long Yan He in your formula.

For this type of neurogenic bladder patient, you must also consider the possibility of psychosomatic factors and bladder damp-heat (infection) pattern. Thus, depending on the etiology and pathomechanism, I would also consider prescribing a center-harmonizing spirit-quieting and stagnation-dissipating phlegm-transforming formula such as Gan Mai Da Zao Tang Combining Ban Xia Hou Po Tang adding heat-clearing toxin-resolving, astringing, and spirit-quieting medicinals such as Pu Huang, Zhi Zi, Huang Bo, Long Dan Cao, Bai Guo, Shan Yao, Long Gu, Mu Li, and Yu Sheng Wan.

Spinal cord injuries may manifest in varying degrees of symptoms from total loss of bladder control (and bowel control), in which the patient is unaware that urine (or feces) has passed or is unable to void (or excrete) without assistance, to the relatively more mild symptoms of urinary incontinence, inability to empty the bladder, urinary frequency, and susceptibility to urinary tract infections (UTIs). The most commonly used general term to describe this pathocondition is neurogenic bladder (or neurogenic bowel).

The reason for this loss of control may be caused by the following: 1) The nerve signals from the *sacral voiding center* to the brain are blocked (or disrupted), resulting in overactive bladder (aka reflex voiding); or 2) The nerve signals from the *micturition ("voiding") center* in the brainstem that instructs the sphincters and bladder (detrusor) muscle to relax when the bladder contracts are being blocked (or disrupted), resulting in involuntary contraction known as detrusor sphincter dyssynergia (DSD).

It is not uncommon for women who have given birth to experience some degree of urinary incontinence, uterine prolapse, bladder prolapse, or other structural abnormalities that affect the bladder and ureter when they get older, which may lead to stress, urge, overflow, or mixed incontinence. In these types of urinary incontinence, the patient is conscience of the voiding sensation and may or may not be able to control it. This type can be identified as qi and yang vacuity pattern.

It is a possibility that at least some of this patient's problems with urinary incontinence may stem from childbearing and are just now manifesting. Treatment for these types of urinary incontinence is the same as I mentioned above, but you should also include Lu Rong. In some patients, urinary incontinence becomes so severe that it may adversely affect cognitive function (e.g., attention span, memory). For these patients specifically, I would consider prescribing a blood-quickening qi-supplementing formula such as Bu Yang Huan Wu Tang adding Shi Chang Pu and Yuan Zhi (open the orifices and quiet the spirit), Yi Zhi (secures essence and reduces urination), and Zi Su Zi (downbears qi and disperses phlegm).

Case Study #2: Urinary Incontinence – Acupuncture and Medicinal Treatment

Q: Recently, I have been treating cancer patients at the affiliated hospital of my alma mater Ajou University. My focus has been on treating urinary incontinence, specifically selecting the acupoints Zhong Ji (CV3), Gui Lai (ST29), and Zu San Li (ST36) for all of these patients. Most of them have experienced either improvement or complete resolution of symptoms after receiving a regimen of treatment.

Many of the gynecologists at the hospital have taken notice of these results, calling me and wondering if this was really true. The Korean Institute of Oriental Medicine (KIOM) has even offered to help me obtain funding from the National Research Foundation. This sounds like an interesting proposition. However, I am concerned that they may choose the most difficult cases or those patients that have undergone surgery without success. What do you think about this situation?

A: Congratulations! You have accumulated a lot of valuable clinical experience already. Don't be afraid to take on challenges. As you have discovered, most cases of urinary incontinence, especially those involving the postpartum phase and related complications of childbearing that develop later in life, are *not* that difficult to treat. In addition to those acupoints, you can also needle San Yin Jiao (SP6) and prescribe Bu Zhong Yi Qi Tang variant.

Effectiveness of treatment can be determined by macroscopically observing the coloration of the vaginal or cervical tissue. Technically, you could use a urethroscope to examine the urethra, but the problem with this approach is that the urethral canal may be too narrow for clear observation and may even irritate the ureter, which results in iatrogenic urinary incontinence. That's why it would be better just to look at the vagina or cervix instead.

You can ask a gynecologist to assist you in examining the vagina or cervix with an endoscopy or speculum to determine whether the coloration is *purplish-red* (i.e., bruised like blunt trauma), *pinkish*, or *pale* in appearance, and if *purulent exudate (pus)* presents. Since we know the root of this pathocondition is qi vacuity pattern, you can prescribe Bu Zhong Yi Qi Tang adding combinations of the following medicinals based on the results of observation:

- *Purplish-red* tissue can be identified as stasis heat or liver channel stasis obstruction pattern—add Chuan Qi, Tao Ren, Hong Hua, Gu Sui Bu, Xu Duan, and Niu Xi.
- *Pinkish* tissue can be identified as qi vacuity pattern—add Li Zhi He, Ju he, Shan Zha, Bai Guo, Qian Shi, Jin Ying Zi, and He Zi.
- *Pale* (non-lustrous) tissue can be identified as qi vacuity with yang vacuity pattern—add the same medicinals as for qi

vacuity pattern plus The Three Great Yang-Supplementers.

- The presence of *purulent exudate (pus)* indicates infection, which can be identified as damp-heat pouring downward pattern—add large doses of Long Dan Cao, Huang Bo, Che Qian Cao, Lian Peng Cao, Lian Xu, and Mu Dan Pi.

Case Study #3: Benign Prostate Hyperplasia – Radiofrequency Ablation Complications

Q: A 63 y/o male Western medicine physician (a colleague I have known for a long time) underwent a radiofrequency ablation (transurethral needle ablation (TUNA)) procedure for benign prostatic hyperplasia (BPH). Following the procedure, he has experienced severe pain in the perineum; and once the urine volume in the bladder reaches about 100 cc, he says "the pain is unbearable."

To maintain independence, he inserts a urinary catheter when necessary on his own (intermittent self-catheritization) and takes analgesics. He asked me if TCM could provide relief and improve these "unbearable" symptoms. What do you think?

A: Difficulty passing urine, incontinence, pain, erectile dysfunction, and urinary tract infection (UTI) (if catheritization is used) are all common complications of these types of ablation procedures, but in most cases they will resolve spontaneously. Naturally, the risk of UTI remains as long as the patient performs catheritization.

These postsurgical complications can be identified as liver channel damp-heat pouring downward and stasis obstruction pattern, requiring administration of a liver and gallbladder repletion fire-draining and lower burner damp-heat-clearing formula such as Long Dan Xie Gan Tang adding Fu Ling, Tao Ren, Mu Dan Pi, Chi Shao, and if necessary, Di Long and Niu Xi.

III. DIABETES

Case Study #1: Diabetes – TCM Provides Effective Treatment

Q: One of the paramount topics in modern clinical medicine right now is figuring out the best way to integrate Chinese medicine and Western medicine for the most effective treatment of diabetes. In most cases, once patients have been diagnosed with diabetes, and are unable to maintain normal plasma glucose levels with lifestyle changes (e.g., diet, exercise) alone, they will begin taking Western medicine drugs.

Only rarely do patients begin TCM treatment (solely or integrative) at the onset, and by the time they decide to seek TCM treatment their conditions have already become very complicated. Since I began studying TCM, one of my aspirations has always been to discover the best possible comprehensive treatment for diabetes patients. My father happened to be my first successful case.

My father was diagnosed with diabetes (diabetes mellitus type 2 (DM2)) last summer, with Glu-AC > 300. He enjoys rich foods and his share of fine liquor and couldn't muster the will power to engage in earnest attempts at lifestyle changes. He told me, "There would be no joy in life without good food and fine liquor." I urged him *not* to take Western medicine, and instead I prescribed Jian Ling Tang variant, administering 1 packet (600 c.c. decoction) 300 c.c./2x/day to be taken in the morning and evening, as is our custom here in South Korea. This formula effectively lowered and has maintained both Glu-AC and Glu-PC within normal levels.

This gave me a great sense of accomplishment and boosted my confidence. After this case, I went on to effectively treat numerous other diabetes patients and discovered that, in some cases, the Xie Xin Tang (Heart-Draining Decoction) variants adding Zhi Mu, Sang Bai Pi, and Ou Jie also provide relatively inexpensive and effective results.

Based on my own clinical experience, there is no question that TCM can play an integral role, either on its own or in an integrative role with Western medicine, for the effective treatment of diabetes. I think it is unfortunate that more patients don't have enough confidence in TCM so they can reap the benefits as well.

Despite gaining some experience and having a bit of success, there are some aspects about the treatment of diabetes that I am still unclear about. Can you help me clarify the following questions?

1) What's the best way to treat type 2 DM involving impaired insulin secretion? During the treatment regimen, if exacerbations in Glu-AC and/or Glu-PC occur, what should I do to bring the glucose levels back down?
2) For patients with asymptomatic diabetes, what's the best approach for lowering glucose levels? Since pill preparations are more convenient for the patient to take, do you think this mode of administration is an acceptable alternative to decoctions?
3) How do you determine when diabetes has been cured and no further treatment is required (especially in the *absence* of noticeable signs and symptoms)?
4) Do you have any advice for lifestyle changes (e.g., diet, exercise)?

A: The pathophysiology of diabetes is extremely complex and modern medicine still doesn't completely understand all of the mechanisms involved, nor the exact extent of the roles genetics, viruses, and environmental factors play in the onset of this pathocondition. Regardless of whether hyperglycemia results from insulin secretion being unable to compensate for insulin resistance, beta-cell dysfunction, or impaired insulin secretion (e.g., loss of normally pulsatile insulin secretion, an increase in proinsulin secretion signaling impaired insulin processing, or an accumulation of islet amyloid polypeptide), the TCM treatment approach will still rely on the same process of signs, symptoms, history, lab test results, and pattern identification as the basis for determining treatment.

Remember! For diabetes patients, you should first reference BUN, CR, and urine protein levels. If these indices are elevated you can consider prescribing a kidney yang-warming and -supplementing, blood-quickening stasis-dissipating, and dampness-eliminating pain-relieving formula such as Shen Qi Wan or You Gui Yin. Just make sure to include Rou Gui, Ren Shen, and Sang Bai Pi. If the above renal function tests are normal, but there are signs and symptoms of cardiovascular and cerebrovascular pathology, then prescribe a blood-quickening qi-supplementing formula such as Bu

Yang Huan Wu Tang adding Chuan Qi, Sang Bai Pi, and possibly even Dai Zhe Shi (powder).

For most cases of asymptomatic diabetes the therapeutic regimen is relatively simple. Just advise the patient to maintain healthy lifestyle habits (e.g., diet, exercise, adequate sleep, weight control) and administer Sang Bai Pi and Dai Zhe Shi. Sang Bai Pi is an essential diabetes medicinal that drains the lung and calms panting, moves water and disperses swelling, and cleans up the metabolic waste that clogs cell membranes throughout the entire body; and Dai Zhe Shi calms the liver and subdues yang, downbears counterflow by heavy settling, and cools the blood and stanches bleeding. Pulverize these medicinals into powder and process this powder into pills that are convenient for the patient to carry around and take orally.

The diabetic should avoid "excessive" intake of refined carbohydrates (e.g., sugars), starches (e.g., grains) and alcoholic beverages. I want to emphasize "excessive" because I do *not* mean strictly "prohibited;" the patient should try their best to minimize intake of these types of foods and beverages. The patient should feel free to consume sensible portions of foods and beverages that encompass the full range of nutrients (e.g., whole grains, fruits, vegetables, nuts, legumes, eggs, meat, seafood). As long as the patient follows these lifestyle habits and takes the TCM medicinals as prescribed, based on my clinical experience, TCM provides a better overall therapeutic approach than Western medicine. TCM effectively regulates the constitution, controls blood sugar levels, and eventually enables the patient to discontinue medication altogether.

In my experience, the quickest and most effective formula for treating diabetes is Jian Ling Tang adding Sang Bai Pi, Zhi Mu, and Huang Bo (or either Huang Qin or Huang Lian); and if constipation presents, then add Da Huang and Sheng Shi Gao (powder). Other good formulas are Zhi Bo Di Huang Tang (subtracting Gan Cao) adding Sang Bai Pi; and Xie Xin Tang (or Huang Lian Jie Du Tang) adding Sang Bai Pi and Dai Zhe Shi (powder). Naturally, regardless of the formula, you would *not* want to include medicinals with a high sugar content, such as The Sweets—Gan Cao, Hong Zao, and Long Yan Rou—into formulas for diabetic patients.

You must explain to the patient in detail about the advantages of TCM medicinals and disadvantages of Western medicine drugs, and encourage the patient to fully comply with your advice and therapeutic regimen. Otherwise, the patient may be indecisive, switching back and forth between TCM medicinals and Western medicine drugs. This mindset may very well lead to the worst-case scenarios of irreversible peripheral nerve, cardiovascular (e.g., angina pectoris, myocardial infarction), cerebrovascular (e.g., transient ischemic attack (TIA), cerebrovascular accident (CVA)), renal, and retinal complications along with a shortened lifespan. No one gains from that type of outcome and the patient really pays the ultimate price!

Case Study #2: Congenital Diabetes (Diabetes Mellitus Type 1)

Q: A young boy who was diagnosed with congenital diabetes in infancy visited me with his parents. He is now 7 years old and must have dialysis performed 2x/week, and on top of the nephropathy, he also has retinopathy with blurry vision.

His parents are determined to do anything possible to help their son live a long, happy and healthy life, and asked me if I think TCM would be able to effectively treat this pathocondition. Please offer your valuable insights and advice. I am not sure about the dosage of insulin units administered.

A: Congenital diabetes is insulin-dependent diabetes (diabetes mellitus type 1 (DM1)). Administration of TCM medicinals regulate the constitution, which allows the body to recalibrate and autonomously regulate glucose metabolism, reduces the dosage of insulin required to control blood glucose levels, and prevents the onset and/or exacerbation of further complications. First, you must examine the patient for the presence of water amassment (e.g., inhibited urination, lower abdominal fullness, lower leg edema).

If *no* water amassment presents, then prescribe You Gui Yin adding Fu Ling, Ze Xie, Sang Bai Pi, Xi Lu Rong, Ding Shu Xiu, Ren Dong Teng, Huang Qi, and Ren Shen/Chuan Qi Powder; and if water amassment *does* present with hasty panting and rapid breathing, then prescribe Wu Ling San (Nephritis Formula) adding Ding Shu Xiu, Ren Dong Teng, Sang Bai Pi, Huang Qi, Rou Gui, and Ren Shen/Chuan Qi Powder.

In some patients, long-term administration of high dose insulin injections may lead to a phenomena called chronic Somogyi rebound (Somogyi effect and posthypoglycemic hyperglycemia), where the patient counterintuitively experiences high blood sugar in the morning as a result of an overabundance of insulin at night.

Case Study #3: Hypoglycemia and Hyponatremia – Confusion, Stupor, and Coma

Q: A 71 y/o male with a 30-year history of diabetes has suffered from periodic episodes of confusion, stupor, and coma caused by hypoglycemia and hyponatremia. This year alone he has had 4 or 5 episodes of confusion and stupor, with each episode only lasting about 1 day, but recently he suffered a paroxysmal attack that put him into a full-on coma, requiring a 10-day hospital stay.

Since then, it's been difficult to maintain blood glucose and sodium levels within a normal range. What is the best approach for treating this patient?

A: For patients experiencing confusion, stupor, and coma (diabetic coma) due to hypoglycemia and hyponatremia, I would consider prescribing a kidney yang-warming and -supplementing, blood-quickening stasis-dissipating, sinew- and bone-strengthening, and dampness-eliminating pain-relieving formula such as Shen Qi Wan (or You Gui Yin) or Shen Fu Tang (or Ren Shen Si Ni Tang) adding Long Yan Rou, Da Zao, and table salt.

The TCM treatment objective should focus on preventing these acute episodes from occurring and gradually reducing the dosage of antihyperglycemic agents, with the goal of eventually discontinuing administration altogether. That's the best approach for completely resolving this pathocondition. This process will take time and require patient compliance, but it provides the best overall approach for controlling blood glucose levels, preventing hypoglycemia unawareness and the potential life-threatening episodes of diabetic coma, and ensuring the patient maintains a high quality and long life.

Case Study #4: Insulin Excess May Induce Hypoglycemia

Q: A 40 y/o male has a family history of diabetes and was diagnosed with this condition 10 years ago. He has incurred several episodes of confusion and loss of consciousness (diabetic coma) over the years. Right now he is taking 12 units of insulin per day and his urine and stool are normal. What should the treatment objective focus on? How would you treat this patient?

A: Actually, diabetes (regardless if it's DM1 or DM2) is not necessarily hereditary. There have been certain susceptibility genes identified, but there may be other epigenetic factors (e.g., diet, obesity, autoantigens, viruses) involved, or it could simply occur idiopathically. In most diabetes patients, I believe the likely causes are either from beta cells of the pancreas becoming infected with a virus (e.g., coxsackievirus, rubella virus, cytomegalovirus, Epstein-Barr virus, retroviruses) or autoimmunity involving autoantigens attacking beta cells and resulting in destruction (insulitis).

As for TCM medicinals, if heat pattern presents, I would consider prescribing formulas such as Bai Hu Tang (clears heat and engenders liquid and disperses thirst and resolves vexation); Huang Lian Jie Du Tang (clears heat and resolves toxin) adding Sheng Shi Gao; Jian Ling Tang (settles the liver and extinguishes wind and enriches yin and subdues yang) adding The Three Yellows and Sang Bai Pi; or Zhi Bo Di Huang Tang (enriches yin, downbears fire, and eliminates steaming) adding Qing Hao, Di Gu Pi, Huang Qin, Huang Lian, and Sang Bai Pi. And if qi- and yin-vacuity pattern present, then make sure to include yin-enriching blood-cooling medicinals such as Tian Men Dong, Mai Men Dong, Tian Hua, Gan Di Huang, Mu Dan Pi, Dan Shen, Dang Shen, Sha Shen, and Yuan Shen.

Some cases of insulin-dependent diabetes (DM1 or DM2) may be due to an insufficiency of factors and hormones in the kidneys that regulate insulin secretion, for which I would prescribe qi-, blood-, or kidney yang-supplementing formulas such as Shen Qi Wan, You Gui Yin, Gui Qi Jian Zhong Tang (either reducing the dose of or subtracting Gan Cao and Da Zao altogether), Zhen Wu Tang, Wu Ling San, or Bu Yang Huan Wu Tang. Just make sure to include Sang Bai Pi, Sheng Shi Gao, Fu Zi, Rou Gui, Huang Qin (or Huang Lian), Huang Bo, and possibly Long Gu and Mu Li. This approach will promote a graduated and sustainable reduction in insulin levels, allowing the patient to reduce his insulin dosage accordingly.

Once the patient begins TCM treatment, if the original 12 units of insulin per day results in blood glucose levels that are too low, then advise the patient to reduce the insulin dose by 2 units (total of 10 units). After 1–2 weeks have the patient test AC (before meals) and HbA1C. The HbA1C estimates plasma glucose levels during previous months (1–3 months) so you can use it as a reference baseline. You want to determine here whether or not AC levels have dropped down below a range of 120 to 80 or below, and *if so*, you should once again advise the patient to reduce the insulin doses by 2 units (total of 8 units). Continue administering the therapeutic regimen in this manner, gradually reducing the dose (by 2 units) of insulin until it can be completely discontinued.

Remember! After blood glucose levels have returned to normal and the patient is no longer dependent on insulin therapy, you must instruct the patient to continue maintaining a healthy lifestyle and closely monitor blood glucose levels. It is *not* uncommon for these types of patients to have an initial hyperglycemic "rebound" back to the "essential state," which can be identified as heat pattern. If this "rebound" occurs, then continue prescribing the appropriate TCM formula for a period of time until blood glucose stabilizes. By regulating the constitution, the ultimate goal of TCM treatment is to wean the patient away from insulin dependency and eventually TCM treatment altogether.

Case Study #5: Diabetic – Neuropathy So Soon?

Q: Mr. Ge came for consultation explaining that the symptoms of his diabetes have been getting worse recently. He said that he has had difficulty "getting it up" (erectile dysfunction) for quite some time and seems to be more forgetful than before. And recently, he has even been having difficulty controlling urination and defecation (urinary and fecal incontinence), occasionally notices a slight "pinkish tint" in his urine (gross hematuria) that was confirmed to be RBCs on lab examination, and feels a lack of strength in both legs.

The good thing is that he has a very positive attitude and optimistic personality! I am considering prescribing Paralysis Formula #3 (including Ma Huang (3 qian) and subtracting Gan Cao and Da Zao) adding Wu Zhu Yu and Sang Bai Pi. Do you think this would be an effective approach?

A: Mr. Ge may be optimistic, but it sounds like he may also be brooding over the possibility of diabetes being the cause of his inability to "get it up" (erectile dysfunction), while the tendency for forgetfulness could be related to aging and the fact that he may be so preoccupied with concerns of health and other matters! The hematuria could be caused by any number of pathoconditions, such as urinary tract infection, bladder or kidney stones, and enlarged prostate, and may have nothing at all to do with diabetes.

Typically, the symptoms of diabetic nephropathy (i.e., urinary and fecal incontinence, lower leg weakness) that you mentioned do not manifest until the patient has had diabetes for at least 25 years, and is more common in people who have problems controlling blood glucose levels. For now, I would focus on making sure blood glucose levels are under control with a TCM diabetes formula, while continuing to evaluate the patient's condition over the next 2–3 months to determine whether it's necessary to prescribe a formula such as Paralysis Formula #3 for diabetic neuropathy.

Now, a good formula for Mr. Ge would be the following: (Yu Sheng) Zhi Bo Di Huang Tang (subtracting Gan Cao) adding Sang Bai Pi (1 liang), Di Long (8 qian), Mu Dan Pi (4 qian), Xi Lu Rong (powder) (1g), and Dai Zhe Shi (powder) (5g). Sang Bai Pi is an essential diabetes medicinal that drains the lung and calms panting, moves water and disperses swelling, and cleans up the metabolic waste that clogs cell membranes throughout the entire body; Di Long is a urinary bladder Tai Yang channel medicinal that clears heat, extinguishes wind, frees the channels, quickens the network vessels, and disinhibits urine; Mu Dan Pi cools the blood and clears heat and quickens the blood and disperses stasis; Xi Lu Rong invigorates kidney yang, boosts essence-blood, strengthens sinew and bone, regulates the thoroughfare and controlling vessels, and promotes hematopoiesis; and Dai Zhe Shi calms the liver and subdues yang, downbears counterflow by heavy settling, and cools blood and stanches bleeding.

Case Study #6: Diabetes with Concomitant Chronic Hepatitis

Q: A 39 y/o male diabetes patient presented with blood glucose levels of AC (ante cibium/preprandial) 250 and PC (post cibium/postprandial) 350, and has a history of chronic active hepatitis with GOT/GPT 60/90. Considering the high glucose levels, I prescribed Zhi Bo Di Huang Tang subtracting Gan Cao and adding large doses of Huang Bo, Huang Qin, Sang Bai Pi, and Dai Zhe Shi. After taking this formula, GOT/GPT decreased to 24/38, but glucose levels remained elevated. The patient's urine and stool are normal and he has no excessive thirst. What's the best approach for treating this patient?

On a related topic, recently a medicinal pill made of Gua Lou Ren and Tian Hua Fen has become popular for the treatment of diabetes. I heard that a South Korean TCM doctor spent a lot of money to purchase the rights to this formula, but afterwards its clinical efficacy has proven disappointing, especially in *maintaining* normal glucose levels over the long term. Have you ever heard about this diabetes pill?

A: Diabetes with concomitant chronic hepatitis involves the excessive secretion of glycogen by the liver and *not* a beta-cell dysfunction issue involving the pancreas. I would continue prescribing Zhi Bo Di Huang Tang (enriches yin, downbears fire, and eliminates steaming) adding Huang Lian for a while longer. If glucose levels do *not* decrease, then change to a liver-settling wind-extinguishing and yin-enriching yang-subduing formula such as Jian Ling Tang (subtracting Gan Cao) adding The Three Yellows and Sang Bai Pi; and if levels still do *not* decrease, then add Sheng Shi Gao.

As for the popular TCM diabetes pill, I believe it was an overseas Chinese U.S. citizen who patented that formula, and it was intended for use as a complimentary therapy taken together with Western medicine drugs. It sounds like a bunch of "snake oil" to me, so to speak, and I wouldn't waste my time or money on it!

Case Study #7: Diabetes Patient – Glomus and Fullness Under the Heart

Q: A 45 y/o male diabetes patient presented with HbA1C 8.6, AC 150–180, and has had a persistent feeling of glomus and fullness below the heart that continues to bother him. How would you treat this patient?

A: It's possible that these symptoms may arise from the side effects of medication. But more likely, it has nothing to do with his diabetes at all, and instead, can simply be identified as stomach heat pattern. I would continue prescribing your original diabetes formula of either Zhi Bo Di Huang Tang or Jian Ling Tang adding The Three Yellows, Sang Bai Pi, and Lai Fu Zi (disperses food and eliminates distention and downbears qi and transforms phlegm).

This should quickly resolve the feeling of glomus and fullness below the heart, allowing the patient to continue making headway in achieving the ultimate goals of lowering blood glucose levels, weaning away from Western medicine drugs, and regulating the constitution so that eventually he can control diabetes through a healthy lifestyle.

IV. MUSCULOSKELETAL DISORDERS

Section 1: Bone, Joints, and Muscle

Case Study #1: Calcific Tendonitis of the Shoulder

Q: A 51 y/o female patient explained that she used to work in a restaurant serving food and clearing tables, which may have led to the pain she now feels in her right shoulder years later. An orthopedist diagnosed her with calcific tendonitis and gave her a local steroid injection to relieve the pain. How would you treat this type of patient?

A: Calcific tendonitis can be classified as congealing cold and cold impediment pattern. First, you must determine whether or not there is *adhesion* by testing her range of motion and the presence of scapular winging.

If so, you can approach this pathocondition like you would fifty-year-old's shoulder (aka frozen shoulder or adhesive capsulitis) by first performing the overhead traction-compression maneuver on the affected shoulder. Then, bleed the well points of the five fingers, needle the acupoints He Gu (LI4), Wai Guan (TB5), Zhong Zhu (TB3), and Hou Xi (SI3), and prescribe heat-clearing toxin-resolving and dampness-disinhibiting medicinals such as San Miao San, Huang Lian Jie Du Tang adding Zhi Mu, Fu Ling and Xe Xie, or Zhi Bo Di Huang Tang for the initial 3 days of treatment.

Following the initial 3 days of treatment, you can prescribe a qi-, blood-, and kidney yang-supplementing formula, such as Gui Qi Jian Zhong Tang, to dispel cold and wind. Plus, perform acupuncture (warm needling) locally on The Three Shoulder Acupoints—corresponding to Jian Yu (LI15), Jian Liao (TB14), and a point snugly wedged between the coracoid process and the humeral head—along with distal points on the arm and hand.

If not, then you can proceed by directly prescribing a qi-, blood-, and kidney yang-supplementing formula such as Gui Qi Jian Zhong

Tang to dispel cold and wind. Plus, perform acupuncture (warm needling) locally on The Three Shoulder Acupoints, along with distal points on the arm and hand.

Case Study #2: Shoulder Joint Pain – Strain, Sprain, or Malalignment?

Q: A patient of mine presented with an odd type of glenohumeral joint pain. When he raises his left arm laterally in full extension above his head there is no pain, but when he lowers his arm back down again he feels pain in his shoulder joint. The hitch is when he lowers his arm *quickly*, *no* pain presents, but only when he lowers his arm *slowly*. What could the reason for this be?

A: Well, you should first determine whether or not a strain, sprain, or subluxation has occurred via thorough history taking and physical examination. Remember! If you have doubts about the type, extent, or severity of an injury, you can always request that the patient have diagnostic imaging tests (e.g., x-ray, MRI)) performed in order to accurately determine your diagnosis and treatment plan.

For most cases, unless there is a fracture or complete dislocation (luxation), you can perform the overhead traction-compression maneuver (shoulder) or recumbent traction maneuver (shoulder) to correct malalignment in the glenohumeral joint cavity. If there is *no* noticeable heat or inflammation, then you can go ahead and prescribe a qi-, blood-, and kidney yang-supplementing formula such as Gui Qi Jian Zhong Tang or Ge Gen Tang adding Gan Jiang, Fu Zi, and Huang Qin.

Case Study #3: Lumbar Scoliosis – TCM Treatment Options

Q: A 16 y/o female patient visited my clinic with a chief complaint of progressively worsening lumbar scoliosis—she had been initially diagnosed with adolescent idiopathic scoliosis (AIS) when she was 14 y/o. She said that an examination 1 year ago showed that her spine was curved to the right (dextroscoliosis) by 15° and this year when she was examined it had increased to 25°.

Her scoliosis has gotten severe enough to the point she cannot come near to touching her toes while doing a forward bend, whereas this was not difficult for her at all a couple of years ago. Is there anything that TCM can do to help this patient?

A: The etiology of scoliosis is unknown, but is thought to involve both genetic and environmental factors. It manifests as unilateral laxity of vertebral ligaments (convex side) at specific locations along the spine, while the opposing side remains normal (concave side).

As for TCM treatment, I would prescribe either Shi Quan Da Bu Tang (quickens and supplements the blood, boosts qi and fortifies the spleen, and supplements kidney yang) or You Gui Yin (warms and supplements kidney yang, quickens the blood and dissipates stasis, strengthens sinew and bone, and eliminates dampness and relieves pain) adding Gan Jiang, Fu Zi, Lu Rong, and Huang Qi (large dose of up to 2 liang). Perform acupuncture (warm needle) locally on Hua Tuo's Paravertebral Points (EX-B2) at the affected site of the spine, along with distal acupoints such as Tian Zhu (UB10), Wei Zhong (UB40), Kun Lun (UB60), and Yang Ling Quan (GB34). Also, advise the patient to do traction stretches (e.g., hanging from a horizontal bar) and forward or backward bend stretches.

You must make sure the patient understands that the therapeutic regimen will require a long period of time in order to strengthen and tighten up the lax vertebral ligaments (results won't appear overnight!). Since the patient is only 16 years old there is still hope that her vertebral ligaments will tighten up and her spine will gradually straighten out, especially if she makes a conscious effort to maintain good posture, gets into the habit of regularly exercising and doing traction type stretching, and sticks to the TCM therapeutic regimen.

If your patient's condition has not improved (or has worsened) after she has physically stopped growing 2–3 years down the road, then she can consider consulting with a neurosurgeon or an orthopedic surgeon to determine if corrective surgery is a feasible option. For patients who do undergo corrective surgery, I would prescribe one of the abovementioned formulas which will promote circulation and the removal of postsurgical metabolic waste buildup, strengthen the surgically corrected sinews (muscles, tendons, and ligaments), expedite the process of osteogenesis for faster fusion, help mitigate the intensity of postsurgical pain, and accelerate the entire recovery process.

As a general rule, for children and adolescents, I would advise *against* using braces or having corrective surgery, because the body still has so much room to grow, develop, and "correct" itself. At this stage, braces and invasive corrective surgery may negatively impact this natural growth process, cause iatrogenic complications, and in the end, may *not* provide overall improvement in quality of life. However, for patients with moderate and severe curvatures of around ≥ 30°, factors such as age and rate of progression may warrant bracing, and corrective surgery may be necessary for an angle of deviation so severe that it dramatically impacts quality of life and/or affects internal organs such as the heart and lungs.

Case Study #4: 'S'-Shaped Scoliosis – You Gui Yin Variant

Q: Recently, a 14 y/o female patient with thoracolumbar scoliosis came for consultation and treatment. She has an 'S'-shaped curve with the largest angle of deviation at 19°. The patient's older sister also has the same type of scoliosis. Can TCM provide effective treatment for this pathocondition?

Wouldn't the administration of yang-supplementing medicinals promote strengthening and development of *both* the healthy and affected sinew (muscles, tendons, and ligaments) and bone that would either negate or even "overcompensate," resulting in an exacerbation of the scoliosis?

A: The therapeutic objective for administration of TCM medicinals in the treatment of scoliosis is primarily focused on stopping the progression, stabilizing the condition, and in the best case scenario offering some slight improvement. But this will take time.

Typically, an orthopedician will recommend simply monitoring a curvature in the spine if it's less than 25°, using a scoliosis brace if it's 25–45°, and undergoing corrective surgery if it's over 45°. Unless the curvature is severe (≥ 45-50°), you should simply advise the patient to do traction stretches (e.g., horizontal bar hanging), get regular exercise, be mindful of maintaining a good posture, and stay on the TCM therapeutic regimen. In the future, if she feels that it is necessary, she can look into the possibility of corrective surgical options.

Right now, the patient is still young and the best option is to prescribe a kidney yang-warming and -supplementing, blood-quickening stasis-dissipating, sinew- and bone-strengthening, and dampness-eliminating pain-relieving formula such as You Gui Yin variant. And if the patient is open to the idea of acupuncture, you can warm needle the following acupoints: Hua Tuo's Paravertebral Points (EX-B2) at the affected site, along with distal acupoints such as Tian Zhu (UB10), Wei Zhong (UB40), Kun Lun (UB60), and Yang Ling Quan (GB34).

Remember! Unless the deviation is severe, it is best for patients to wait until the spine is fully matured. If a patient does undergo corrective surgery at some point in time, it is best to take TCM medicinal decoctions afterwards to strengthen the sinew and bone, otherwise there is a good chance that some time after the surgery a "spinal drift" (deviation) may recur.

In regards to your question about yang-supplementing medicinals somehow having an "overcompensating" effect, the pharmacodynamics of TCM medicinals have *adaptogenic* and *targeted therapy* actions, with formula compositions containing conductor medicinals that enter specific channels, organs, regions and parts of the body. For instance, in this case, a formula that supplements kidney yang, such as You Gui Yin, which contains medicinals that enter the kidney—governs the bones and engenders marrow—channels (Tu Si Zi, Di Huang, Gou Qi Zi, Shan Zhu Yu, and Shan Yao) and serve as a conductor to the lumbus (spine) and lower limbs (the medicinal pair Niu Xi and Du Zhong), can be prescribed as the main formula. This formula composition is designed to focus on targeting the spine (and lower limbs) and compensating for the deficiencies in the "affected" sinew and bone. Oral administration of this formula decoction promotes the synthesis and metabolism of amino acids and manifests in the anabolism of sinew and bone at the sites of dyshomeostasis!

Case Study #5: Osteoporosis

Q: A few days ago, a friend of mine brought his mother in to see me explaining that tests, including a DXA scan (dual-energy x-ray absorptiometry), revealed the presence of decreased bone mineral density (BMD). She has tried both prescription medication (i.e., biphosphonates and SERMs (selective estrogen receptor modulators)), over-the-counter vitamin supplements, and attempted to make healthy lifestyle changes over the past 6 years, but her condition has gotten worse.

She wants to try taking TCM medicinals in hopes of halting BMD loss and lowering the risk of incurring fragility fractures in the future. I requested she have an MRI performed and it showed pronounced porosity throughout many bones in her body including vertebrae. What is the best approach for treating this type of pathocondition?

A: Typically, osteoporosis can be effectively treated by prescribing TCM formulas that nourish kidney yin and supplement kidney yang. Just make sure to include medicinals such as Gui Ban Jiao (Tortoise-Plastron Gelatin), Lu Jiao Jiao (Deer Antler Gelatin), Cu Lu Rong (Coarse-Haired Deer Antler), or Xi Lu Rong (Fin-Haired Deer Antler).

High-dose vitamin D intake and the administration of antiresorptive drugs (e.g., biphosphonates, SERMs) inhibit the rate of bone resorption, but do *not* promote healthy bone formation, resulting in the accelerated production of brittle bone even more susceptible to fracture. It is like adding on a coating of superglue to the leg of an old antique chair; the wood (bone) inside is still weak (fragile) and withering away (losing density) as time passes by, and if it happens to break (fracture) it still won't be easy to fix (heal). Add to this the very real problem of having patients who overdo it by taking a veritable smorgasbord of "health" supplements that include calcium and vitamin D, unwittingly "overcompensating" and running the risk of toxicity (i.e., hypercalcemia).

Osteoporosis can be classified into four main pattern types:

1) Spleen qi vacuity—elderly patients with poor appetite, nutritional intake, and intestinal absorption;
2) Static blood—inflammation or obstruction of exchange pathways connecting microvasculature and bone marrow, resulting from inhibited circulation and leading to insufficient blood perfusion and the chronic depletion of existing bone marrow and collagen;
3) Kidney yin vacuity—patients with a history of osteomyelitis or tuberculosis, those who have received chemotherapy or radiotherapy, and those with nutritional deficiencies that leads to either insufficient intestinal absorption of calcium or

accelerated break down of bone by osteoclasts; and

4) Kidney yang vacuity—insufficient kidney hormone levels disrupt the kidney-parathyroid hormone (PTH) feedback mechanism, resulting in insufficient bone marrow and collagen that leads to a vicious cycle of increasingly brittle vertebrae.

Case Study #6: Vertebral Osteomyelitis – Lower Limb Paralysis

Q: Two months ago, a 70 y/o male slipped and fell while jogging. After the fall, he didn't feel like there was anything wrong at all and went on with his daily routine up, until about 3 weeks later, when all of the sudden he couldn't move both lower limbs.

After being admitted into the hospital he was first administered high-dose intravenous corticosteroid therapy to relieve symptoms, and then an MRI was performed which revealed vertebral osteomyelitis in the spinal cord extending from T8 down to the lumbar spine.

Right now he is still in the hospital receiving corticosteroid infusions in hopes of stabilizing his condition and preventing deterioration. His family just contacted me saying that he can only move the first and second toes on his right foot, while the left foot is completely paralyzed. What role can TCM play in the treatment of this transverse myelitis case?

A: It sounds like the administration of high-dose corticosteroid infusions have *not* been able to effectively resolve the inflammation and the resulting metabolic waste buildup continues blocking the nerve conduction pathways of the lower limbs. In the majority (at least 2/3) of these types of cases, the administration of corticosteroids (or TCM heat-clearing toxin-resolving (anti-inflammatory) medicinals for that matter) during the acute stage will effectively resolve the inflammation and enable the patient to make either a partial or complete recovery.

Since the patient has already been administered corticosteroids to resolve inflammation, this condition can be identified as yang vacuity pattern and can be treated with one of the formulas in the Paralysis Formula Series—Paralysis Formula #1 (Di Long San Variant), Formula #2 (Shi Quan Da Bu Tang Variant), or Paralysis Formula #3

(You Gui Yin Variant). As you administer your formula, you should advise the patient to gradually reduce the dose of corticosteroids up until complete discontinuation.

Once he has been weaned away from corticosteroids, the patient will likely present with exterior heat with repletion constipation pattern. At this time, if exterior pattern (i.e., fever) presents in the *absence* of neurological symptoms (i.e., paresis, paralysis, and/or paresthesias), you can consider prescribing formula variants such as Da Qing Long Tang, Ma Huang Tang, Gui Zhi Tang, or Ge Gen Tang. Just make sure to include large doses of The Three Yellows, Sheng Shi Gao, Di Long, Da Huang, and if necessary Pu Xiao. If *both* exterior pattern and neurological symptoms present, then you should consider prescribing Paralysis Formula #1 (Di Long San Variant). In the *absence* of exterior pattern symptoms (or once they have resolved), you can prescribe either Paralysis Formula #2 or Paralysis Formula #3.

This type of pathocondition can be identified as vacuity-repletion complex pattern with the presentation of signs, symptoms, and diagnostic tools (e.g., laboratory tests, imaging studies) ultimately determining your choice of therapeutic regimen. As always, your capacity to accurately conduct pattern identification as the basis for determining treatment will make it possible to achieve effective results over time, gradually relieving symptoms and putting the patient on the path to recovery.

Case Study #7: Vertebral Osteomyelitis – Epidural Abscess and Bacteremia

Q: A 65 y/o female explained that about 6 months ago she suffered a T12 vertebral fracture from an automobile accident and subsequently underwent a surgical procedure involving spinal fusion (spondylodesis) to join the vertebrae through internal fixation.

Infection resulted as a complication following surgery, resulting in the development of an epidural abscess and bacteremia. The patient underwent two more surgeries in order to drain the pus from the abscess and was prescribed antibiotics and corticosteroids.

Now, the patient still has mild paresis in her right arm and hand. How would you treat this patient?

A: In my opinion, this sounds like a case of vertebral osteomyelitis with subsequent development of an epidural abscess. Once the abscess broke open it failed to heal and the inflammation resulted in metabolic waste buildup that has blocked nerve conductance in the right upper extremity. That's why the patient now presents with paresis.

At this stage, further surgical debridement will *not* improve the condition and the best approach would be to take antibiotics along with TCM medicinals. The most important thing for you to do is accurately identify the pattern and begin administering your formula as soon as possible.

In Chinese medicine, osteomyelitis can be identified as steaming bone taxation heat pattern and Shao Yang heat pattern, requiring administration of formula variants such as Hyperactive Immune Formula, Xi Jiao Di Huang Tang, Zhi Bo Di Huang Tang, Di Gu Pi Yin, Xiao Chai Hu Tang, or Qin Lian Si Wu Tang.

Just make sure to include the following medicinals: Huang Bo (as the sovereign medicinal to clear heat and resolve toxin); Qing Hao, Zhi Mu, and Di Gu Pi (enrich yin and downbear fire, cool the blood and clear vacuity heat, and eliminate steaming bone); Ma Huang and Di Long (nervous system conductor medicinals); and Niu Xi (quickens the blood and frees the channels, supplements the liver and kidney, strengthens sinew and bone, disinhibits water and frees strangury, and conducts fire (blood) downward).

You can also consider adding small doses of either Wan Ling Dan (contains a small dose of Xiong Huang, thus *mild* toxin-resolving actions) for less severe cases of bacteremia or Xiong Huang (*potent* toxin-resolving action) for severe cases of sepsis.

Case Study #8: Tuberculosis Spondylitis – More Common in the Elderly

Q: A 68 y/o male has been suffering from chronic lumbar pain for many years now. At the onset he thought it was just a part of aging, and at times when the pain was really bad he would seek treatment from a physiotherapist.

Recently, the pain has been so unbearable that he couldn't even walk, prompting him to go see a neurologist for a thorough examination (e.g., MRI, blood culture), which revealed a tuberculous growth at L3. His neurosurgeon advised against undergoing surgery, thus the patient decided to give TCM a try. At his initial clinical visit he presented with severe lumbar pain and difficulty walking, but *no* external contraction exterior pattern-type symptoms (i.e., fever). Would it be accurate for me to classify this patient's condition as paralysis (paresis)?

A: The elderly are the demographic who most commonly present with tuberculous spondylitis (Pott's disease), resulting from either reactivation of latent tuberculosis or new infection due to relatively compromised immune systems. And it may simply go undiagnosed for many years such as in the case of your patient.

The first step in your therapeutic regimen should be to prescribe an yin-enriching fire-downbearing, vacuity heat-clearing and steaming bone-eliminating formula such as Zhi Bo Di Huang Tang, Ba Xian Chang Shou Wan, or Bai He Gu Jin Tang. Just make sure to include Di Long, Qing Hao, Zhi Mu, Di Gu Pi, Sheng Du Zhong, and Niu Xi. If repletion heat presents, then add The Three Yellows; and if water swelling (edema) presents, then add The Four Lings. This approach should provide effective relief of symptoms and an improved quality of life.

Case Study #9: Hallux Valgus (Bunion)

Q: Is it advisable to directly needle A Shi (ouch) acupoints (阿是穴 □ shì xué) on the big toe for the treatment of hallux valgus (aka bunion)?

A: Acupuncture typically will *not* provide very effective treatment for hallux valgus (aka bunion). However, if the malalignment (incongruency) of the first metatarsophalangeal (MTP) joint is *not* too extreme, and it is still *possible* to do a traction-manipulation maneuver on the big toe to restore alignment (congruency), you may consider directly needling into the MTP joint adding moxa cones on the tail (warm needle). This approach may provide better results.

Remember! The force of the traction-manipulation maneuver may result in acute inflammation and thus you should bleed the spleen and liver channel well points on the big toe and prescribe a formula variant such as Zhi Bo Di Huang Tang (enriches yin, downbears fire, and eliminates steaming) or Zuo Gui Yin (warms and supplements kidney yang and replenishes essence and supplements blood), making sure to include a large dose of Huang Bo (clears heat and resolves toxin).

After the inflammation resolves, you can change to a kidney yang-warming and -supplementing, blood-quickening stasis-dissipating, sinew- and bone-strengthening, and dampness-eliminating pain-relieving formula such as You Gui Yin. If pronounced pain presents, then also add Huo Luo Dan (dispels wind and eliminates dampness, transforms phlegm and frees the network vessels, and quickens the blood and relieves pain).

If the degree of malalignment is too extreme to effectively perform the traction-manipulation maneuver, then warm needle above, below, and along the sides of the joint space as a means of preventing further deterioration. If the degree of deformity and/or pain is too much for the patient to bear, then another option would be to consult a podiatrist for surgical realignment. Surgery may resolve the problem, but also comes with the possibility of complications (e.g., deformities, avascular necrosis, hallux varus, nonunion, malunion) and recurrence.

Regardless of the therapeutic approach, you should advise the patient to avoid wearing tight shoes and high-heeled shoes with a tight toe box. This will reduce the likelihood of exacerbation and recurrence.

Case Study #10: Pseudohypoparathyroidism – Hypocalcemic Seizures

Q: A mother and father brought their 5 y/o boy to my clinic explaining that their son had been born with low calcium levels (hypocalcemia) and subsequently had been diagnosed with pseudohypoparathyroidism (i.e., hypocalcemia, hyperphosphatemia, and secondary hyperparathyroidism). The patient has been taking medication to control the condition and has exhibited no physical or cognitive abnormalities other than mild attention deficit problems.

A few days ago he suddenly passed out, but then quickly regained consciousness. Then, later that same day in the evening at around 11 p.m., he passed out again when he was watching television. His parents rushed him to the emergency room where he eventually regained consciousness. Upon coming to, he presented with mild generalized spasms (tetany) and vomiting, prompting a nearly 3-week stay in the hospital to stabilize his condition and conduct evaluations.

He has been taking Western medicine drugs to control his condition since then. He still vomits several times each day, usually after eating meals and at nighttime, but he doesn't have seizures or spasms. How would you approach this case?

A: This is a complicated case for sure and really tough on the child (and parents). I am aware of another related phenotype of this congenital disorder called Albright hereditary osteodystrophy (Martin-Allbright syndrome), but it also presents with even more severe physical and cognitive abnormalities. Generally, I classify all types of congenital conditions (e.g., hemophilia, cerebral palsy) involving compromised physical, cognitive, and physiological development as wilting pattern (痿證 w□ i zhèng).

For the treatment of wilting pattern, I would typically prescribe a kidney yang-warming and -supplementing, blood-quickening stasis-dissipating, sinew- and bone-strengthening, and dampness-eliminating pain-relieving formula such as You Gui Yin or Shen Qi Wan. However, for your patient, you could even consider prescribing a simpler approach such as Si Ni Tang (warms the channels and expels cold and returns yang and stems counterflow) or Zhen Wu Tang (warms kidney yang and disinhibits water qi). Just make sure to add Sheng Shi Gao in order to promote the release of calcium from the bones, calcium synthesis and reabsorption by the kidney, and the absorption of vitamin D in the large intestine. And if vomiting persists, then also include Ban Xia and Fu Ling in your formula.

This therapeutic approach will help increase calcium levels and resolve the symptoms induced by hypocalcemia.

Case Study #11: Fractured Ribs in Car Accident – Chest and Rib Distention and Pain

Q: Three weeks ago, a 45 y/o male got into an automobile accident, fracturing two of his ribs on the left side. Since the accident he has experienced frequent cough, shallow breathing, wheezing after a deep breath, and distention and pain on the left side of the chest that worsens with deep breaths and certain movements. X-ray shows fracture lines without any noticeable displacement.

I prescribed Chai Ling Tang (including large doses of Fu Ling, Bai Zhu, and Ze Xie) adding Ma Huang and Xing Ren. Do you think this is a good formula?

A: This sounds like a stereotypical case of fractured ribs. For these types of patients, it is important to always advise them to get x-rays, and if necessary, a CT scan to rule out potential complications in the thorax (e.g., pneumothorax, hemothorax, atelectasis, pulmonary contusion, pneumonia). In the case of floating rib fractures, you need to rule out potential complications in the abdomen (e.g., laceration of liver, spleen, and kidneys). Most simple fractures will mend on their own within 1 to 2 months, but TCM therapeutic intervention will expedite the healing process and effectively mitigate and resolve symptoms.

Chai Ling Tang (clears heat and transforms phlegm-damp, disinhibits water, moves qi and quickens the blood, and relieves pain) is a great formula for this patient. However, it's *not* necessary to increase the doses of Bai Zhu, Fu Ling, and Ze Xie, but I would add Yu Sheng Wan. You should also consider needling acupoints such as Nei Guan (PC6), Chi Ze (LU5), and Tai Chong (LI3) for even faster results at resolving the frequent cough, shallow breathing, and distention and pain. Once the patient's cough resolves, then you know that the fracture has healed.

However, in some patients the pain and distention may persist even after the fracture has healed, and I classify this as intercostal nerve "phantom pain." "Phantom pain" most commonly presents in people who are under a lot of stress or unable to handle pressure well and also those with posttraumatic stress disorder (PTSD) (which includes traffic accidents!).

Even for these types of patients, just stay the course by continuing to administer Chai Ling Tang variant, performing acupuncture, and if necessary, simply consider incrementally increasing the dose of Yu Sheng Wan. This should provide effective results over time. It has been my experience that for patients with "phantom pain," adding in blood-quickening stasis-transforming medicinals such as Chuan Qi, Ru Xiang, and Mo Yao really does *not* improve the overall treatment outcome.

Case Study #12: Calf Tightness and Cramping After Only 20 Minutes of Jogging

Q: A 52 y/o male patient visited me explaining that recently he suffers from excruciating tightness and pain in his left calf (Cheng Jin (UB56) and Chang Shan (UB57)) after only 20 minutes of jogging. Do you think that the cause of this condition is vascular or neural? And how would you treat it?

A: This sounds like peripheral vascular disease (PVD) (aka peripheral arterial disease (PAD)), which involves narrowing of the peripheral arteries due to atherosclerosis. Atheroslerotic plaques may lead to narrowing of the arteries and ischemia of the lower extremities. Mild cases of ischemia present with intermittent claudication, such as in your patient here, while severe cases may cause rest pain, skin atrophy, cyanosis, ulcers and gangrene. Typically, this type of condition can be classified as either stasis heat or cold stasis pattern, which results in vascular spasm of the lower extremities.

You can consider prescribing a blood-quickening stasis-dispelling and qi-supplementing pain-relieving formula such as Ru Mo Si Wu Tang, Bu Yang Huan Wu Tang, or Sheng Yu Tang adding other medicinals based on the presenting signs, symptoms, and pattern. If the patient presents with edema, then add The Four Lings and Chuan Qi. If the patient presents with pain upon sitting (rest pain), then add The Three Great Yang-Supplementers, Niu Xi, Huang Bo, and Chuan Qi. Make sure to perform acupuncture as well, needling (or warm needling) the distal acupoints corresponding with the site of tightness and pain. This approach should provide noticeable relief of symptoms in a short period of time.

You should advise your patient to try brisk walking instead of jogging for a while, which provides the same type of cardio workout with less stress on the lower extremities. It's best for the patient to get on their feet and keep moving as much as possible—do *not* just sit around and do *not* sit cross-legged! These simple habits will help prevent the feeling of tightness and cramping. Naturally, a healthy diet, getting enough sleep, stress reduction, and quitting smoking are equally important.

V. NEUROLOGICAL DISORDERS

Case Study #1: Sinew Wilting Following Lumbar Spine Surgery

Q: A 30 y/o female patient visited me explaining that back during her college days she was diagnosed with lumbar spinal disc herniation and underwent surgical treatment. Following surgery she suffered from paresis, myasthenia, and muscle atrophy in her left leg, making it impossible for her to stand and walk on her own. About 6 months after surgery, she also began experiencing mild upper extremity weakness in both arms, which has progressed over the years.

Now, she has slow motor responses in her arms and difficulty raising her arms. I understand that the lower extremity problems could have been due to the severity of the original injury or possibly a complication of surgery, but why would she also begin to have upper extremity weakness? She has lived with this disability for many years now and expressed her frustration. It was obvious that she really feels depressed about her condition. Do you think this weakness in her upper arms could be asthenia caused by depression? What is the best approach for treating this patient?

A: The progressive upper extremity limb weakness has nothing to do with lumbar spine surgery. Psychosomatic asthenia is a possibility, but the more likely causes that you must rule out are myasthenia gravis, motor neuron disorder, muscular dystrophy, and occipital foramen stenosis. She should see a neurologist for a thorough examination to verify the etiology.

As for TCM treatment, these types of pathoconditions can be classified as sinew wilting (筋痿 j□ n w□ i) and identified as dual qi and yang vacuity pattern. Thus, I recommend prescribing a formula such as Bu Yang Huan Wu Tang, Bu Zhong Yi Qi Tang, or Gui Qi Jian Zhong Tang adding The Three Great Yang-Supplementers, Huang Qin, Di Long, Ma Huang (small dose), and Ren Shen/Chuan Qi Powder.

Later on during the therapeutic regimen, as her condition begins to improve, you can begin adding incremental doses of Xi Lu Rong (powder), which will produce noticeable improvements in strength and function and further accelerate the healing process.

Case Study #2: Myasthenia Gravis – Atrophy of the Thenar Eminence

Q: Over the past 3 months, a middle-aged male patient first started feeling weakness and then later on noticed muscular atrophy in his left hand. Upon examination, there was pronounced atrophy of the thenar eminence (He Gu (LI4) and Yu Ji (LU10)) on his left hand, but no other significant signs, symptoms, or complaints.

Suspecting this patient may have myasthenia gravis, I prescribed Gui Qi Jian Zhong Tang adding Ma Huang and Di Long. The patient took this formula for two weeks, but decided to discontinue treatment because he didn't notice any "immediate" improvement. I explained to him that results may take some time to appear and encouraged him to continue taking this regimen for at least 3 months before deciding whether or not to give up. He thanked me for my concern and efforts, but seemed to think his condition wasn't that serious and he didn't really need to treat it.

This was a particularly frustrating case for me, because I am confident that I can help him resolve symptoms and effectively manage this pathocondition. Do you have any suggestions on this case?

A: These symptoms suggest myasthenia gravis, but to confirm the diagnosis you should advise your patient to see a neurologist for a thorough examination (i.e., EMG, AChR antibodies, chest CT, Edrophonium test (Tensilon test)). This will be beneficial for both you and the patient and may even persuade him to start treating the condition now, before it progresses into more generalized and complex symptoms.

In the early stages of myasthenia gravis, prior to the administration of immunosuppressants (e.g., glucocorticoids, azathioprine) and depending on presenting signs and symptoms, this pathocondition can be identified as a type of wilting—heat, muscle heat, damp-heat, stomach heat, Yang Ming heat, or lung heat scorching the lobes—pattern. Thus, to effectively remedy symptoms and control disease progression, you can consider prescribing a corresponding formula, such as one of the Miao San (Mysterious Powder) variants (e.g., Er Miao San, San Miao Wan, Si Miao Wan), Wen Dan Tang, Zhi Bo Di Huang Tang, Qing Wei San, or Bai Hu Tang.

If the patient has already been administered immunosuppressants, then the pathocondition can be identified as qi vacuity wilting or dual qi and yang vacuity wilting pattern. That's when it is appropriate to prescribe a qi-, blood-, and kidney yang-supplementing formula, such as Gui Qi Jian Zhong Tang (incrementally increasing the dose of Huang Qi up to a maximum of 2 liang), or a spleen-fortifying qi-supplementing and yang-upbearing formula, such as Bu Zhong Yi Qi Tang adding Ma Huang and Di Long. Acupuncture is also an important part of the therapeutic regimen and you should warm needle acupoints along the corresponding channels of the affected sites.

Remember! The rate of progression for myasthenia gravis is variable. Symptoms may remain relatively mild for some patients, while others may go through periods of improvement and then suddenly present with progressive exacerbations. Muscle weakness worsens throughout the day with increased activity and improves after rest. Typical symptoms are ocular muscle weakness (e.g., ptosis, diplopia), bulbar muscle weakness (e.g., slurred speech, difficulty chewing and swallowing), proximal limb weakness (e.g., difficulties standing up, climbing stairs), and respiratory muscle weakness. Some patients may even experience myasthenic crisis that results in acute respiratory failure and death.

The best approach for treating myasthenia gravis is with long-term administration of TCM medicinals (and if necessary, concomitant Western medicine therapeutic intervention), follow-up examinations, and subsequent formula modifications. Once the symptoms have resolved and the condition has stabilized, you can then begin tapering down the dosage and eventually discontinuing treatment.

For patients who are *not* compliant and/or do *not* recognize the need to treat their pathocondition, all we can do as doctors is try our best to fulfill our responsibility of providing the most accurate medical information possible, including details about symptoms, progression, and prognosis. Make sure to write down the key points of the information and advice discussed with the patient in his medical record and let the patient (and family) decide for themselves. In this way, patients gain a positive impression of your candor and professionalism, and if their conditions persist and/or exacerbate, they may very well decide to come back again for treatment in the future!

Case Study #3: Myasthenia Gravis – Atrophy, Fatigue, and Heaviness

Q: Recently, a 51 y/o male patient visited me explaining that he began feeling generalized weakness and fatigue about 2 years ago, and after undergoing a thorough examination he was diagnosed with myasthenia gravis. He was initially treated with pyridostigmine (cholinesterase inhibitor) and then corticosteroids, which seemed to control the progression for a while, but over the past 3 months he has had muscle atrophy, generalized fatigue, and a feeling of heaviness throughout his entire body.

I tried the treatment approach you told me about, prescribing Gui Qi Jian Zhong Tang (including a large dose of Huang Qin (8 qian)) adding Ren Shen (powder). Results have been good so far. The patient said that he began feeling more energy and strength after only 4 days of administration. Is there anything I should be aware of as the treatment regimen continues?

A: Great! That formula will provide effective treatment for dual qi and yang vacuity wilting pattern, but you should also incrementally increase the dose of Huang Qi up to a maximum of 2 liang. In the future, you must continue conducting the four examinations to identify any changes in the pattern that may warrant modifications to your therapeutic approach.

Over time, if the patient continues regaining muscle strength and tone, without any other symptoms arising, and appears to have stabilized, this is a sign the condition has returned to the "essential (root) state" of heat—muscle heat, damp-heat, stomach heat, Yang Ming heat, or lung heat dryness—pattern. At that time, you should consider either modifying your original formula or changing to a new formula accordingly.

The Yellow Emperor's Inner Canon mentions lung heat scorching the lobes (i.e., thymoma, thymic hyperplasia) as the principle etiology of wilting disease and identifies Yang Ming channel as the focus of treatment. I like to classify this pathocondition as muscle wilting (肌痿

j□ w□i) myself, which tends to present concomitantly with either damp-heat, phlegm-rheum, stubborn phlegm and strange rheum, qi vacuity, cold phlegm, or cold rheum.

It doesn't have to be that complicated though. You can use this simplified pattern guideline as a reference for treating the various manifestations of wilting pattern in myasthenia gravis:

1) Lung heat scorching the lobes pattern—Patients whose myasthenia gravis is caused by a thymoma almost always undergo surgical resection (thymectomy), and thus I have never treated this type of patient.
2) Damp-heat and phlegm-rheum with qi vacuity pattern—In these patients, skeletal muscle weakness and fatigue results from an autoimmune induced production of acetylcholine receptor (AChR) antibodies, leading to impaired signal transduction in the neuromuscular junction (NMJ) and resulting in skeletal muscle weakness and fatigue. The trigger for autoantibody production is unknown, but the disorder may be associated with abnormalities of the thymus, autoimmune hyperthyroidism, and other autoimmune disorders. For this pattern type, you can prescribe formulas such as the Miao San (Mysterious Powder) variants (e.g., Er Miao San, San Miao Wan, Si Miao Wan), Wen Dan Tang, or Zhi Bo Di Huang Tang.
3) Dual qi and yang vacuity pattern—In these patients the disease has further progressed, presenting with generalized weakness, fatigue, and muscle atrophy. For this pattern type, you can prescribe formula variants such as Gui Qi Jian Zhong Tang, Bu Zhong Yi Qi Tang, and Bu Yang Huan Wu Tang. Just make sure to include The Three Great Yang-Supplementers and large doses of Huang Qi.

Remember! As a general rule, when prescribing a patient medicinals over a long period of time, it is good practice to switch up your formula every now and then. Naturally, for many patients the process of pattern identification as the basis for determining treatment may naturally lead you to choose different formulas and/or extensively modify your main formula. However, in the treatment of many types of chronic conditions, you may not necessarily need to change your formula or even make that many modifications.

For these patients who receive long-term administration of the same formula variant, you should *periodically* switch over to another formula that includes similar actions, but with a different emphasis. For instance, if you prescribe a qi-, blood-, and kidney yang-supplementing formula, such as Gui Qi Jian Zhong Tang variant, continually for a long duration (say 6 months to 1 year), then you could switch over to a blood-quickening qi-supplementing formula such as Bu Yang Huan Wu Tang variant for a period of time (say 1 month) and evaluate the patient's progress. If you determine that your original formula (e.g., Gui Qi Jian Zhong Tang) is still the best option, then switch back to it.

This approach will alleviate the potential for the patient building up tolerance to the medicinals, and depending on the types of medicinals prescribed, will reduce the chances of developing deleterious side effects.

Case Study #4: Lower Extremity Weakness and Ankle Adduction – Wilting Pattern

Q: A 64 y/o female patient explained that 1 year ago she suddenly incurred weakness in both legs and both ankles shifted laterally (adduction) away from the midline by approximately 20° to 30° degrees. She walks with a limp now and feels self-conscious about it, so she rarely goes out of the house anymore unless it's absolutely necessary.

She underwent a thorough physical examination by a neurologist that included an MRI and EMG, but was not given a definitive diagnosis. Her doctor told her that the only thing they can do for her is perform surgical correction. She decided against surgery and instead sought treatment from a traditional Korean medicine (TKM) doctor, receiving 6 months of treatment that included medicinals and acupuncture.

A friend of hers recommended me and now she hopes to try TKM again. I really want to help her get back in stride. I suspect this patient may have myasthenia gravis. What do you think?

A: Hmm!...Paroxysmal weakness of the lower extremities and ankle adduction causing the patient to walk with a limp. I would suspect myasthenia gravis as one possibility as well, but it seems odd that this condition would go undiagnosed following a thorough medical examination. Regardless if there is a definitive diagnosis or not, in classical TCM pathological terms this condition can be identified as wilting pattern. Wilting pattern can present with concomitant damp-heat, phlegm-rheum (phlegm heat, cold phlegm, stubborn phlegm and strange rheum), stomach heat, qi vacuity, dual qi and yang vacuity, and kidney yang vacuity.

First, you should examine her lower extremities to determine the presence of heat or cold pattern. If heat and/or swelling present, then prescribe formula variants such as Di Long San and Zhi Bo Di Huang Tang; and if muscle weakness (myasthenia) and atrophy present in the *absence* of heat and/or swelling, then you must consider the possibility of a progressive neurodegenerative disease, such as amyotrophic lateral sclerosis (ALS).

For ALS patients, once the disease has progressed to the point of urinary and fecal incontinence and paresis or paralysis of the lower extremities, then you can apply the "paralysis" therapeutic approach prescribing either Paralysis Formula #2 or Paralysis Formula #3.

Case Study #5: Thenar Eminence Atrophy and Forearm Weakness – Wilting Pattern

Q: A 63 y/o female patient explained that years ago she began noticing atrophy in the "fatty part" between her right thumb and index finger (thenar eminence) and weakness in her right arm. She went to see a specialist for an examination that revealed a "pinched nerve" in her neck (cervical radiculopathy) for which she underwent a surgical procedure (posterior cervical laminoforaminotomy) to decompress the C6 spinal nerve. But after surgery the patient's condition did not improve and her doctors told her that it was "too late for treatment."

She has trouble using chopsticks to eat and can't grip or lift heavy objects with her right arm. What I don't really understand is that if this is a case of cervical radiculopathy, why doesn't the patient feel any numbness or pain, just atrophy and weakness? Do you think there could be some other underlying cause?

A: That does seem odd. If the decompression surgery did *not* improve the symptoms at all, then you should consider the possibility of myasthenia gravis or radial neuropathy. At this stage, regardless of whether these symptoms are being caused by the thymus gland (thymic hyperplasia), autoreactive antibodies (acetylcholine receptor (AChR) antibodies), spinal nerve compression, or peripheral neuropathy, you can prescribe a qi-, blood-, and kidney yang-supplementing formula such as Gui Qi Jian Zhong Tang, Shi Quan Da Bu Tang, or Bu Yang Huan Wu Tang. Just make sure to include The Three Great Yang-Supplementers, Huang Qin, and Ren Shen/Chuan Qi Powder.

As for acupuncture, you can warm needle acupoints locally at and distally along channels that correspond with the location of atrophy and weakness. Remember! Acupuncture alone will likely *not* be very effective in helping the patient regain muscle strength, but it will definitely help promote a tauter and fuller appearance of muscle tonicity for the sake of aesthetics.

You should remind the patient that this therapeutic regimen will take some time (3–6 months) before noticeable results appear. But even after that, you should continue administering treatment for at least 1 year (sometimes longer depending on the case) in order to ensure the patient has completely regained muscle strength and motor function. In the future, if the patient feels any weakness in her arm or hand, she should come back for follow-up treatment to prevent the potential of further exacerbation.

Case Study #6: Cholinergic System Dysfunction – Acetylcholine Dysregulation and Demyelination

Q: A 46 y/o male patient visited me with the following history: Recently, every time he gets emotionally excited or agitated his left arm feels weak and limp, his tongue feels numb, his speech becomes slurred, and at nighttime in bed he feels an aching distention-type pain in his back. He went for a medical examination, but the results of an MRI and MRA revealed nothing abnormal. Do you think this could be caused by anxiety?

A: No, this pathocondition does *not* sound like it is caused by emotional excitability and agitation, but by some type of cholinergic system dysfunction—dysregulation of acetylcholine (ACh) that causes symptoms of excitability, agitation, and demyelination.

It can be classified as a type of wilting pattern. In the post-acute stage, it can be identified as wilting with phlegm-heat pattern, requiring the prescription of a Shao Yang depressed (or residual) heat-clearing and inner body harassment phlegm turbidity-dispelling formula, such as Wen Dan Tang variant. If corticosteroids have been administered, then it can be identified as wilting with dual qi and yang vacuity pattern, requiring the prescription of a spleen-fortifying qi-supplementing and yang-upbearing formula such as Bu Zhong Yi Qi Tang combining Si Ni Tang, Gui Qi Jian Zhong Tang, or Ban Xia Tian Ma Bai Zhu San. Just make sure to include large doses of Huang Qi and Gan Jiang.

Remember! If your patient visited you right at the onset (acute stage), then this could be identified as externally contracted exterior pattern and you could consider prescribing a sweat-promoting, exterior-resolving and channel-coursing formula such as Ge Gen Tang variant. However, the acute stage therapeutic window for this exterior pattern is very short (3–4 days), so you must catch the pathocondition right at the onset in order for this type of formula to be effective. After the acute stage, this pathocondition will then evolve into the post-acute stage, which can be identified as a type of depressed (or residual) heat pattern as mentioned above.

Case Study #7: Amyotrophic Lateral Sclerosis – Is There Anything I Can Do?

Q: A 59 y/o female presented with severe weakness in both legs, numbness in both big toes, and mild weakness in her left arm. After telling me her symptoms she immediately broke down crying, telling me, "the doctors told me that I couldn't be cured," and went on asking me repeatedly, "Can I be cured, can I be cured…?" Once she calmed down, she told me that she had been diagnosed with amyotrophic lateral sclerosis (ALS). Is there anything I can do for her?

A: ALS is tough, full of hardship and heartache. You should tell the patient straight up that this really is a difficult condition to effectively treat. What makes it even worse is that all of the available drugs administered to mitigate the symptoms and provide temporary relief, *paradoxically*, will accelerate the process of neural degeneration and exacerbate the progression of motor dysfunction and cognitive impairment.

You can prescribe a kidney yang-supplementing, qi- and blood-supplementing, and dampness-eliminating pain-relieving formula such as You Gui Yin or Paralysis Formula #3 (You Gui Yin Variant), which will help slow down the rate of disease progression and improve quality of life. Even more importantly, you must provide ongoing emotional support and encouragement throughout what will inevitably be a downward spiraling progression up until the end. It is essential that "you" stay positive as well, because your attitude will have an impact on how the patient deals with the condition!

Case Study #8: Amyotrophic Lateral Sclerosis – Try Paralysis Formula #2 or #3

Q: Recently, I have been treating several amyotrophic lateral sclerosis (ALS) patients. One case in particular involves a 49 y/o female with the following history: At the onset, she incurred weakness from the knee down in her right leg, causing her to frequently lose balance and fall down. She was examined by a neurologist at a local hospital who misdiagnosed her as having lumbar radiculopathy, for which she underwent surgery that failed to resolve the symptoms. Eventually, she underwent further tests at a major medical center and was diagnosed with ALS and immediately began receiving treatment.

Despite treatment, her condition continues to deteriorate. Now, her right lower leg is completely paralyzed, she cannot flex or extend her right wrist (but can still move her fingers), her left lower limb is paralyzed except for some movement in her toes, but fortunately she can still use eating utensils with her left hand to eat. She also has constipation and an occasional dry cough. The only drug she is taking now is Riluzole (sodium-channel blocker). Please offer your advice and guidance on this case.

A: ALS is a motor neuron disease (MND) that is extremely difficult to treat and tends to be a torturous experience for patients to live through—I have heard some say a "living hell." This is a progressive neurodegenerative disease that affects both upper and lower motor neurons, and most patients eventually develop one or both of the life-threatening symptoms of respiratory impairment and dysphagia. Both doctors and the patient are powerless.

There really isn't much doctors can do for the patient, while the patient is relegated to watching themselves gradually wither away on a hijacked path inevitably leading to an early death. This may sound callous, but the truth is, towards the end patients are literally so powerless that they couldn't even commit suicide if they wanted to. Most patients will eventually end up dying from respiratory failure or foreign body airway obstruction that induces a fatal bout of pneumonia or simply choke to death.

If the disease has already progressed to the stage of dry cough, that may be a sign of imminent respiratory failure. You must be careful. Riluzole does not offer any significant efficacy in the treatment of ALS, and in fact, long-term administration may even cause the nerves to degenerate even faster. There are no other available drugs or procedures, so conventional medicine must make do with what they have.

For this patient, I would consider prescribing either Paralysis Formula #2 (Shi Quan Da Bu Tang Variant) (supplements qi, the blood, and kidney yang, frees the channels and quickens the network vessels, and disinhibits water by bland percolation) or Paralysis Formula #3 (You Gui Yin Variant) (warms and supplements kidney yang, frees the channels and quickens the network vessels, strengthens sinew and bone, and quickens the blood and transforms stasis). Make sure to incrementally increase the doses of Ma Huang, Di Long, Ren Shen (powder), and Da Huang (up until the patient maintains 2–3 stools/day).

At some point, the patient will likely receive enterostomy feeding, have a tracheostomy tube inserted and/or be put on mechanical ventilation. In the late stage of ALS, TCM can only relieve symptoms and possibly improve the overall condition for a period of time. When the symptoms really become too much to endure, then it may be best for the patient to be administered both corticosteroid and TCM medicinal therapy in efforts to improve quality of life up until the end.

Case Study #9: Distal Extremity Numbness and Lower Leg Weakness

Q: A 45 y/o patient presented with a history of bilateral numbness in three fingers (3rd, 4th, and 5th), the heart (center) of soles, and the occipital region, along with bilateral lower leg weakness. A neurologist conducted tests and had an MRI taken, which provided *no* conclusive results, and she was administered medication, which was *not* effective. In fact, her condition has continued to get worse! Particularly troubling is that sometimes both lower legs suddenly "give out," causing her to fall down. Urine and stool, appetite, and sleep are all normal.

A: The symptoms you have described suggest pathology of the cervical spine or brain, and could possibly be some type of motor neuron disease (MND). In TCM, the manifestation of these symptoms can be identified as wilting pattern.

As for treatment, first, I would try prescribing a spleen- and stomach-supplementing, phlegm-damp-transforming, and blood-nourishing wind-stabilizing formula such as Ban Xia Tian Ma Bai Zhu San variant (including a large dose of Huang Qi) adding Ma Huang, Di Long, and Niu Xi. You can also perform acupuncture (warm needling) as well, selecting dual qi- and blood-supplementing acupoints (e.g., Shou San Li (10) and Zu San Li (ST40), brain-arousing acupoints (e.g., Tian Zhu (UB10) and Feng Chi (GB20)), and other acupoints on channels that correspond with the affected sites. Acupuncture serves as an adjuvant therapy that will accelerate the recovery process.

You can evaluate the results of your treatment during ensuing follow-up visits and determine whether or not you need to change course or continue with this therapeutic approach. This will promote blood perfusion, nerve innervation, and improve muscle strength; and in the worst case scenario of MND, it can help promote nerve regeneration and reduce the overall rate of disease progression.

Case Study #10: Phantom Cold – "Water Droplets Flowing Up My Back"

Q: A 68 y/o male who has worked a lifetime in the maritime industry visited me recently. Starting about three years ago, every time he went out to work at sea he would frequently feel a strange sensation that he described as "water droplets flowing up my back." This sensation eventually spread over his entire body and was even more pronounced after eating and at nighttime when he was trying to sleep. This was particularly troublesome because he couldn't get a good night's sleep. Do you think this a neurological or psychosomatic disorder?

A: I would diagnosis this condition as phantom cold, which I believe is a type of neuropsychological disorder that shares some similarities to phantom itch and phantom pain. These four potential pattern types with accompanying formula suggestions come to mind (but you will also need to conduct further examination to distinguish for yourself):

- Yang vacuity externally contracted exterior cold pattern—Ma Huang Fu Zi Xi Xin Tang combining Si Ni Tang adding Huang Qin
- Wind-cold settling in the exterior pattern—Xiao Qing Long Tang adding Gan Jiang and Fu Zi
- Exterior depression with static blood obstructing the network vessels pattern—Di Long San adding Gan Jiang and Fu Zi
- Kidney yang vacuity pattern—You Gui Yin adding Ma Huang, Xi Xin, and Di Long

Regardless of which formula you choose, it is essential to add Gan Cao (boosts qi and supplements the center and relaxes tension and relieves pain), Long Yan Rou (supplements and boosts the heart and spleen and nourishes blood and quiets the spirit), and Yu Sheng Wan (promotes cerebral collateral circulation and recalibrates autoregulation in the brain). Plus, you should also perform acupuncture (warm needle) on acupoints along the urinary bladder channel. And if you wanted to, you could try infrared light therapy, by rubbing Mugwort Leaf (Artemisia) Ointment on the patient's back and directing the beam of an infrared lamp over the surface.

Remember! Making the necessary lifestyle modifications is essential for achieving therapeutic success. You should advise the patient to regularly exercise (preferably in the sunshine). Adequate amounts of exercise will jumpstart the qi dynamic, getting the juices flowing and activating the sweat glands, which will promote perspiration and make the body feel like it needs rest at night. This will be beneficial for both remedying the phantom cold sensation and sleeping problems. Also, remind the patient to eat a healthy, well-balanced diet that includes fresh fruits, vegetables, grains, nuts, meat, fish, mushrooms and eggs.

For patients with sleeping problems, especially yin vacuity sleeplessness (不寐 bù mèi), you can also recommend that they eat an egg yolk (enriches yin and nourishes the blood, quiets the heart, and supplements the spleen and stomach) right before bedtime to help get a good night's sleep!

Case Study #11: Phantom Itch – "Ants Crawling" Sensation Is Quite Common!

Q: A 60 y/o male patient explained that he always feels like there are "ants crawling" around the front of his right ear (near Er Men (TB21)) or that there is something sticking on it. There is a persistent, subtle, mild itchy feeling, not the type of itch that makes you want to scratch it for relief, but a gnawing type that *continuously* annoys the patient. He has seen many doctors and been administered both TCM and Western medicine treatment without effective results. Do you think this could be a trigeminal nerve (CNV) problem?

A: The "ants crawling" sensation of this patient is likely a psychoneurological symptom that can be classified as phantom itch. I would consider prescribing either Xian Fang Huo Ming Yin (clears heat and resolves toxin and quickens the blood and relieves pain), Wen Dan Tang (clears Shao Yang depressed heat and dispels phlegm turbidity harassing the inner body), or Bu Yang Huan Wu Tang (quickens the blood, supplements qi, and transforms stasis) variants. Just make sure to include The Three Insects and Yu Sheng Wan in your formula. Naturally, you could also needle acupoints locally at the affected site and distally along the corresponding channels to enhance efficacy.

Case Study #12: Phantom Pain – Heavy, Sagging Sensation in the Anus

Q: A 29 y/o male came for a clinical visit describing a history as follows: Two years ago, after sitting on the cold, frozen ground for an extended period of time, he felt a heavy, sagging sensation in the anus, which eventually progressed into painful distention. An anorectal specialist suspected it was hemorrhoids and decided to perform laser hemorrhoidoplasty, but the symptoms remained, and now he even feels distention and pain around the anus, especially after defecating.

I identified this pathocondition as center qi fall vacuity pattern, in which qi vacuity resulted in poor blood circulation to the anal sphincter and perianal area, and thus prescribed a 2-week dosage of Bu Zhong Yi Qi Tang (including a large dose of Huang Qi). The patient said that he felt a little bit of improvement, with slightly less distention and pain.

Is it possible that sitting on a cold surface for long durations could have caused some type of nerve damage or is this just a severe case of hemorrhoids?

A: *Internal* hemorrhoids may cause pain, especially upon defecation, due to anal sphincter spasm, and thrombosed *external* hemorrhoids may also cause sudden onset pain. However, in most cases of hemorrhoids there will be a stereotypical clinical picture that involves a progression of symptoms, including an itching sensation and recurrent bleeding, particularly after such a long period of time has elapsed.

That's why I would classify this patient's pathocondition as a type of phantom pain, likely caused by damage to the cauda equina and resulting in neurological deficits affecting the anus and anal sphincter. Prescribing the spleen-fortifying qi-supplementing and yang-upbearing fall-raising formula Bu Zhong Yi Qi Tang variant should be fine, but you must also make sure to add Ma Huang, Di Long, Bai Zhi, Fang Feng, Huang Qin, and Yu Sheng Wan. If necessary, you can even consider adding in The Three Insects.

Plus, I would perform acupuncture on Bai Hui (GV20), Ren Zhong (CV26), Ba Liao (UB21 to UB34), The Perianal Acupoints*, He Gu (LI4), Shen Men (HT7), Er Bai (EX-UE8), and Chi Ze (LU5); and bleed the large intestine channel well point (Shang Yang (LI1)) as well as Er Jian (LI2) and San Jian (LI3).

This therapeutic regimen will provide effective relief of symptoms and over time will help to completely resolve the phantom pain.

*Note: The Perianal Acupoints are four acupoints roughly corresponding with Hui Yin (CV1) and Chang Qiang (DU1) longitudinally along with two accompanying latitudinal acupoints, which are all located at a distance of approximately 0.5 cun on each side of the anus and together form symmetrical x-y axis coordinates. Needle perpendicularly, parallel with the anal canal, at a depth of approximately 1.8 cun.

Case Study #13: Flu-Like Symptoms Evolve into Guillain-Barre Syndrome!

Q: Recently, I have had two patients diagnosed with Guillain-Barre Syndrome (GBS) make clinical visits.

One is a 38 y/o male who began feeling bilateral weakness of the four limbs about 4 months ago and has shown improvement following administration of corticosteroids, but still has mild muscle weakness in the extremities and difficulty walking (walks tentatively and at a slower pace). Urine and stool are normal, there are no other presenting symptoms, and he has *not* been administered corticosteroids since the initial treatment (2 months ago).

The other is a 51 y/o male who came down with flu-like symptoms about 9 months ago, thinking that it was simply a gastrointestinal tract infection. However, as these flu-like symptoms resolved, he began having weakness in both arms and legs, becoming so severe that he was bedridden for the next 8 months. He presented with the following clinical picture: inhibited tongue movement, but he *can* still speak clearly enough to communicate; left-sided facial paralysis; bilateral atrophy and weakness of the muscles between the fingers, but he *can* still move his fingers enough to use utensils for eating; and right thigh muscle atrophy and weakness, making it difficult to lift his leg. Right now, he is still being administered oral corticosteroids and digestants.

How would you treat these patients?

A: GBS is a postinfectious inflammatory and demyelinating polyneuropathy in which the patient is hospitalized during the acute stage to provide symptomatic and supportive management and administration of drugs such as analgesics, antispasmodics, corticosteroids, and in some cases intravenous immunoglobulin (IVIG) and plasmapharesis.

About 2/3 of patients (like the 51 y/o patient!) present with exterior heat pattern symptoms at the onset and 70% have a positive prognosis of remission without any lingering sequelae. Patients who have already been administered immunosuppressants (i.e., corticosteroids) can be identified as wilting (yang vacuity) pattern.

For the 38 y/o patient, considering that only 4 months have elapsed since the onset of infection, that he is *no* longer taking corticosteroids, and that he still presents with neurological symptoms suggesting the presence of inflammation, I would classify this condition as being in the *post-acute* stage (≤ 6 months). In this *post-acute* stage, I would prescribe an yin-enriching fire-downbearing formula such as Zhi Bo Di Huang Tang, San Miao San, or Si Miao Wan. Just make sure to add Ma Huang and Di Long (nervous system conductor medicinals).

After you start noticing improvement in symptoms following administration of this formula, then you can begin incrementally increasing the dose of The Three Great Yang-Supplementers (Gan Jiang, Fu Zi, and Rou Gui), starting out at a combined total dose of 1 liang. As symptoms improve and there are *no* signs of inflammation flare-ups, you can increase the doses of The Three Great Yang-Supplementers up to 5–8 qian each.

Once the condition has stabilized, you can consider changing to a qi-, blood-, and kidney yang-supplementing formula such as Shi Quan Da Bu Tang, You Gui Yin, Shen Qi Wan, Bu Zhong Yi Qi Tang, or Bu Yang Huan Wu Tang adding Ma Huang, Di Long, Niu Xi, Du Zhong, The Three Great Yang-Supplementers, and Ren Shen/Chuan Qi Powder. And if hypertonicity or spasm presents, add The Three Insects.

For the 51 y/o patient, considering that your patient is being administered corticosteroids to suppress the inflammation and that 9 months have elapsed since the onset of infection, I would classify this condition as being in the *chronic* stage. Once the disease has entered the *chronic* stage, then it can be identified as qi vacuity, dual qi and blood vacuity with kidney yang vacuity, or kidney yang vacuity pattern. In the *chronic* stage, you should consider prescribing formulas such as Gui Qi Jian Zhong Tang, Bu Yang Huan Wu Tang, Paralysis Formula #2 (Shi Quan Da Bu Tang Variant) or Paralysis Formula #3 (You Gui Yin Variant). Just make sure to include the The Three Great Yang-Supplementers, Ma Huang, Di Long, and Huang Qin. And if spasm presents, add The Three Insects.

The clinical manifestation of GBS is highly variable. Some patients will go into remission and make a complete recovery without any problems; some patients will incur rapid, progressive deterioration from the onset and then go on to make partial recovery with the presence of lingering symptoms; some will go into remission following treatment and then after a period of time begin to relapse with a gradual, progressive deterioration; some will stabilize rather quickly after the *acute* onset and then later on incur sudden, severe deterioration; and some will go directly from the *acute* onset stage into the *chronic* stage of progressive deterioration.

Thus, we must stay vigilant of ongoing developments in our patients' conditions, paying particular attention to any sudden manifestations of *heat* (e.g., fever, malaise). If *heat* pattern does present, then you should add the appropriate doses of The Three Yellows (clear heat and resolve toxin) and Qing Hao, Zhi Mu, and Di Gu Pi (enrich yin and downbear fire, cool the blood and clear vacuity heat, and eliminate steaming bone) based on the specific signs, symptoms and pattern.

Case Study #14: It's An Inflammatory Demyelinating Polyneuropathy

Q: Today, a 24 y/o male diagnosed with Guillain-Barre syndrome (GBS) came for a clinical visit. The first episode occurred when he contracted a respiratory tract infection at the age of 10 y/o, which unexpectedly progressed into tingling sensations (paresthesia) that affected the distal extremities, prompting a stay in the hospital for treatment and a thorough examination. He was diagnosed with GBS, but the symptoms completely resolved without any problems.

Then, at the age of 15 y/o, he suddenly began having a similar type of paresthesia in the limbs, warranting a lengthier 3-month hospital stay. This time treatment was *not* effective in resolving the symptoms, as the patient was discharged from the hospital with weakness (reduced muscle tone) of the arms and legs, bilateral atrophy of the muscles between the fingers (still capable of finger abduction and adduction though inhibited and weak), and bilateral leg weakness (he is able to walk with the assistance of a walker).

Over the years, his condition has seemed to stabilize for the most part, but I *did* notice bilateral muscle atrophy of the extremities below the wrists and ankles. Do you think TCM medicinals could effectively treat his condition? Please offer your invaluable insights!

A: Guillain-Barre syndrome (GBS) and its subtypes and variants are postinfectious pathoconditions, resulting in inflammatory and demyelinating polyneuropathy. This patient has apparently incurred a relapse, one of the merely 3% of GBS patients who do.

At the onset (*acute* stage), it can be identified as exterior pattern. In the *post-acute* stage (≤ 6 months) with*out* administration of immunosuppressants (i.e., corticosteroids, intravenous immunoglobulins (IVIG)) and in the presence of inflammation, it can be identified as yin vacuity fire pattern, requiring administration of yin-enriching fire-downbearing medicinals. In the *post-acute* stage, following the administration of immunosuppressants, and in the *chronic* stage, it can be identified as dual vacuity of qi and blood with kidney yang vacuity pattern or kidney yang vacuity pattern.

Your patient's condition can definitely be classified as in the *chronic* stage, requiring the administration of formula variants such as Shi Quan Da Bu Tang, Ren Shen Yang Rong Tong, You Gui Yin, Shen Qi Wan, Bu Yang Huan Wu Tang, or Gui Qi Jian Zhong Tang. Just make sure to include The Three Great Yang-Supplementers, Ma Huang, Di Long, and Ren Shen/Chuan Qi Powder. If tetany (periodic painful muscular spasms, tremors, and hypertonicity) presents, then add The Three Insects, and if anal sphincter paralysis presents with constipation, you should consider prescribing either Paralysis Formula #2 (Shi Quan Da Bu Tang Variant) or Paralysis Formula #3 (You Gui Yin Variant).

Ttreatment of acute postinfectious demyelinating pathoconditions, such as GBS, during the "golden period" (*acute* stage ≤ 2 weeks) will inevitably provide the best outcome. For patients presenting with exterior pattern symptoms of fever, generalized malaise, and heaviness and painful distention of the limbs at the early onset of infection, you should prescribe heat-clearing exterior-effusing formulas such as Yang Dan Tang, Da Qing Long Tang, and Ge Gen Tang. Just make sure to include The Three Yellows, Sheng Shi Gao, Ma Huang, and Di Long. TCM can still offer effective treatment during the *post-acute* stage (≤ 6 months), but the results will take longer with a less likely chance of complete recovery.

TCM offers excellent therapeutic efficacy for the treatment of GBS. However, your patient has already entered the *chronic* stage. Intervention now will first involve preventing further deterioration and muscular atrophy, and then working towards progress in the future. Let's put it this way: if it takes 1 month to stabilize the condition and 2 months to start showing signs of progress, then you could consider yourself well on the way to becoming a "master" physician.

Typically, for most patients like this, it will take anywhere from 6 months to 1 year to achieve significant improvement in symptoms. That's why it is important from the outset to clearly explain your therapeutic regimen and the likely timeframe for progress. And by all means to have patience!

Remember! GBS may also cause cardiovascular autonomic dysfunction (arrhythmia) and even respiratory failure that leads to death. So stay vigilant and be prepared to respond!

Case Study #15: Peripheral Neuropathy – "The Pain Is Still Killing Me"

Q: A 35 y/o male patient visited me explaining that 2 weeks ago he began feeling general malaise and fatigue, and not long after these symptoms resolved, he began having an intense "pins and needles" sensation in his arms and legs that felt like someone was stabbing him with a sharp needle. He said that at times the pain was almost unbearable. Right now he is taking vitamin B complex and corticosteroids, but he said "the pain is still killing me."

A: Your patient's history suggests a peripheral neuropathy of infectious etiology. The *acute* stage exterior pattern or "golden period" (≤ 2 weeks, within 3–4 days after onset even more ideal!) has already passed. And since your patient *has* been administered corticosteroids, this pathocondition can be identified as dual qi and blood vacuity with kidney yang vacuity or kidney yang vacuity pattern. Thus, I would prescribe either Gui Qi Jian Zhong Tang or Bu Yang Huan Wu Tang adding The Three Insects, Zao Jiao Ci, Ci Ji Li, The Three Great Yang-Supplementers, Huang Qin, and Yu Sheng Wan.

For patients still in the *acute* stage, who have *not* been administered immunosuppressants (e.g., corticosteroids, IV immunoglobulins (IVIG)), this condition can be identified as exterior wind-heat pattern, for which you can prescribe a sweat-promoting exterior-resolving formula such as Ge Gen Tang adding The Three Yellows.

Case Study #16: Anxiety Induces "Stiff Tongue" Sensation

Q: A 45 y/o male patient came into my clinic explaining that about 6 months ago he began experiencing periodic (every 2 or 3 day intervals) tongue stiffness, like it was cramping up and contorting. He recently underwent a thorough lab workup and examination (including an MRI), but *no* abnormalities (blood pressure normal and *no* vascular or neurological deficits) were found.

Do you think this sensation could suggest that the patient has a cerebrovascular disorder or space-occupying lesion?

A: Hmm…periodic tongue stiffness occurring roughly every 2 to 3 days and no other specific signs or symptoms found after thorough examination. It sounds to me like this could be a case of anxiety or psychosomatic etiology. Typically, if there was a problem with the cranial nerves (hypoglossal nerve (CN XII) or vagus nerve (CNX)), the "stiff tongue" would not present sporadically, but remain persistent and progressively evolve, with concomitant difficulty swallowing (dysphagia) or inability to swallow (aphagia).

That's why I think this patient may have a case of visceral agitation (臟躁 zàng zào), manifesting as wooden tongue (木舌 mù shé) or swollen tongue hard as wood.

I would prescribe a center-harmonizing agitation-calming and stagnation-dissipating phlegm-transforming formula such as Gan Mai Da Zao Tang Combining Ban Xia Hou Po Tang adding Long Yan Gan and Yu Sheng Wan. You should also advise your patient to get enough sleep (at least 8 hours of sleep each night), exercise regularly, eat small portions of sweet foods (e.g., natural sweets like dates, raisins, jujubes, sugar cane, longan), and possibly a little bit of alcohol as a mild sedative. This therapeutic regimen, along with lifestyle and dietary adjustments, should put your patient on the path to a limber tongue!

Case Study #17: Phantom Heat – Heat Sensation in Upper Back

Q: This 80 y/o female patient has felt a constant heat sensation day and night in her upper back region—near Fei Shu (UB13) and Gao

Huang Shu (UB43)—for more than 10 years now. Urine and stool are normal, blood pressure and blood glucose are in the normal range for her age, and she doesn't suffer from any other chronic illnesses. Would you identify this as yin vacuity pattern?

A: This sounds like a typical case of phantom heat rooted in neuropsychological etiology.

Yes, I would identify this as a dual yin and blood vacuity pattern, requiring the prescription of a blood-nourishing yin-enriching and heat-clearing blood-cooling formula such as (Yu Sheng) Di Gu Pi Yin adding Qing Hao and Zhi Mu (enrich yin and downbear fire, cool the blood and clear vacuity heat, and eliminate steaming bone), Sheng Mu Li and Sheng Long Gu (subdue yang and quiet the spirit), and Yu Sheng Wan (quiets the spirit and calms the nerves, promotes cerebral collateral circulation, and recalibrates autoregulation in the brain). Give it a try!

Case Study #18: Tidal Heat and Spontaneous Sweating Upon Urination and Defecation

Q: A 60 y/o female visited me with a chief complaint of feeling a mild heat sensation throughout her entire body every time she urinated or defecated, which initially started about 10 years ago. She has undergone thorough Western medical lab workups and examinations without any significant findings and tried both Western medicine and TCM treatment without efficacy.

I am considering prescribing Gan Mai Da Zao Tang for this patient. Do you think this is a good approach?

A: A generalized heat sensation upon urination and defecation suggests an autonomic reflex arc disorder, resulting in the disruption of normal thermoregulation functions. This pathocondition can be identified as yin vacuity with mild exterior pattern.

As for Gan Mai Da Zao Tang, sure, you could take that approach, but you would definitely need to add in Qing Hao, Zhi Mu, and Di Gu Pi (enrich yin and downbear fire, cool the blood and clear vacuity heat, and eliminate steaming bone), and Sheng Mu Li and Sheng Long Gu (calm the liver and subdue yang, quiet the spirit, and astringe and secure). If it were my patient, I would likely prescribe a blood-nourishing yin-enriching and heat-clearing blood-cooling formula such as Di Gu Pi Yin adding Qing Hao and Zhi Mu.

For some people, as they get up there in age, this type of reflex arc disorder may progress to the point where they develop urinary and fecal incontinence accompanied by tidal heat and spontaneous sweating. Once they have "relieved" themselves, thermoregulation returns to normal. Paralysis patients have a tendency to respond like this too. They feel nervous and have anxiety when they have to urinate or defecate and their blood pressure may rise, but after they "relieve" themselves, blood pressure returns to normal.

Case Study #19: Chronic "Twitches" of the Inner Thighs and Upper Arms

Q: This 66 y/o female visited me with a chief complaint of what she calls "twitches" of the inner thighs and upper arms, which makes it difficult for her to walk with a steady gait. She also has symptoms of dizziness, palpitations, constipation, and dry mouth. Oddly, despite going through the gamut of tests (i.e., CT scan, MRI, nerve conduction velocity (NCV), and electromyography (EMG)), *no* abnormalities were found.

Could this be a longstanding undiagnosed Tourette syndrome (TS), Huntington disease (HD), Parkinsonism, or some type of demyelinating disease? Please offer your advice and suggestions.

A: First of all, how long has she had these "twitches"?

If these symptoms have been around sense adolescence, then this strange case of yours could be *TS*, which is a neurological disorder characterized by involuntary, repeated, intermittent movements and/or vocalizations (motor and vocal tics).

HD is a neurodegenerative disorder characterized by rapid, jerky, arrhythmic and sporadic uncontrollable muscle movements (chorea) that are only noticeable when the patient moves. The choreiform movements of *HD* are similar to *essential tremor* in that they only occur upon movement, and is in direct contrast with the characteristic resting tremor of *Parkinson's disease (PD)* that disappears upon movement. Plus, if it were a case of *HD* with well-established symptoms, the CT scan and MRI should have picked up atrophy in the basal ganglia by now.

There is a possibility that it could be an *inflammatory demyelinating disease* (i.e., *Guillain-Barre syndrome (GBS)* or one of its variants), which is not that easy to diagnose. If flaccidity develops, then you must definitely consider the involvement of postinfectious complications resulting from an *inflammatory demyelinating disease*, and modify your formula accordingly.

Another possibility is chronic muscle twitching (aka *benign fasciculation syndrome (BFS)*), which, like *GBS*, is thought to be caused by a microbial infection, but may also result from drug side effects, anxiety (stress) or depression, and a deficiency of magnesium or calcium.

Most likely, this is a case of chronic muscle twitching (aka *BFS*) or some type of *demyelinating disorder*. Thus, I would consider prescribing either an yin-enriching fire-downbearing and steaming bone-eliminating formula, such as Zhi Bo Di Huang Tang, or a Shao Yang harmonizing heat-clearing and fright-settling spirit-quieting formula, such as Chai Hu Jia Long Gu Mu Li Tang. Just make sure to include Long Gu, Mu Li, The Three Insects, The Three Yellows, Tian Ma, and Da Huang in your formula.

You should try to suss out more clearly the age of onset, whether there are precipitating factors, if she is taking other medication, and any other details that may be helpful in making a more definitive diagnosis.

VI. HEMATOLOGIC DISEASES

Case Study #1: Myelodysplastic Syndrome – Steaming Bone Taxation Heat Pattern

Q: A 62 y/o male patient has been having ongoing problems with low hemoglobin (Hb) levels for the past two years. At the onset, he had been feeling extremely fatigued and weak, so his doctor recommended a thorough physical examination and blood workup. Lab test results revealed Hb 2.1 (normal range 14–18 g/dL). He was referred to a hematologist who diagnosed him with myelodysplastic syndrome (MDS). Following administration of cytotoxic chemotherapy, his Hb increased back up to 11.0; but after 6 months, it dropped back down to extremely low levels again.

Since then, the patient has continued efforts to treat this condition with both Western medicine and TCM, but neither has been effective at maintaining Hb levels anywhere near the normal range. It has gotten to the point that he must receive erythropoietin (EPO) injections to stimulate RBC production and increase Hb levels. But even with EPO, he can only maintain Hb levels at around 4.3.

I am not sure what I can do for him. What would you prescribe for this patient?

A: Hmm!...Unable to adequately elevate and maintain Hb levels even after the administration of chemotherapy and EPO.

MDS is a diverse group of bone marrow disorders that hematologists refer to as a "smouldering" of the bone marrow and is sometimes referred to as "preleukemia." Similarly, in TCM, MDS can be identified as "steaming bone" taxation heat pattern, for which you can prescribe (Yu Sheng) Zhi Bo Di Huang Tang adding Qing Hao and Di Gu Pi (enrich yin and downbear fire and cool the blood and eliminate steaming bone) and Gu Sui Bu, Xu Duan, and Qian Cao (quicken the blood and transform stasis, break blood and stanch bleeding, and free the channels and mend breakages).

If this is ineffective, then add The Three Great

Yang-Supplementers, starting out at small doses (e.g., 0.5 qian each) and gradually increasing the doses (e.g., 1 qian□ 1.5 qian□ 2 qian□ 2.5 qian each) in an incremental manner, while also increasing the dose of Huang Bo in proportionally larger doses (e.g., 5 qian□ 8 qian□ 1 liang) to counterbalance the heat and avert the potential for an iatrogenic "overcompensation" effect.

Initially, this approach will effectively elevate Hb levels. However, you may find that after 3 to 5 weeks of administering this formula, Hb levels *fail* to continue elevating. That's when you should once again incrementally increase the doses. And if this still is *not* effective at elevating and maintaining Hb levels, then try adding Lu Rong. But remember! You must use either Cu Lu Rong (Lu Jiao Jiao or Lu Jiao Shuang), *not* Xi Lu Rong.

Case Study #2: Acute Myeloid Leukemia

Q: A friend of mine who is also a TCM doctor had been feeling extremely fatigued and looked really pale (pallor) for about 6 months, prompting him to go in for a thorough medical examination to find out if there was anything wrong. That's when he was diagnosed with acute myeloid leukemia (AML).

Initially, he received a regimen of chemotherapy followed by granulocyte colony-stimulating factor (G-CSF) and granulocyte-macrophage colony-stimulating factor (GM-CSF) to stimulate production and maturation of neutrophils. Unfortunately, these therapies were *not* effective in remedying the cytopenias (i.e., □ RBCs, □ neutrophils, and □ platelets) and elevated myeloblast count.

The bone marrow failure persisted without any signs of making headway. Thus, his hematologist advised that the best option would be to choose the path of undergoing either autologous or allogeneic stem cell transplantation. He already underwent the stem cell transplantation (SCT) and is now receiving a regimen of prophylactic antibiotics to prevent graft-versus-host disease (GVHD).

This patient (TCM doctor and close friend of mine!) has heard of your reputation and achievements, and asked me to get your opinion on how to treat this condition. Please offer your guidance and advice.

A: AML can be identified as steaming bone taxation heat (骨蒸勞

熱 gu zh□ ng láo rè) pattern and Shao Yang depressed heat (少陽鬱熱 shao yáng yù rè) pattern. Following induction chemotherapy, patients are susceptible to suppressed hematopoiesis that can lead to cytopenias.

Typically, once a patient has been diagnosed with suppressed hematopoietic function and low WBC count, Western medicine will administer induction chemotherapy and either G-CSF or GM-CSF (biologic response modifiers (aka immunotherapy). The problem is that in addition to neutrophils, G-CSF and GM-CSF also activate the proliferation of immature stem cells and cancer cells, which results in further dysplasia and more obstacles in the way of achieving successful stem cell transplantation. In this regard, administering TCM medicinals offers a potentially better outcome.

A recent patient of mine, whom I'll call Mr. Wen, is a case in point. Following thorough testing and examination, Mr. Wen was diagnosed with AML, received the initial induction chemotherapy, and then followed the advice of his hematologist to receive an SCT. Not only were the results *un*successful, but 6 months later the poor guy suffered a cerebrovascular accident (CVA). After about 1 year of supportive therapy, that included blood transfusions of erythropoietin (EPO) and platelets, he finally came in to see me.

After only 4 months of administering TCM medicinals, he regained hematopoietic function, and after 5 months, he discontinued transfusions and artificial ventilation—successfully going into remission. He continued taking my formula, while undergoing speech and physical therapy as well, and has made vast improvements in the ability to speak and walk. The patient has now gone 1 1/2 years without a relapse.

A while ago, he underwent a bone marrow aspiration, which confirmed that the blood type and antigen of the bone marrow cells were all of the transplants. This case provides clear clinical evidence that, even after stem cell transplantation failure, the administration of TCM medicinal therapy for 1 1/2 years effectively promoted the autoregulatory capacity of the body's bone marrow stem cell replication mechanism. This is just another example of the remarkable efficacy and vast potential of TCM medicinals.

If the patient is currently being administered chemotherapy or has already completed a chemotherapeutic regimen, you must closely monitor the lab test results (i.e., WBC/DC) to determine which medicinals to prescribe. For instance, if lymphocyte and neutrophil counts are elevated, then make sure to include Shan Ning Ma Gen (cools the blood and stanches bleeding, quiets the fetus, and resolves toxin) and Zhang Hu (disinhibits the gallbladder and abates heat, clears heat and resolves toxin, quickens the blood and dispels stasis, and dispels phlegm and suppresses cough).

Typically, for patients who have already received chemotherapy, I would prescribe an yin-enriching blood-cooling formula such as Zhi Bo Di Huang Tang, Di Gu Pi Yin, Ba Xian Chang Shou Wan, Zuo Gui Yin, Dang Gui Liu Huang Tang, or Xi Jiao Di Huang Tang. Just make sure to include the essential medicinals Qing Hao, Zhi Mu, Di Gu Pi, and Huang Bo along with Niu Xi, Mu Dan Pi, Chi Shao, and Chai Hu. If suppression of hematopoiesis presents, then add Ren Shen/Chuan Qi Powder; and if this is *not* effective, then add The Three Great Yang-Supplementers (starting out with small doses and increasing incrementally).

And in cases of severely suppressed hematopoiesis, you should add Cu Lu Rong (8 qian–1 liang). Cu Lu Rong can inhibit the replication of abnormal cells and proliferation of cancer cells and accelerate the elimination of aging cells (apoptosis), whereas Xi Lu Rong promotes an increase in new stem cell production (proliferatrion). Remember! The actions and indications of these two medicinals are different. Make sure you know when to use them!

Case Study #3: Polycythemia Rubra Vera

Q: Dr. Kim, one of my professors from university whom I have maintained contact with over the years, recently referred 2 patients with polycythemia rubra vera (PRV) to me. One patient has increased red blood cell (RBC) count and the other has both increased RBC and platelet (PLT) count.

How would you treat this type of chronic myeloproliferative disorder (MPD)?

A: Simply put, PRV involves the malignant transformation of stem cells that leads to an excess production of RBCs (and may also include other cell lines such as white blood cells (WBCs) and PLTs) in the bone marrow (and possibly other sites of hematopoiesis such as the spleen and liver). These cells accumulate in the bone marrow and blood stream where they increase the blood volume and viscosity. It is the most common of the myeloproliferative disorders. The clinical symptoms tend to develop gradually and include thrombotic episodes (e.g., stroke, retinal vascular occlusion, deep vein thrombosis), gout, headaches, dizziness, tinnitus, hypertension, hypermetabolism (e.g., weight loss), hepatomegaly, and splenomegaly

Elevated RBC and PLT counts can be identified as Shao Yang depressed heat with steaming bone and blood heat pattern. Thus, I would prescribe a formula such as Xiao Chai Hu Tang or Di Gu Pi Yin, making sure to include Qing Hao, Zhi Mu, Mu Dan Pi, Di Gu Pi, and Zhi Zi. If heat is pronounced, consider adding Huang Bo; to prevent the development of thrombotic episodes, consider adding a small dose of Da Huang (drains precipitation and attacks accumulations and quickens the blood and dispels stasis); and if symptoms of hyperactivity of liver yang present, then consider adding Sheng Mu Li (calms the liver and subdues yang).

I have treated a patient with an extremely high PLT of 1.5 million (normal range 150,000–400,000 μL)! This patient developed thrombocythemia (high PLT count) after undergoing chemotherapy (CT), and developed drug-induced neurological symptoms following repeated regimens of CT. At first, these symptoms manifested as early signs of cognitive deficit (e.g., memory loss, forgetfulness, mood swings) and eventually evolved into the inability to recognize others and engage in conversation. Then, he suffered a cerebrovascular accident (CVA), which resulted in generalized paralysis, and eventually the feeble-mindedness (凝呆 ch□ d□i) developed into the complete withdrawal of full-on dementia.

So you must be vigilant when treating these types of chronic MPDs! You have to know what you are up against.

Case Study #4: Aplastic Anemia

Q: A 41 y/o female patient was diagnosed with aplastic anemia 6 years ago. Her most recent lab tests are as follows: Hb 6 (normal range 12–16 g/dL) and PLT 40,000 (normal range 150,000–400,000 μL).

Over the years, she has received blood transfusions when necessary, a course of anti-thymocyte globulin (ATG) with cyclosporin to modulate the immune system, and even underwent a bone marrow transplant that resulted in graft failure. After the antibody therapy (i.e., ATG), initially her condition improved, but eventually her blood counts dropped back down again.

How would you treat this patient?

A: Aplastic anemia involves damage to the hematopoietic stem cells in the bone marrow that inhibits the stem cells ability to generate healthy (mature) blood cells. This causes a deficiency in all three blood cell types (pancytopenia)—red blood cells (anemia), white blood cells (leucopenia), and platelets (thrombocytopenia).

If this aplastic anemia patient has already undergone an unsuccessful bone marrow (multipotent stem cells) transplant, then this can be identified as kidney yang vacuity pattern. You can consider prescribing You Gui Yin or Shen Qi Wan adding Gan Jiang, Ren Shen/Chuan Qi Powder, and Xi Lu Rong (powder) (incrementally increasing the dose by 5 fen every 3–5 weeks).

Remember! Some patients may experience loose stools from taking these types of blood-supplementing yin-nourishing medicinals (e.g., Di Huang), so if necessary, make sure to add Shan Zha, Ji Nei Jin, and Cang Zhu (disperse food and promote digestion and fortify the spleen and open the stomach).

This therapeutic approach will promote the accelerated production of all three blood cell types (RBCs, WBCs, and PLTs), gradually regulate the constitution to restore the multipotent stem cell function in the bone marrow, and over time, reconstitute all three blood lines so that mature blood cells can be autonomously generated once again.

VII. DERMATOLOGICAL DISORDERS

Section 1: Atopic Dermatitis

Case Study #1: It's Tough for Children with Atopic Dermatitis

Q1: My youngest son has an atopic constitution and it's been tough for everyone in the family to try to deal with the condition. I remember at the beginning when I first noticed tiny maculopapular lesions that looked like "chicken skin" on the toes of his right foot and around his mouth; then it soon spread over his entire body, and he had a mild fever and runny nose almost like the common cold.

My wife was disturbed about it so she took him to see a dermatologist who prescribed topical corticosteroids. Well, the topical corticosteroids did quickly suppress the spread and provided a pleasant respite from the itchiness and discomfort, but after a while the effects wore off. One day when I was applying the ointment to his chest, I discovered that his skin had turned pale white and was still itchy. That's when I decided it was time to try using Chinese medicine instead!

The first time I really closely inspected his eczematous skin, I could only describe it as "horrific." He presented with tiny, pinpoint maculopapular lesions (looks like "chicken skin") and scaling on the four bends (四彎 sì w□n)*, abdomen, back, front and back of the neck, and face. Plus, he also had oozing (lymphatic fluid) around the periphery of his ears.

I was reading up on some information related to eczema and atopy and saw that the human herpesvirus (HHV-6 and HHV-7) may cause a dry eczematous rash around the mouth. Do you think this type of viral infection could have been an initiating factor that triggered the allergic reaction?

I prescribed Atopic Dermatitis Formula adding Qing Hao, Zhi Mu, Di Gu Pi, and Huang Qin, which I plan on administering up until the atrophied skin returns to its moistened luster and then change to Seborrheic Dermatitis Formula adding Huang Qin. Do you think this is a good treatment plan?

A: Yes, I think that is a good formula. I would continue prescribing it!

I believe that almost all allergic reactions, including four bends wind (四彎風 sì w□ n f□ ng) (aka atopic dermatitis), are caused by the common cold (i.e., external contraction, microbial infection) in which the pathogen has not been completely eradicated.

Dry eczematous rash around the mouth is very common in children and usually simply caused by dry skin from repeated lip and perioral licking, which may result in an allergic reaction or infection that is limited to the area around the mouth. This is different from the generalized maculopapular, erythematous lesions of four bends wind (atopic dermatitis).

For the differentiation of similar types of eczematous skin manifestations, you can reference this general pathomechanistic guideline:

- Facial eczema—dampness pattern
- Four bends wind (atopic dermatitis)—blood desiccation pattern
- Seborrheic dermatitis (wandering wind of the face (面游風 miàn yóu f□ ng) and glossy scalp wind (油風 yóu f□ ng)—exterior wind-heat pattern
- Wind papules (urticaria)—exterior wind-heat, blood desiccation, or exterior stasis with frenetic blood heat pattern
- Pompholyx (dyshidrotic eczema)—exterior wind or exterior wind heat with dampness (Yang Ming heat) pattern
- Folliculitis of the head and body—Yang Ming exterior heat pattern
- Dry lichen (psoriasis)—exterior blood desiccation with heat or yang vacuity with true cold false heat pattern

Q2: Thanks for your guidance. My child's atopic dermatitis (four bends wind) has improved and his skin color is gradually returning to normal again from what had been large, itchy maculopapular patches with dry thickened skin and scaling that he had scratched red and raw.

When I first started treating pediatric patients with atopic dermatitis, I always thought it was too much of a hassle and would take too long time to treat, and even then, may not produce as effective results as Western medicine. Thus, I would refer these patients to a dermatologist, including my own son! However, through this personal experience, I realized that the topical and oral corticosteroids prescribed by dermatologists would indeed quickly get the condition under control, but after about three weeks of administration, the effectiveness noticeably diminishes and the condition even worsens. In my son's case, the erythema around his eyes and the flexural creases of the extremities worsened, scaling over the affected areas increased, the itch intensified, and oozing appeared on his neck after scratching.

That's when I decided to prescribe Atopic Dermatitis Formula adding Qing Hao, Zhi Mu, and Di Gu Pi. After taking the formula for only 2 days, his condition showed dramatic improvement (about 2/3 of a turnaround!). It was very effective. Thank you for your advice and encouragement!

A: Congratulations on the successful initial results! However, do *not* get too excited yet! Atopic dermatitis will take time to treat, with inevitable progressions and regressions along the way. So you must have patience and stay the course. Atopic dermatitis can be identified as blood desiccation with exterior wind-heat (at the onset and during flare-ups) or exterior cold pattern (post-acute). In most patients, it's not that tough of a case, with gradual improvement occurring over time.

Q3: My son took my formula for about 4 months and his condition seemed to have completely resolved. Our whole family was ecstatic about it. We could go about our lives as normal again. Well…that was up until I took him to the park a few days ago to get outdoors and have some fun. Unfortunately, he caught a cold with a runny nose and sticky white nasal mucus, and then bam!...the atopy flared up again with intense itchiness on the four bends (flexural creases of the limbs), chest, back, and face that turned erythematous upon scratching. What is the best way to treat this flare-up?

A: Ahh!…The external contraction (microbial infection) triggered a flare-up! Simply prescribe Atopic Dermatitis Formula (nourishes the blood and enriches yin, resolves the exterior and dispels wind, and supplements the spleen, liver, and kidney) adding Huang Qin. And if pronounced runny nose and nasal congestion present, then also add Lai Fu Zi (downbears qi and transforms phlegm and precipitates qi and stabilizes panting), Bai Zhi (resolves the exterior and dissipates wind and frees the orifices), or Xing Yi (effuses and dissipates wind-cold and frees the nasal orifices). After the external contraction resolves, you should continue prescribing this formula up until he has incurred 2–3 external contractions or after going through 1 full winter without a flare-up. That's when you can feel assured that this pathocondition has been cured.

*Note: The four bends (四彎 sì w□n) refer to the flexural creases of the limbs, specifically the elbow (antecubital) and knee (popliteal fossae), but can be broadly interpreted as flexural creases over the entire body (e.g., wrists, ankles, neck).

Case Study #2: Atopic Dermatitis Takes Time to Treat – Stay the Course!

Q: In the past year, I have treated several atopic dermatitis patients. It has taken continuous administration of formulas such as Da Qing Long Tang, Atopic Dermatitis Formula, and Wen Dan Tang to resolve the eczema (itchy maculopapular, erythematous patches) over the cheeks and around the eyes, and the dark red, dry and itchy cracked skin on the neck and flexural creases of the extremities. Have you observed a similar manifestation in your clinical experience in Taiwan?

A: Due to climate and lifestyle factors (e.g., cold weather, preference for spicy foods, indoor heating), the majority of patients in South Korea will likely present with exterior wind-heat and blood heat pattern or blood desiccation with either exterior heat or cold stasis pattern.

In Taiwan, most of the patients that come visit me can be identified as blood desiccation with either exterior heat or cold stasis pattern. Thus, I tend to prescribe either Blood Desiccation Formula (enriches yin and emolliates the liver and nourishes the blood and moistens dryness) or Atopic Dermatitis Formula (nourishes the blood and enriches yin, resolves the exterior and dispels wind, and supplements the spleen, liver, and kidney). Just make sure to include The Three Great Yang-Supplementers and Huang Qin. If oozing is pronounced, then I will include large doses of Huang Qin and add Sheng Shi Gao and Bai Xian Pi. And for those patients who present with concomitant asthma, I will include Ma Huang and Xing Ren; and for those who present with concomitant tearing on exposure to wind, I will include Ma Huang, Bai Zhi, Xin Yi, and Xi Xin.

I cannot emphasize this concept enough, for atopic dermatitis patients, it is essential to continue prescribing the formula up until the skin appears completely normal upon physical observation. After that, it is necessary for patients to continue taking TCM medicinals up until they incur 2–3 common colds (external contraction) or get through an entire winter free from a flare-up. That's when you know it is time to gradually discontinue administration of TCM medicinals and the patient has been cured.

And remember! Once the manifestation of symptoms (e.g., lichenification, eczema, pruritis) of atopic dermatitis resolve, adolescents and young adults in particular, have a tendency to incur breakouts of acne and folliculitis. This is simply a therapeutic response (瞑眩反應 míng xuàn fan yìng) as the underlying heat toxin at the root of the pathocondition is being drawn out and effused from the body. For patients with these "breakouts," I typically will prescribe Xian Fang Huo Ming Yin (clears heat and resolves toxin, disperses swelling and breaks hardness, and quickens the blood) variant.

Case Study #3: Treating Atopic Dermatitis in Late Adolescence

Q: Now that I have gained quite a bit of experience treating atopic dermatitis, I can say that I have had good results treating children and young kids, and fairly good results with adults who present in the acute (or flare-ups) and post-acute stages. But for patients in *late adolescence* and *young adults* as well as *adults* in the *chronic stage*, I had never seemed to be able to make much progress in resolving their conditions. This had left me feeling frustrated and mystified for quite some time.

However, recently I have been treating two atopic dermatitis patients, a 16 y/o male and an 18 y/o female, whose histories and clinical presentations are almost identical: initial onset at a young age with subsequent periodic flare-ups and exacerbations, who now have red, cracked, thickened and scaly skin on the four bends and intensely itchy skin, especially at night, on the front and back of the neck, face, abdomen, and knees. They have also tried the gamut of Western, Chinese, and folk medicine remedies, but nothing has been ultimately effective.

Normally, I would prescribe either an yin-enriching liver-emolliating and blood-nourishing dryness-moistening formula such as Blood Desiccation Formula or a sweat-effusing exterior-resolving with internal heat-clearing formula such as Da Qing Long Tang. But since I have *not* had too much success with those approaches for this age group in the past, I have always wanted to try a different approach.

With this in mind, I decided on prescribing the liver-settling wind-extinguishing and yin-enriching yang-subduing formula Jian Ling Tang combining Huang Lian Jie Du Tang (including up to 8 qian of the essential medicinals) adding Sheng Shi Gao. I also advised the patients to avoid eating spicy foods (e.g., chili peppers, raw garlic). Well, so far so good...the male patient is coming along well and the parents of the girl called me in tears of joy expressing how grateful they all were. Naturally, I also felt a great sense of accomplishment.

I have a couple of related questions that I would like to ask. First, if a patient has already taken corticosteroids (topical or oral), are they likely to present with a "rebound effect" once they discontinue using the medication? And second, traditional Korean medicine (TKM) doctors tend to group pompholyx (dyshidrotic eczema), hidradenitis suppurativa, and nummular eczema (discoid eczema and nummular dermatitis) together as having the same underlying pathomechanisms as atopic dermatitis and thus treat them the same way. Do you think this is the right mentality and approach?

A: Congratulations on your growing understanding of etiology and pathomechanisms and identifying the pattern as the basis for determining treatment! This requires an open mind and the ability to continuously adapt to change. Humans are organisms that coexist with a myriad of other organisms in a perpetual dynamic continuum—the constantly changing external environment affects a myriad of other organisms that continuously adapt and evolve, mutually affecting each other, directly and indirectly impacting our body, mind and spirit.

Using a less metaphysical analogy, but no less relevant, you could say that doctors are like chefs. A chef must be willing to learn new culinary concepts and be responsive to new challenges. A chef can't just rely on a handful of the same old dishes, because after a while, diners will gradually get tired of the menu and the restaurant will fail. Being a traditional Chinese medicine doctor, and especially one that operates her/his own private clinical practice, it is essential to constantly learn new things, stay abreast of the latest advancements in biomedicine, and be aware of current trends in our society as a whole. Only in this way can we keep our fingers on the pulse of patients and their pathoconditions, as they continuously evolve amidst our ever-changing environment.

Many doctors remain contented with treating the same types of patients whom generally present with a narrow scope of pathoconditions. In that paradigm, it becomes easy to rest on your laurels and convince yourself that nothing in this world is difficult. However, that is a lazy mentality with finite ends. We must be continuously open to new ideas and concepts and adapt to change. It's not so much "out with the old and in with the new" as it is building on the traditional foundations of the past, adapting to our changing environment in the present, and evolving into the future!

As for prescribing Jian Ling Tang variant for the treatment of chronic recalcitrant atopic dermatitis, I have had to do this on very rare occasion, and specifically for patients whose mood and emotional factors become the trigger that "fuels the fire." It's as if the patient becomes "embroiled" in their unfit skin, "boiling" away in itchy, fissured, weeping (oozing), crusting, lichenified angst. This obsession further exacerbates the vicious pathological cycle. For these types of patients, I will first try Blood Desiccation Formula combining Ma Xing Gan Shi Tang (including a large dose of Sheng Shi Gao (up to 2 liang)). And if that is *not* effective, then I will go ahead with Jian Ling Tang. But remember! Jian Ling Tang only suppresses the emotional trigger, and once that trigger has been adequately resolved, you must go back to prescribing a formula that actually addresses the skin problem proper.

This just reminded me of a seborrheic dermatitis patient of mine from more than 20 years ago. It was the weirdest thing, every time the woman went back home to her parent's house, the itchy erythematous plaques on her skin would immediately take a turn for the better. Could this be because of environmental, dietary, or psychological factors? My guess is that it was likely psychological, with less stress and a sense of emotional security this patient's mind and spirit opened up the pathway for a healthy body.

In response to your two questions:

1) The discontinuation of *topical* corticosteroids will likely *not* cause a "rebound effect," but repetitive application over even moderate periods may result in common side effects, including epidermal thinning, dermal atrophy, hypopigmentation, delayed wound healing, acne, and folliculitis, just to name a few.

   However, the administration of *oral* corticosteroids, with its potent systemic anti-inflammatory and immunosuppressive actions, *does* lead to adrenal insufficiency, which can be identified as kidney yang vacuity pattern. Once administration has been discontinued, then the inflammation and hyperactive immune responses revert back to the root or "essential state," which can be identified as repletion heat pattern.

   So, in a sense, this "rebound effect" is more like turning off the water while the embers are still flaring. If patients are concomitantly administered Chinese medicine during this weaning away process, then this "rebound effect" can be either mitigated or completely avoided.

2) As for the tendency to group certain types of pathoconditions together, the key here is for the doctor to conduct a thorough examination of the patient, including history, presenting signs and symptoms, diagnostic tests, and a list of the medications that the patient is currently taking. Once this has been done, the doctor can then conduct pattern identification to determine the treatment.

   Sure, it is possible that the application of TCM diagnostic principles will result in identification of the same (or similar) pattern for different pathological conditions and thus result in the same (or similar) corresponding TCM treatment. However, it is *not* a "one shoe fits all" approach, and as you know, any given pathocondition may manifest differently throughout the various stages of disease and even differently from patient to patient.

Case Study #4: How Long Does Treatment of Atopic Dermatitis Take?

Q: My patients with atopic dermatitis always ask me: "How long will it take before I am cured?" Based on my experience, I tell them it could take anywhere from 6 months to 4 years or more. It depends on the severity of the condition. What would you say? Please offer your advice and guidance.

A: That is a pretty good rough estimate. It really does depend on the patient. If the eczematous rash is limited to just a few locations, such as the face and four bends (antecubital fossa and popliteal fossa), then it may only take about 6 months for complete resolution back to natural, supple luster. Naturally, there will be refractory cases in which the condition is really severe. In these patients, the only thing we can do is try our best: sometimes we can make a phenomenal breakthrough and sometimes we can just hope to control the symptoms as much as possible so the patient can go on with their lives relatively unencumbered.

The most effective formulas I have found so far are my Atopic Dermatitis Formula (nourishes blood and enriches yin, resolves the exterior and dispels wind, and supplements the spleen, liver and kidney) and Blood Desiccation Formula (nourishes blood, enriches yin, and moistens dryness), depending on the presentation and stage of the pathocondition.

In chronic cases, for male patients in particular, who tend to present with kidney yang vacuity pattern, I may prescribe You Gui Yin adding exterior-resolving conductors for the skin (e.g., Ma Huang and Xing Ren); and for female patients, who tend to present with liver channel blood vacuity pattern, I may prescribe Atopic Dermatitis Formula (including large doses of Dang Gui, He Shou Wu, Tu Si Zi, and Sha Yuan Zi), which also includes the exterior-resolving conductors for the skin (e.g., Ma Huang and Xing Ren).

Section 2: Lichen

In classical TCM pathologic terminology, there was not always a definitive etiological or pathophysiological distinction made for the usage of certain terms. Lichen (癬 xian) happens to be one of those nonspecific terms that describes the physical appearance of a scaly, well-circumscribed pathological lesion manifesting on the skin. Generally, the various pathological terms that include lichen in their names—e.g., coin lichen (圓癬 yuán xian, coin lichen (金錢癬 j□n qián xian), dry lichen (乾癬 g□n xian), oxhide lichen (牛皮癬 niú pí xian), and pine bark lichen (松皮癬 s□ng pí xian)—correlate with the modern pathological terms of either tinea, eczema, dermatitis, or psoriasis. The usage of these classical TCM terms is often based on individual preference, rather than indicating a specific etiology or pathology. The key, as always, is to accurately identify the pattern as the basis for treatment.

Case Study #1: Jock Itch (Tinea Cruris)

Q: Five years ago, this 32 y/o male had suffered from anal abscesses and fistulas and underwent a fistulotomy that successfully resolved the condition. After the surgery, he began noticing a papular rash on his buttocks. He has been to see several dermatologists who have prescribed both topical and oral medication, but nothing has been ultimately effective.

Upon inspection, I observed a dark red-colored rash of ring-like plaques on his buttocks (left side more pronounced) with raised borders and pustules that weeped clear (serous) exudate along with a little clear, blood-streaked (serosanguinous) exudate. He also said it was itchy. The patient explained that when he sits for long periods of time, he sweats a lot on his buttocks, especially the left side where the rash is more pronounced. Sometimes he sweats so much that it soaks through his underwear onto his pants.

I decided to prescribe Xian Fang Huo Ming Yin combining Huang Lian Jie Du Tang adding Xiong Huang (minute dose) and Long Dan Cao. Do you think this is a good approach?

A: From your description, this sounds like a classic case of jock itch (tinea cruris), and likely has nothing to do with the surgical procedure (fistulotomy). Tinea cruris is caused by a fungal (dermatophyte) infection, and it is possible that scratching in combination with the damp compressive force of sitting could have caused a secondary infection (e.g., *S. Aureus*, *Candida albicans*, or *Malassezia*) that resulted in folliculitis (localized inflammation of hair follicles or sebaceous glands that present as pustules or papules).

I can kind of see where you are coming from by prescribing the heat-clearing toxin-resolving, swelling-dispersing hardness-breaking, and blood-quickening pain-relieving formula Xian Fang Huo Ming Yin combining Huang Lian Jie Du Tang adding Xiong Huang (minute dose) and Long Dan Cao. But based on this logic, you may as well simply go ahead and approach this pathocondition as liver channel damp-heat pattern and prescribe Long Dan Xie Gan Tang variant.

I would identify this as more of an exterior dampness with heat pattern. For exterior dampness with heat pattern, you can prescribe medicinals for both oral administration and topical application as follows:

For oral administration, you could consider prescribing an exterior-resolving dampness-eliminating and lung qi-diffusing and -disinhibiting formula, such as Ma Xing Yi Gan Tang adding Sheng Shi Gao (a composition that comprises the essential medicinals of Seborrheic Dermatitis Formula!), or a fleshy exterior-harmonizing and evil-expelling itch-relieving formula, such as Gui Zhi Ma Huang Ge Ban Tang adding Sheng Shi Gao, Yi Yi Ren, Bai Xian Pi, and Huang Qin.

But if it were me, I would prescribe Seborrheic Dermatitis Formula (resolves the exterior, dispels wind and eliminates dampness, diffuses and disinhibits lung qi, clears heat and resolves toxin, and dispels wind) adding Ci Ji Li (calms and courses the liver and dispels wind) and Zao Jiao Ci (quickens the blood, disperses swelling, and expels pus)—serve as pore conductors with the capacity to regulate opening and closing (開闔 k□i hé) of the pores and promote dermal circulation), Bai Xian Pi (clears heat and dries dampness and dispels wind and resolves toxin), and Huang Qin (clears heat and dries dampness and drains fire and resolves toxin).

For topical application, you could prescribe Body Soothing Powder (resolves toxin and itch with clearing coolness, dissipates wind and dispels dampness, closes sores and engenders flesh, clears heat and kills worms, and checks sweating) to dab on the itchy sweat-prone area. You could also prescribe an immersion and wash therapy, such as Antimicrobial Wash (clears heat and resolves toxin, kills worms and relieves itch, dispels wind and eliminates dampness, and closes sores and engenders flesh), making sure to double the dose of each medicinal for better efficacy; or even Liu Yi San (clears summerheat and disinhibits dampness), which is simply a 6:1 ratio of Hua Shi and Gan Cao, a less expensive method that may be just as effective. Have the patient decoct the medicinals in a large pot, wait for the liquid decoction to cool, put it into a tub, and then immerse and soak the affected area(s) (i.e., buttocks).

If these approaches are *not* effective, then I would prescribe Tinea/Pompholyx Immersion (clears heat and resolves toxin (antimicrobial), removes the old and institutes the new (exfoliant), and closes sores and engenders flesh). Typically, all it takes is to soak the affected area(s) in this potent infusion as described above 1 or 2 times for it to resolve the infection, dry up, scab over, and heal the lesions (plaques).

Oh! And don't forget, if heat (inflammation) pattern is pronounced, then also bleed Da Zhui (GV14) (above, on, and below) and Wei Zhong (UB40). You can also needle those same two acupoints throughout the administration of your therapeutic regimen even if the heat (inflammation) has resolved, thinking of it as a kind of channel conductor that guides the medicinals to the affected site.

Taiwan has a hot, humid subtropical climate, so tinea cruris is very common here. South Korea has a cool, dry temperate climate, so this condition will likely be much less common except for those who exercise a lot, participate in athletics, work hard labor, and serve in the military. And also for people who sweat a lot! People have to bundle up to go outside in the cold weather and have the heater on inside during cold weather, so for those with sweaty body constitutions this provides a hospitable warm, damp environment for dermatophytes to nestle into the skin, take residence (colonize), and have offspring (proliferate).

For these types of "sweaty" patients, you must advise them to wear clothing made of breathable fabric such as cotton and down. It should be all right to eat spicy foods and drink alcohol if they want to, since it likely won't make any difference. The key for this condition is to keep the groin and buttocks area dry and well ventilated!

Case Study #2: Tinea – Exterior Dampness Pattern

Q: A 10 y/o boy has had stubborn lichen (tinea) (頑癬 wán xuan) on his groin area for four years now. His mom said, "It just won't go away!" Every winter is gets worse, with red pustules that itch like crazy. After administering Long Dan Xie Gan Tang for 3 weeks, the pustules disappeared but it still itches, though not as bad.

A: All types of tinea, also known as dermatophyte infection—pedis (athlete's foot), corporis (ringworm), capitis, unguium (onychomycosis), and cruris (jock itch)—can typically be identified as exterior dampness pattern. Thus, I would prescribe an exterior-resolving dampness-eliminating and lung qi-diffusing and -disinhibiting formula such as Ma Xing Yi Gan Tang adding Sheng Shi Gao.

You should also prescribe a dab-on topical application such as Body Soothing Powder (resolves toxin and itch with clearing coolness, dissipates wind and dispels dampness, closes sores and engenders flesh, clears heat and kills worms, and checks sweating). It is possible that more severe cases of tinea may be identified as liver channel damp-heat pattern, thus requiring administration of Long Dan Xie Gan Tang variant; and if extremely severe, then also consider adding a small dose of Xiong Huang. And make sure to advise the patient to keep the affected area dry at all times!

Sexually transmitted diseases (STDs) (e.g., gonorrhea, syphilis, genital herpes, trichomonas vaginalis, pediculosis pubis (aka pubic lice or "crabs")), bobble wind (scrotal folliculitis) (繡球風 xiù qiú f□ ng), louse-bourne diseases (e.g., epidemic typhus), Behcet's syndrome, and Bartholin's cysts can be identified as liver and gallbladder damp-heat, liver channel repletion fire, and damp-heat in the lower burner pattern, for which you could prescribe Long Dan Xie Gan Tang variant.

However, if the oral administration of Long Dan Xie Gan Tang turns out to be effective, then you can continue prescribing it if you want. But if it were me, I would make sure to combine it with Ma Xing Yi Gan Tang and the topically applied Body Soothing Powder.

Case Study #3: Psoriasis – Pattern Identification and Treatment

Q: In my clinical practice, I have treated several patients with psoriasis and have a fundamental understanding of the etiology, pathophysiology, clinical presentation, and diagnosis of this condition, along with a basic formula that can be prescribed for treatment—Blood Desiccation Formula adding The Three Great Yang-Supplementers, Huang Qin, and Sheng Shi Gao.

However, I still don't have a clear understanding of how to modify my formula in response to fluctuations in the clinical presentation (which medicinals to add or subtract, the right doses, and when to make the move) after I begin administering treatment.

All of the TCM (TKM) doctors in South Korea that I have talked to don't really have too many ideas about this. The common reply is that psoriasis can*not* be effectively treated, so that is basically the end of the conversation. Has that been your experience as well?

A: About 95% of my dry lichen (psoriasis) (乾癬 g□n xian) (aka psoriasis (銀屑病 yín xiè bìng)) patients can be identified as having variations of blood desiccation pattern. Many present as either blood desiccation yang vacuity with heat pattern or blood desiccation with heat pattern, and some as blood desiccation with exterior wind-heat or exterior wind-heat and dampness pattern. That's why I would prescribe a blood-nourishing yin-enriching and dryness-moistening formula, such as Blood Desiccation Formula, adding the following medicinals based on the specific pattern type:

- Blood desiccation yang vacuity with heat—Blood Desiccation Formula adding Bai Xian Pi (clears heat and dries dampness and dispels wind and resolves toxin), Sheng Shi Gao (clears heat and drains fire), Gan Jiang and Fu Zi (return and reinforce yang, "boost" the metabolism and immune system, and bolster right qi), and Huang Qin (clears heat and resolves toxin)
- Blood desiccation with heat—Blood Desiccation Formula adding Sheng Shi Gao and Huang Qin
- Blood desiccation with exterior wind-heat—Blood Desiccation Formula adding Sheng Shi Gao, Huang Qin, Ma Huang and Xing Ren (exterior-resolving conductors for the skin), and Yi Yi Ren (disinhibits water and percolates dampness and clears heat and expels pus)

- Blood desiccation with exterior wind-heat and dampness—Blood Desiccation Formula adding Bai Xian Pi

The remaining 5% of my patients present as exterior wind-heat with varying degrees of dampness. That's why I would prescribe an exterior-resolving dampness-eliminating and lung qi-diffusing and -disinhibiting formula, such as Ma Xing Yi Gan Tang adding Sheng Shi Gao, Huang Qin, and Bai Xian Pi , or possibly even Bai Zhu, Fu Ling, and Ze Xie.

However, I have found that it is becoming more common for dermatologists to prescribe topical corticosteroids and orally administered immunosuppressants (e.g., corticosteroids) together, which may result in a greater tendency for the presentation of blood desiccation yang vacuity with heat pattern as I mentioned above.

Additionally, for patients with blood desiccation with exterior wind-heat and dampness pattern who present with pruritis, you can include a topically applied ointment, such as Body Soothing Ointment (Body Soothing Powder mixed in petroleum jelly), in your therapeutic regimen. And for patients with dry, lichenified skin, you can also advise them to apply topical medications (e.g., moisturizers, corticosteroids, vitamin D derivatives, tar preparations, retinoids/vitamin A) prescribed by a dermatologist.

Remember! Though very rare, the administration of oral corticosteroids may result in the adverse affect of generalized erythroderma in people with certain constitutions. For these patients, you can continue prescribing Blood Desiccation Formula, making sure to add Qing Hao, Zhi Mu, and Di Gu Pi (enrich yin and downbear fire, cool the blood and clear vacuity heat, and eliminate steaming bone), and if the generalized erythroderma is severe with intense itch, peeling (exfoliation), lichenification, and possible lymph swelling, then you can prescribe Blood Desiccation Formula combining Jian Ling Tang.

Case Study #4: Nummular Eczema

Q: A 38 y/o female patient of mine came back to see me about her recurring nummular (discoid) eczema. A few years ago, I had administered medicinals over a period of about 1 year for the treatment of this condition, and it completely resolved.

About 1 month ago, she came back with folliculitis (localized inflammation of the hair follicles and/or sebaceous glands) on both lower legs. I prescribed Xian Fang Huo Ming Yin variant, which quickly resolved most of the papules and pustules, except for the spot on her right leg near Yang Fu (GB38), which developed into an itchy, coin-shaped erythematous plaque about 2 cm in diameter, with oozing and crusting. I prescribed Seborrheic Dermatitis Formula adding Pu Gong Ying and a large dose of Huang Qin. Do you think this is the right approach?

A: Nummular (discoid) eczema is a hypersensitivity reaction (dermatitis) that may be caused by multiple factors, such as dry skin, infection, drug side effects, and irritants. The pathomechisms and pattern identification for this pathocondition are the same as psoriasis: exterior wind-heat with dampness, blood desiccation yang vacuity, blood desiccation with exterior wind-heat, and blood desiccation with wind-heat-damp pattern.

For patients who have *not* been administered oral corticosteroids, you can simply prescribe Ma Xing Yi Gan Tang (resolves the exterior and eliminates dampness and diffuses and disinhibits lung qi) adding Sheng Shi Gao, Bai Xian Pi, and Huang Qin; or Seborrheic Dermatitis Formula (resolves the exterior, dispels wind and eliminates dampness, diffuses and disinhibits lung qi, and clears heat and resolves toxin, and dispels wind) adding Pu Gong Ying, Jing Jie, Fang Feng, and Zao Jiao Ci. If oozing (weeping) is pronounced, then make sure to include large doses of Huang Qin and Sheng Shi Gao; or consider changing your formula to Xian Fang Huo Ming Yin (clears heat and resolves toxin, disperses swelling and breaks hardness, and quickens the blood and relieves pain) variant.

Seborrheic Dermatitis Formula resolves the exterior, dispels wind and eliminates dampness, diffuses and disinhibits lung qi, and clears heat and resolves toxin. So, yes, for this particular patient, who clearly presents with exterior wind-heat and dampness, you could prescribe Seborrheic Dermatitis Formula. If itch is pronounced, then you could also prescribe the topically applied Body Soothing Ointment (resolves toxin and itch with clearing coolness, dissipates wind and dispels dampness, closes sores and engenders flesh, and clears heat and kills worms). If heat (inflammation) is pronounced, then first bleed Da Zhui (GV14) (above, on, and below) and the well points (on the toes or fingers corresponding with the affected area). Plus, you can perform acupuncture on Feng Chi (GB20), Tian Zhu (UB10), He Gu (LI4), San

Yin Jiao (SP6), and Yin Ling Quan (SP9).

In my experience, most patients will first go to see a dermatologist who administers topical corticosteroids, and if the condition is severe and extensive, then oral corticosteroids. Over time, the administration of oral corticosteroids will result in what can be identified as blood desiccation yang vacuity pattern along with varying degrees of heat and dampness. This will require administration of Blood Desiccation Formula (nourishes the blood, enriches yin, and moistens dryness) adding The Three Great Yang-Supplementers, Ma Huang, Sheng Shi Gao, Huang Qin, and Bai Xian Pi (or possibly Xing Ren, Yi Yi Ren, and Gan Cao).

Case Study #5: Coin Lichen – Blood Desiccation Formula

Q: Eight months ago (earlier this year in April), a 42 y/o female patient developed coin lichen—a single round, itchy, raised erythematous eczematous patch—on her lower leg (about 2 cun above Jie Xi (ST41)). After taking Chinese medicine, the lesion began to improve and eventually completely disappeared.

Recently, during the cold of December, the patient returned with the same type of coin lichen at about the same spot as last time. Well, I prescribed the same formula—Seborrheic Dermatitis Formula adding Huang Qin and Pu Gong Ying—but after taking the formula for 2 weeks now, there has not been any improvement whatsoever. In fact, the lesion has expanded to about 5 cm in diameter and the oozing and crusting persists. I decided to continue with the same formula, but increased the doses of Huang Qin (1 liang), Pu Gong Ying (1 liang), and Sheng Shi Gao (3 liang).

Do you think this is a good approach and would it be advisable for her to use the medication prescribed by her dermatologist?

A: In my experience, it should be all right if the patient wants to use topical applications (e.g., emollients, corticosteroid ointments, and creams), but just remember, if the patient takes oral corticosteroids and/or antifungal drugs, then the condition will transmute into blood desiccation, blood desiccation with exterior heat (or heat-damp), or blood desiccation with yang vacuity pattern.

This "coin lichen" patient sounds like a case of nummular (discoid) eczema. Depending on the specific manifestation of symptoms, you can prescribe an yin-enriching liver-emolliating and blood-nourishing dryness-moistening formula such as Blood Desiccation Formula. Just make sure to add medicinals that correspond with the specific pattern, such as Ma Huang and Xing Ren (exterior-resolving conductors for the skin), Huang Qin, Bai Xian Pi, Sheng Shi Gao, Yi Yi Ren, The Three Great Yang-Supplementers, and Lu Lu Tong.

Or, you could also consider prescribing Ma Xing Yi Gan Tang (resolves the exterior and eliminates dampness and diffuses and disinhibits lung qi), Ma Xing Gan Shi Tang (drains heat, diffuses the lung and calms panting, and suppresses cough), or Seborrheic Dermatitis Formula (resolves the exterior, dispels wind and eliminates dampness, diffuses and disinhibits lung qi, clears heat and resolves toxin, and dispels wind).

However, for this patient, it sounds like the best approach would still be to prescribe Blood Desiccation Formula adding Ma Huang, Xing Ren, Yi Yi Ren, Sheng Shi Gao, and Bai Xian Pi. And if that doesn't provide positive results, then consider adding The Three Great Yang-Supplementers along with a topically applied formula such as Body Soothing Powder (for dry lesions) or Body Soothing Ointment (for oozing and crusting lesions).

Case Study #6: Not Sure About Diagnosis? – Prescribe Xian Fang Huo Ming Yin Variant

Q: About one month ago, this 11 y/o boy began noticing redness, heat and swelling of the skin on his left elbow with a pronounced papule bulging from the core of the follicle, which gradually flattened and then enlarged in diameter. A dermatologist prescribed topical and oral corticosteroids, but it was *not* effective.

Based on the clinical presentation of papules and pustules arising from the follicles, I diagnosed this as folliculitis and prescribed Xian Fang Huo Ming Yin variant. Do you think this is a good approach?

A: From your description, it is difficult to provide a definitive diagnosis of folliculitis.

Generally speaking, if the pruritic erythematous maculopapular patches present on the flexural crease (e.g., antecubital fossa), then this would suggest atopic dermatitis. It could be sweat rash (miliaria), but the climate in South Korea is not as damp and hot as Taiwan, and thus this condition would likely not be as prevalent there.

Another possibility is impetigo, but this condition is much like miliaria in that it more commonly occurs in hot and humid climates. You also need to rule out herpes zoster—also known as girdling snake cinnabar (蛇丹 shé d□n), fire-girdle sore (缠腰火丹 chán y□o huo d□n), and snake cinnabar (蛇纏腰 shé chán y□o) in classical TCM pathologic terminology—but it rarely presents on the elbow.

However, I think it is most likely a case of psoriasis—also known as dry lichen (乾癬 g□n xian), oxhide lichen (牛皮癬 niú pí xian), and pine bark lichen (松皮癬 s□ng pí xian)—which further makes sense because after applying topical steroids the lesion would typically turn a dark red color. You can take the above differential diagnosis possibilities into consideration when you reevaluate and make your final diagnosis during subsequent follow-up visits.

As for treatment, it may be just fine to prescribe Xian Fang Huo Ming Yin at first. This is a multiaction, all-purpose "go-to" formula that clears heat and resolves toxin, disperses swelling and breaks hardness, and quickens the blood and relieves pain for the treatment of all types of skin conditions, innominate toxin swelling, malignant tumors, and autoimmune diseases.

On a similar note, here are some more examples of "go-to" formulas to prescribe if you are unable to make a definitive diagnosis of internal medicine pathoconditions. For cases of external contraction (microbial infection) that present with cough and wheezing, you can prescribe either Da Qing Long Tang (effuses sweat and resolves the exterior and clears heat and eliminates vexation) combining Huang Lian Jie Du Tang (clears heat and resolves toxin); or Ma Xing Gan Shi Tang (drains heat, diffuses the lung and calms panting, and suppresses cough) adding Huang Qin. For conditions such as lymphadenitis, Shao Yang disease pattern, liver depression and qi stagnation pattern, and stereotypical symptoms that commonly present in psychosomatic disorder, you can prescribe Xiao Chai Hu Tang (courses and rectifies the liver and disinhibits the gallbladder). Similarly, for cases of foot Tai Yin channel disease pattern, phlegm-cold-damp obstruction pattern, and stereotypical symptoms that commonly present in psychosomatic disorder, you can prescribe Ban Xia Tian Ma Bai Zhu San (supplements the spleen and stomach, transforms phlegm-damp, and nourishes the blood and stabilizes wind). And for patients presenting with Shao Yang depressed heat pattern, phlegm-rheum and damp-heat pattern, mood disorders, and stereotypical symptoms that commonly present in psychosomatic disorder, you can prescribe Wen Dan Tang (clears Shao Yang depressed heat and dispels phlegm turbidity harassing the inner body).

Sometimes the pathocondition has either not fully manifested and/or is difficult to make a definitive diagnosis. More time is needed to observe the patient until the pathocondition fully manifests and/or you can confidently identify the pattern. You can always modify or change the formula if necessary. These "go-to" formula variants that I have just mentioned above can be prescribed initially to serve the dual mind-body function of both calming the patient's anxiety and making headway on the path towards resolving the condition.

Case Study #7: Psoriasis – Has Nothing to Do with the Laundry Detergent!

Q: A 52 y/o male laundry service store owner suspects that frequent exposure to detergents over the years (estimates washing tens of thousands of customers' clothes!) has resulted in allergic contact dermatitis. He has itchy, red, scaly plaques dispersed over his entire body, a generalized heat sensation, and the skin on his palms looks a lot like pompholyx, with oozing blisters, crusting, and fissures.

Over the years, he has been to see a number of TCM and Western medicine doctors, but nothing has been able to cure his condition. In fact, it just keeps getting worse! The plaques on his body look a lot like psoriasis to me and since he doesn't have any joint-related symptoms, I went ahead and prescribed Huang Lian Jie Du Tang adding a large dose of Sheng Shi Gao. Do you think this sounds like a good approach?

A: Hhm…scaly plaques dispersed over his entire body and a generalized heat sensation…That sounds like psoriasis (a chronic inflammatory skin disorder) to me, which can be identified as blood desiccation with exterior wind-heat pattern. It doesn't have anything to do with the laundry detergent! However, it *is* possible that the blistering on the hands may be caused by irritant contact dermatitis (a Type IV hypersensitivity reaction).

For the *acute* stage and during *flare-ups*, Huang Lian Jie Du Tang (clears heat and resolves toxin) adding Sheng Shi Gao (clears heat, drains fire, and eliminates vexation) may be effective, but you should also add Ma Huang and Xing Ren (exterior-resolving conductors for the skin), and Lu Lu Tong (expels wind, frees the network vessels, and relieves itch). Or, you could consider changing the formula to either Ma Xing Yi Gan Tang (resolves the exterior and eliminates dampness and diffuses and disinhibits lung qi) or Gui Ma Ge Ban Tang (harmonizes the fleshy exterior, expels evil, and relieves itch) adding Sheng Shi Gao, Huang Qin, and Bai Xian Pi.

In the *post-acute* and *chronic* stage, I would consider prescribing Blood Desiccation Formula (nourishes the blood, enriches yin, and moistens dryness) adding Sheng Shi Gao, Huang Qin, Ma Huang, Xing Ren, and Yi Yi Ren. Plus, you can prescribe the topically applied Body Soothing Powder (for dry lesions) or Body Soothing Ointment (for oozing and crusting lesions) to resolve toxin and itch with clearing coolness, dissipate wind and dispel dampness, close sores and engender flesh, clear heat and kill worms, and check sweating.

If necessary, you could also consider prescribing Antimicrobial Wash (clears heat and resolves toxin, kills worms and relieves itch, dispels wind and eliminates dampness, and closes sores and engenders flesh). After a soaking session, this medicinal wash should be put back into a container and stored for reuse. The next day, the patient can reboil this same decocted medicinal infusion for about 5 minutes and proceed with the soaking process as before.

If this still does *not* quickly improve the symptoms, then you can advise the patient to apply topical medication (e.g., corticosteroids, antihistamines) prescribed by a dermatologist. These topical medications can serve as adjuvant therapy that effectively relieves the symptoms, giving the TCM medicinals time to work on treating the root and resolving the condition.

Section 3: Pustules

Case Study #1: Pompholyx vs. Tinea Manuum

Q: A 44 y/o female visited me explaining that over the past 8 years she has suffered from itchy red palms, dryness, thickened skin, scaling, and sometimes cracks and fissures open up on her fingertips. During this time, she has visited several different dermatologists and tried all types of medications, including oral and topical corticosteroids, but nothing has proven effective.

I identified this condition as blood desiccation pattern and thus prescribed Blood Desiccation Formula adding The Three Great Yang-Supplementers (3 qian each) and Dai Zhe Shi (8 qian). After taking this formula for 1 month, she came back for a follow-up, presenting with relatively softer skin of pinkish color instead of bright red. There seems to be a slight improvement.

Based on the presentation of symptoms, it looks to me like this is a case of either *pompholyx* or *tinea manuum*? Do you have any advice on treatment?

A: For patients with dry, fissured (cracked) hands, you can differentiate *pompholyx* (*dyshidrotic eczema*) and *tinea manuum* by determining the answers to these questions:

Are there small, deep-seated dot-like vesicles that appear beneath the skin at first and eventually erupt as blisters (vesiculation) on the surface? Is there an intense itch or burning sensation? After scratching, do the lesions ooze and crust? And after crusting, does the skin thicken and turn dry and scaly textured. If *so*, then the condition is likely *pompholyx*.

In the *absence* of small, deep-seated dot-like vesicles, you need to answer these questions: Is there a blistering rash on the surface of the skin (in particular the edges of the fingers or palm) that appear in crops, break, ooze, peel and burn? Is there itchy, scaly, fissured skin that fails to grow new skin at the site of peeling? Or, are there circular (or ovular) lesions with elevated borders? Is it only on one hand? Are both feet affected as well? And in the chronic stages, do the creases of the skin appear as whitened lines? If *so*, then the condition is likely *tinea manuum*.

However, depending on the specific manifestation of symptoms throughout the various stages (i.e., acute, post-acute, and chronic), both of these pathoconditions may present as identical patterns (i.e., exterior wind-heat (-damp), exterior wind-heat (-damp) toxin, damp-heat accumulated toxin, or blood desiccation with wind heat or with yang vacuity).

Considering the cold climate of South Korea, I suspect that most patients with *tinea manuum* would present with blood desiccation pattern. Regardless if the patient presents in the acute stage or during flare-ups (i.e., exterior wind-damp pattern) or in the post-acute or chronic stages (i.e., damp-heat accumulated toxin or blood desiccation pattern), you can still prescribe Tinea/Pompholyx Immersion. Soaking the affected areas in this immersion therapy will clear heat and resolve toxin (antimicrobial), remove the old and institute the new (exfoliant), and close sores and engender flesh.

Case Study #2: Pompholyx – Keep Your Hands Dry!

Q: I often use the (Yu Sheng) Seborrheic Dermatitis Formula variant for the treatment of pompholyx (dyshidrotic eczema). This formula is initially effective at improving symptoms. However, I have found that if these patients come into frequent contact with water, the condition readily relapses, and they tend to become entrenched in a recalcitrant, hyperkeratotic state that is extremely difficult to treat. How would you treat this condition?

A: Dyshidrotic eczema (pompholyx) can be identified as Yang Ming heat pattern. Although you may have gotten positive results from Seborrheic Dermatitis Formula, I think you will get even better results by prescribing oral administration of Xian Fang Huo Ming Yin (clears heat and resolves toxin, disperses swelling and breaks hardness, and quickens the blood and relieves pain) and an immersion therapy of Tinea/Pompholyx Immersion (clears heat and resolves toxin (antimicrobial), removes the old and institutes the new (exfoliant), and closes sores and engenders flesh). Plus, bleed Da Zhui (GV14) (above, on, and below) and the well points on the fingers, and needle the acupoints Feng Chi (GB20), Tian Zhu (UB10), He Gu (LI4), Zhong Zhu (TB3), and Zu San Li (ST40).

Chronic conditions presenting as a vicious cycle of recurrent blistering, intense itch, peeling, redness, pronounced thickening of the stratum corneum (horny layer), and deep fissures (cracks) in the skin can be identified as blood desiccation pattern. Thus, for these patients, you can prescribe Blood Desiccation Formula. If heat *is* pronounced (e.g., the patient presents with an eruption of vesicles, intense itch, or secondary infection manifesting as pustules with a red border), then add Sheng Shi Gao and Huang Qin (or Pu Gong Ying); and if heat is *not* pronounced, then consider adding The Three Great Yang-Supplementers.

Since South Korea is a cold climate, especially along the coasts where it is cold *and* damp, you must also consider the possibility of chilblain (pernio, chill burn). Thus, for these patients, besides Blood Desiccation Formula, you could consider prescribing a blood-nourishing, kidney yang-supplementing, and channel-warming formula such as Gui Qi Jian Zhong Tang, Dang Gui Si Ni Tang, Di Huang Yin Zi, and Qi Bao Mei Ran Dan; or a pus-expelling flesh-engendering formula such as Tuo Li Xiao Du San or Qian Jin Nei Tuo San. Regardless of the formula you choose, make sure to include The Three Great Yang-Supplementers and Huang Qin; and if heat *is* pronounced, add Sheng Shi Gao. Also, advise these patients to dress warmly and wear gloves in the cold weather, and by all means, try to keep the hands dry, having as little contact with water as possible.

Remember! For dyshidrotic eczema (pompholyx) patients who present with itchy, dry and/or fissured skin, you can also recommend the topical application of Purple Cloud Ointment or simply Ma You (麻油/Sesame Oil).

Case Study #3: Chronic Acne Vulgaris with Pockmarks

Q: I have a male patient with a 30-year history of acne vulgaris. The left side of his face from in front of his ear down to his neck is covered with scarring (pockmarks), interspersed with papules and nodules of different sizes and brown marks (postinflammatory pigmentation) in some spots. This is clearly a case of inflammatory acne with hyperpigmentation and scarring.

He has tried the gamut of topical and oral medications prescribed by both dermatologists and Chinese medicine doctors, including a chemical peel, but nothing has proven ultimately effective at resolving the condition. What would you do for this patient?

A: Acne can be classified into two categories: *inflammatory*—manifesting as closed comedones (whiteheads), papules, pustules, nodules, and cysts; and *noninflammatory*—manifesting as open comedones (blackheads) and pseudocysts.

Mild cases of *inflammatory* acne can be identified as wind-heat toxin congestion in the lung and stomach pattern; and moderate to severe cases that present with a large number of inflammatory lesions can be identified as wind-heat toxin congestion in the lung and stomach with blood aspect heat toxin pattern.

As for treatment, I would first bleed Da Zhui (GV14) (above, on, and below) and Li Dui (ST45); and then needle Feng Chi (GB20), Tian Zhu (UB10), He Gu (LI4), Zhong Zhu (TB3), and Zu San Li (ST40). For wind-heat toxin congestion in the lung and stomach pattern, I would prescribe a heat-clearing toxin-resolving formula that includes Huang Qin (or Huang Lian), such as Yang Dan Tang, Qing Shang Fang Feng Tang, Qing Yan Li Ge San, or Gua Lou Niu Bang Zi Tang. For exterior wind damp-heat toxin accumulating and blood aspect heat toxin pattern, I would prescribe Xian Fang Huo Ming Yin variant.

Noninflammatory acne can be identified as spleen qi or kidney yang vacuity pattern. Thus, for treatment I would prescribe Xiang Sha Liu Jun Zi Tang, Bu Zhong Yi Qi Tang, Gui Qi Jian Zhong Tang, Shi Quan Da Bu Tang, Shen Qi Wan, or You Gui Yin. Just make sure to include The Three Great Yang-Supplementers, Huang Qin, and Jin Yin Hua.

For this patient with *chronic* acne that has been severe enough to result in scarring (pockmarks), treatment will require administration of a qi-, blood-, and kidney yang-supplementing formula such as Gui Qi Jian Zhong Tang (including a large dose of Huang Qi) adding Zi He Che and Jin Yin Hua. If the acne is severe, with a large number of inflammatory lesions (i.e., whiteheads, papules, pustules, nodules, and cysts), then you should include large doses of Huang Qin and Jin Yin Hua, or consider changing to the *inflammatory* acne therapeutic approach above until the condition stabilizes. And during the cold winter months, as long as the inflammatory lesions are not severe—you can also consider including large doses of The Three Great Yang-Supplementers.

This formula will promote the excretion of the sebum, debris, and bacteria in the pores (pilosebaceous units); facilitates the suppuration and discharge of comedones (whiteheads), papules, pustules, nodules, and cysts; and expedites the healing of sores and tissue so that no scarring is left behind.

Case Study #4: Impetigo and Ecthyma

Q: A 15 y/o girl who is now in 9th grade said that she has had sensitive skin and been prone to allergic reactions since she was a child. Her skin is so sensitive even a mosquito bite will result in local infection, erythema, swelling, and pus formation that sometimes leaves behind a scar. She is more susceptible to develop these types of inflamed vesicles and pustules that crust over and become ulcerated during the hot summer months. What's the best way to treat this patient?

A: Oh!...This sounds like a stereotypical case of impetigo (膿痂疹 nóng ji□ zh□n). Impetigo is a common superficial skin pathocondition that is typically caused by *Staphylococcus aureus*, and presents as vesicles or pustules that evolve into crusted erosions or plaques which heal slowly in 2–4 weeks without scarring. If indurated ulcers present that result in scarring, then this is called ecthyma.

Ecthyma causes deeper erosions (ulcerations) of the skin that extend into the dermis and is usually caused by *Staphylococcus aureus* or *Streptococcus pyogenes*. It presents with the same clinical features as impetigo, but underneath the hard crust an indurated ulcer develops which takes longer to heal and tends to leave behind a scar. Staphylococcal and streptococcal skin infections are much more common in the hot, humid summer months; and yes, for people with "sensitive" skin, even insect bites are predisposing factors for this pathocondition.

In TCM, these types of bacterial skin infections can be identified as exterior wind with damp-heat toxin accumulating and blood aspect heat toxin pattern. Thus, I would prescribe a heat-clearing toxin-resolving and swelling-dispersing hardness-breaking formula such as Xian Fang Huo Ming Yin adding Huang Qin (clears heat and dries dampness, drains fire and resolves toxin, and cools the blood), Pu Gong Ying (clears heat and resolves toxin, disperses welling-abscesses and dissipates binds, and disinhibits dampness), and Jing Jie (effuses the exterior and dissipates wind, outthrusts papules and heals sores, and rectifies the blood).

Case Study #5: Milium

Q: A 12 y/o boy presented with numerous pearly-colored bumps under the surface of the skin that appear around the eyes and eyebrows and on the forehead. They look a bit like the pustules presenting in acne, with*out* the yellow-colored pus inside and erythema surrounding the borders of the bumps. He has had these for about 6 months now, so his mother decided to bring him in to see if the condition could be treated.

I prescribed Wen Dan Tang combining Ma Xing Yi Gan Tang (including a large dose of Ma Huang) adding Rou Gui (large dose). After taking this formula for the past 10 days, there has been *no* improvement in the condition. Do you think there is a better approach for treating this condition?

A: Based on your description, this definitely sounds like milium (pl. milia). Milia are small cysts containing keratin. They do *not* have an opening on the skin's surface so they can*not* be extruded easily ("popped") just by simply squeezing them.

This condition can be identified as exterior dampness pattern or phlegm-rheum pattern. For exterior dampness pattern, I would prescribe either Ma Xing Yi Gan Tang or Gui Zhi Ma Huang Ge Ban Tang; and for phlegm-rheum pattern, I would prescribe Wen Dan Tang adding Ma Huang, Xing Ren, and Gui Zhi.

In many patients milia will spontaneously resolve after a period of time. However, in some patients the condition persists indefinitely. This patient has only taken your formula for 10 days. It sounds like you are on the right track, but it may take some time and patience for this condition to resolve. Chinese medicine can promote local circulation of the dermis, transform phlegm, soften hardness, and outthrust papules, thus expediting the process of keratin reabsorption and resolution.

Actually, since this is a purely cosmetic condition, it is*n't* imperative that you treat it. You should mention this to the patient and his family. If they decide to forgo treatment, you can still advise the patient to eat lots of Yi Yi Ren, mixing it in steamed rice, soups, or in other dishes. Yi Yi Ren disinhibits water and percolates dampness, fortifies the spleen, and clears heat and expels pus—plus, it tastes great!

Case Study #6: Keratolysis Exfoliativa

Q: I have seen several patients with keratolysis exfoliativa (aka exfoliative keratosis). The typical clinical picture is as follows: Initially, the patient presents with air-filled blisters on the surface of the skin along the edges of the fingers and on the palms. After the blisters break open, the peeled skin remains tethered and scaly, and the underlying skin of the peeled areas appears pink or reddish-colored. The round peeled areas become dry and may crack open.

Right now, I am treating a patient who also presented with peeling on the tips of his fingers in which the underlying skin of the peeled areas becomes hard, dry and cracks open. I prescribed Ma Xing Yi Gan Tang for oral administration and also had the patient soak his hands in Tinea/Pompholyx Immersion. After a 3-day regimen of immersion therapy and 2 weeks of taking the formula, his hands have shown marked improvement. It seems like I am on the right track. What do you think?

A: I would classify this condition as a type of goose-foot wind (鵝掌風 é zhang f□ng). At the onset or during flare-ups, this can be identified as exterior wind-damp pattern (e.g., presenting with air-filled blisters that break open and reveal the underlying skin). As the condition evolves into prolonged episodes or becomes persistent (e.g., dry, possibly itchy, skin with repeated episodes of peeling, lichenification, and fissures eventually opening up), this can be identified as blood desiccation pattern.

Ma Xing Yi Gan Tang is a good formula for treating exterior wind-damp pattern, and the immersion formula (clears heat and resolves toxin (antimicrobial), removes the old and institutes the new (exfoliant), and closes sores and engenders flesh) will promote exfoliation and expedite the process of skin regeneration. If your therapeutic regimen has been working, then by all means continue. For skin conditions that present with peeling and pronounced dryness and cracking, you could also advise the patient to topically apply Purple Cloud Ointment, Sesame Oil, or fresh Ji Zi Bai (雞子白/Chicken Egg White/aka Albumen).

Remember! Both modern biomedical and classical TCM pathological terminology simply describe a particular set of presenting symptoms at a specific point in time. Oftentimes, there may be ambiguity in the use of terminology, especially when a definitive cause is unknown (e.g., hypersensitivity reactions, genetic predisposition, autoimmune response, microbial infections) and/or there are overlapping symptoms that present in the various phases of pathological manifestation. The key is for you to apply the eight-principle pattern identification method and have a clear picture of how you define the use of various terms. Don't get too caught up in the terminology or else you can't see the forest for the trees! You'll either run into a tree or get lost! Hahaha…!

In TCM, the term goose-foot wind (鵝掌風 é zhang f□ng) is a prime example. The broad definition of goose-foot wind describes the presentation of symptoms on the hands (palms and light-colored skin along the borders of the palms and fingers) and feet (soles and light-colored skin along the borders of the feet and toes). These symptoms manifest as itchy skin that peels and leaves behind a sensitive layer of underlying erythematous skin that grows back slowly, becomes dry, and lichenifies, with fissures eventually opening up. Over time, the skin may thicken, with fissures occurring more frequently, thus increasing the possibility of secondary infection.

Section 4: Macules, Papules, and Wheals

Case Study #1: Bluish-Purple Macule on the Lower Extremity – "Just Appeared All of a Sudden"

Q: A 40 y/o female patient visited me explaining that about 1 week ago she noticed a flat, round cloud-shaped macule on her right shin that "just appeared all of a sudden" for no apparent reason. The macule is bluish-purple colored on the perimeter and at the center the skin is normal colored. It does *not* itch, but occasionally turns reddish colored at the center.

I administered a 1-week prescription of Di Gu Pi Yin variant, and she is scheduled to come back next week for follow-up. Does this sound like a good formula for this clinical presentation?

A: Based on the description, the bluish-purple cloud-shaped macule on her shin can be identified as blood heat pattern. Unless there are other presenting signs, symptoms or details in her history that would make it necessary to rule out other possibilities, this sounds to me like it could simply be a "normal" physiological manifestation of vascular dilation.

If this is the case, then it is *not* even necessary to provide treatment. But, if the patient wants to take medicinals, then yes, a blood-nourishing yin-enriching and heat-clearing blood-cooling formula such as Di Gu Pi Yin variant is a good choice!

Case Study #2: Round Erythematous Patches – Looks Like an "Alcohol Rash"

Q: A 26 y/o female patient explained that she has had sensitive skin ever since suffering from a bout of gastroenteritis in high school. She frequently breaks out in a rash that she says looks like an "alcohol rash" that some people whom are allergic to alcohol get.

The rash presents as red, cloud-shaped, mildly itchy patches (as opposed to plaques and wheals which are raised) on her back and abdomen. The strange thing is that she has a large, round, grayish-tinted patch on her back that has never gone away. How would you treat this type of skin condition?

A: These patches can be identified as blood heat with exterior wind pattern or exterior wind with blood heat pattern. Thus, depending on which pattern is more pronounced, you could consider prescribing one of the following formulas:

- A heat-clearing blood-cooling and blood-nourishing yin-enriching formula such as Di Gu Pi Yin adding Fang Feng, Jing Jie, and Lian Qiao (course wind and dissipate heat)
- An exterior outthrusting with coolness and acridity and heat-clearing toxin-resolving formula such as Yin Qiao San adding Qing Hao, Zhi Mu, and Di Gu Pi (enrich yin and downbear fire and cool the blood and clear vacuity heat)

And during cold weather, you could also consider adding Ma Huang (promotes sweating, resolves the exterior, and relieves itch) and Gui Zhi (promotes sweating and resolves the exterior, warms and frees the channel vessels, and assists yang and transforms qi).

Case Study #3: Itchy Skin After Moving House

Q: A patient visited me explaining that he, his wife, and kindergarten-aged child all have had itchy skin after moving house a couple of weeks ago. When they scratch their skin, red marks (erythematous wheals) swell up along the sites of contact (dermatographism).

In addition to dermatographism, their child also has sores that form crusty scabs (impetigo) on the backs of her fingers and abnormal keratinization of the skin (keratosis pilaris) on her upper arms and outer thighs that appears as dark purple-colored scaly spots. How would you treat these patients?

A: Sounds to me like the house moving rustled up lots of dust, dander, mildew, and mites, which has caused a hypersensitivity reaction (*urticaria*) with concomitant *dermatographism.*

At the onset, during the acute stage, *urticaria* can be identified as exterior wind-heat pattern, for which you could prescribe a sweat-effusing exterior-resolving and lung-diffusing wind-dispelling formula such as Da Qing Long Tang, Yue Bi Tang, Yang Dan Tang, or Gui Zhi Ma Huang Ge Ban Tang. If the condition persists into the post-acute or chronic stage, then it typically can be identified as blood desiccation pattern.

In severe cases (e.g., wheals extend deeper into the tissue and may spread over a large area), you can prescribe a heat-clearing toxin-resolving, swelling-dispersing hardness-breaking, and blood-quickening pain-relieving formula such as Xian Fang Huo Ming Yin adding Jing Jie (effuses the exterior and dissipates wind, outthrusts papules and heals sores, and rectifies the blood), Huang Qin (clears heat and resolves toxin), and Ma Huang and Gui Zhi (promote sweating and resolve the exterior, disinhibit water and disperse swelling, outthrust papules, and relieve itch).

Additionally, during the acute stage (or flare-ups) when heat and wheals are pronounced, you should bleed Da Zhui (GV14) (above, on, and below), Wei Zhong (UB40), and the stomach channel well point (Li Dui (ST45)); and needle Feng Chi (GB20), Tian Zhu (UB10), Wei Zhong (UB40), He Gu (LI4), Chi Ze (LU5), and Zu San Li (ST36).

Impetigo results from bacterial infection and can be identified as exterior wind with damp-heat toxin accumulating and blood aspect heat toxin pattern, for which Xian Fang Huo Ming Yin adding Huang Qin, Pu Gong Ying, and Jing Jie will provide effective treatment.

Keratosis pilaris results from keratin scales depositing in the follicle as opposed to exfoliating as normal. If there is simply discoloration that appears as spots (with*out* pus-filled fluid) at the site of follicles, then this can be identified in two ways. If the spots (follicles) are bright red colored, then this can be identified as exterior wind-heat pattern, for which you can prescribe Ma Xing Yi Gan Tang. If the spots (follicles) are pink-colored or skin-colored, then this can be identified as either blood desiccation pattern, for which I would prescribe Blood Desiccation Formula; or blood desiccation with yang-vacuity pattern, for which I would add The Three Great Yang-Supplementers and Huang Qin. If pustules (*with* pus-filled fluid) present at the sites of follicles, then this indicates heat and inflammation; thus, I would prescribe Xian Fang Huo Ming Yin adding Huang Qin.

Since you said the child has *urticaria* with concomitant *dermatographism*, *keratosis pilaris* (i.e., "dark-purple colored scaly spots"), and *impetigo*, I would consider prescribing Xian Fang Huo Ming Yin combining Gui Ma Ge Ban Tang. This therapeutic approach will effectively resolve these types of skin pathoconditions.

Case Study #4: Dermatographism – Blood Desiccation Pattern

Q: I have had several cases of young adults who come in explaining that they have "oddly" sensitive skin. Most of the time, the skin appears normal without any noticeable abnormalities. But once they happen to scratch their skin or rub up against some object, anywhere from 5–10 minutes later itchy marks (wheals) appear that either remain skin-colored or turn pinkish or red-colored, and may even spread beyond the initial site of irritation after continued scratching.

These wheals eventually fade away within about 15–20 minutes, without leaving behind any trace that they had been there. Some patients muse that they can write their names and draw pictures on their skin, essentially initiating an acute flare-up. But for some patients these flare-ups can be more severe, presenting with intense itch, sensation of heat, and wheals that extend down to deeper levels of the skin and spread over larger portions of the body.

I used to have this same problem as a kid up until high school and then it just stopped happening, and has never occurred since then. My mother took me to a dermatologist at that time who diagnosed me with dermatographism (aka inducible urticaria). As the old saying goes, I was "in the same boat" as these patients, so I know how annoying and discomforting it can be. How do you treat this type of urticaria?

A: Dermatographism (aka dermatographia, dermatographic urticaria, inducible urticaria, urticaria factitia) literally means "to write on the skin." It is an exaggerated whealing tendency that appears after slight pressure or stroking is applied on the skin and is likely mediated by local histamine release, other chemical mediators, or possibly some type of autoantibody to an unknown cutaneous protein. The capillaries become dilated and erythematous, further arteriolar dilation occurs, and a wheal is then formed through fluid transudation. This type of urticaria is most common in young adults, but can occur at any age, and in many patients it may resolve spontaneously.

The root of this pathocondition can be identified as blood desiccation pattern, requiring administration of a blood-nourishing liver-emolliating and yin-enriching dryness-moistening formula such as Blood Desiccation Formula variant. A simple guideline can be used to differentiate the presence of concurrent patterns based on observation of color and extent of edema (e.g., the deeper the edema in the dermis and the larger the wheal) are as follows:

1) Skin-colored wheals—blood desiccation pattern: Administer Blood Desiccation Formula adding exterior-resolving conductors such as Ma Huang (small dose), Gui Zhi, Fang Feng, and Jing Jie. Perform acupuncture on the acupoints He Gu (LI4), Chi Ze (LU5) Xue Hai (SP10), San Yin Jiao (SP6), and Yin Ling Quan (SP9).
2) White-colored wheals—blood desiccation with yang vacuity pattern: Administer Blood Desiccation Formula adding exterior-resolving conductors as above, The Three Great Yang-Supplementers, and Huang Qin; and perform acupuncture (warm needle) on the acupoints He Gu (LI4), Chi Ze (LU5) Xue Hai (SP10), San Yin Jiao (SP6), and Yin Ling Quan (SP9).
3) Dark red-colored wheals—blood desiccation with exterior wind-heat and blood heat pattern: Administer Blood Desiccation Formula adding exterior-resolving conductors as above, blood-cooling medicinals such as Mu Dan Pi and Di Gu Pi, and heat-clearing toxin-resolving and dampness-disinhibiting swelling-dispersing medicinals such as Pu Gong Ying and Feng Wei Cao. Bleed Da Zhui (GV14) (above, on, and below) and Cun Kou (Tai Yuan (LU9)); and perform acupuncture (needle) on the acupoints Feng Chi (GB20), Tian Zhu (UB10), He Gu (LI4), Chi Ze (LU5), Zu San Li (ST36), San Yin Jiao (SP6), Yin Ling Quan (SP9), and Xue Hai (SP10).
4) Severe, acute flare-ups (manifesting as pronounced heat, swelling and intense itch): You should consider changing to a heat-clearing toxin-resolving, swelling-dispersing hardness-breaking, and blood-quickening pain-relieving formula such as Xian Fang Huo Ming Yin (including a large dose of Sheng Shi Gao) adding heat-clearing toxin-resolving and dampness-disinhibiting swelling-dispersing medicinals. Bleed Da Zhui (GV14) (above, on, and below), Cun Kou (Tai Yuan (LU9)), and Wei Zhong (UB40); and perform acupuncture (needle) on the acupoints Feng Chi (GB20), Tian Zhu (UB10), He Gu (LI4), Chi Ze (LU5), Zu San Li (ST36), San Yin Jiao

(SP6), Yin Ling Quan (SP9), Wei Zhong (UB40), and Bai Hui (GV20).

As I mentioned above, this pathocondition can typically be identified as blood desiccation pattern. And during the cold weather season, it commonly manifests as blood desiccation with yang vacuity pattern. Just make sure to keep an eye out for acute flare-ups, manifesting as exterior wind-heat (or wind-damp-heat), and modify your formula accordingly.

Remember! In the vast majority of cases, this is a benign condition. However, there is a correlation between dermatographism, autoimmune diseases (e.g., Bechet disease), and hypereosinophilic syndrome, so you must conduct a comprehensive patient interview and examination in order to rule out the unexpected!

Section 5: Folliculitis

Case Study #1: Chicken's-Droppings Welling-Abscess

Q: A 17 y/o female visited me with a case of scalp folliculitis that presented as redness around the hair follicles, excessive sebaceous secretions, itchiness, and hair loss at the sites of the lesions. Pus can be extracted by squeezing the inflamed pustules that have come to a head.

After prescribing a 4-week regimen of (Yu Sheng) Seborrheic Dermatitis Formula, her condition has not improved very much except for that she does*n't* feel itchiness anymore. How should I proceed from here?

A: Scalp folliculitis can be identified as chicken's-droppings welling-abscess (雞屎癰 j□ shi y□ng) in classical TCM pathology. Seborrheic Dermatitis Formula (resolves the exterior, dispels wind and eliminates dampness, clears heat and resolves toxin, and diffuses and disinhibits lung qi) is an effective formula for treating scalp folliculitis.

I would consider including large doses of Huang Qin and Jin Yin Hua and adding a large dose of Pu Gong Ying as well. Also, bleed Da Zhui (GV14) (above, on, and below), Wei Zhong (UB40), and the urinary bladder channel well point (Zhi Yin (UB67)); and needle Feng Chi (GB20), Tian Zhu (UB10), He Gu (LI4), Chi Ze (LU5), Wei Zhong (UB40), and San Yin Jiao (SP6).

Just focus on resolving the inflammation. Once the inflammation has resolved, the hair will grow back!

Case Study #2: It's Folliculitis, *Not* "Heat Rash"

Q: My son has tiny pinhead pustules on his forehead (near Yin Tang (EX-HN 3). It looks like miliaria (heat rash) to me.

I have tried prescribing both Da Qing Long Tang combining Wen Dan Tang and Ma Xin Yi Gan Tang combining Wen Dan Tang, but these formulas have not been effective. What would you prescribe for this condition?

A: It is the dead of winter in South Korea. This cannot be "heat rash" for goodness sake, it must be folliculitis! I recommend that you prescribe Xian Fang Huo Ming Yin, bleed Da Zhui (GV14) (above, on, and below), and needle Feng Chi (GB20), Tian Zhu (UB10), He Gu (LI4) and Zu San Li (ST36).

Case Study #3: Folliculitis on Buttocks

Q: This female patient has had problems with folliculitis on the buttocks for 5 years now. She said that she usually breaks out with a new batch (30 or more!) of mostly superficial pustules, and occasionally inflammatory nodules, on her buttocks every time her period comes. The superficial pustules resolve eventually, but the nodules can linger on causing soreness when sitting down.

I prescribed Xian Fang Huo Ming Yin (including large doses of Sheng Shi Gao (2 liang) and Bai Zhi (1 liang)) adding Pu Gong Ying (1 liang), Huang Qin (8 qian), Di Yu (3 qian), Huai Hua (3 qian), and Hua Shi (4 qian). After taking this formula for about 1 month, during her next menstruation, she only broke out with 2 pustules and the lingering nodules from before were almost completely healed. How would you proceed from here?

A: Great! Xian Fang Huo Ming Yin (clears heat and resolves toxin, disperses swelling and breaks hardness, and quickens the blood and relieves pain) has been recognized as a "sage formula for the treatment of sores" since antiquity. If you have been having success with this formula, then by all means continue prescribing it! Typically, I would continue administering this formula for 2–3 more months in order to ensure complete resolution and reduce the chance of recurrence.

Aside from this formula, for some patients, I have also had effective results prescribing either Yang Dan Tang or Ge Gen Huang Qin Huang Lian Tang adding Pu Gong Ying, Lian Qiao, and Jin Yin Hua (clear heat and resolve toxin and disperse welling-abscesses and dissipate binds). If there is pronounced redness and inflammation, then you can bleed Da Zhui (GV14) (above, on, and below), Wei Zhong (UB40), and the well points on the channels that correspond with the site(s) of the lesions. Plus, you can needle distal points that greatly supplement qi and blood (e.g., He Gu (LI4) and Zu San Li

(ST36)) and points that correspond with the site(s) of the lesions (e.g., Tian Zhu (UB10), Wei Zhong (UB40)).

Case Study #4: Dry, Itchy Skin and Folliculitis

Q: A 53 y/o male patient visited me with extremely dry and intensely itchy skin over virtually his entire body, which is more pronounced during the winter months and at nighttime. It looks like he also has folliculitis on his back and neck. I prescribed Blood Desiccation Formula adding Huang Qin (8 qian), Pu Gong Ying (1 liang), Sheng Di Huang, Zhi Mu, and Di Gu Pi.

Over the past few years of treating patients, I have observed that most South Koreans with dry, itchy skin can be identified as yin vacuity pattern. I am not sure if this is because we eat lots of kimchi and drink our share of soju or not. However, this patient said that he really does*n't* eat that much kimchi or drink very much hard liquor in general. What do you think?

A: Well, I do*n't* think kimchi or soju have anything to do with the dry, itchy skin or folliculitis. Only when the liver is severely damaged (e.g., cirrhosis) do patients begin to present with itchy skin.

Typically, in the acute stage, folliculitis can be identified as exterior wind-heat pattern, but in more severe manifestations patients may receive long-term administration of topical steroids (e.g., eosinophilic folliculitis) or antimycotics (e.g., malassezia folliculitis), which will result in yang vacuity pattern.

You have a lot of cold weather in the northern hemisphere, and cold windy weather alone may cause dry, itchy skin in some people. If the patient does not drink enough water or eat fruits and vegetables, then this could manifest as yin vacuity pattern.

It looks like you are focusing on treating the dry skin mainly (Blood Desiccation Formula variant) and adding some heat-clearing toxin-resolving medicinals (Huang Qin and Pu Gong Ying) to address the folliculitis. If you want to focus on treating the folliculitis, then you could consider prescribing Xian Fang Huo Ming Yin, Ma Xing Yi Gan Tang, or Ma Xing Gan Shi Tang, adding other medicinals accordingly.

Case Study #5: Postinflammatory Hyperpigmentation – "It Keeps Spreading!"

Q: A 45 y/o female patient visited me yesterday with dark brown spots (macules) and some larger patches on her upper chest, back and neck. It does*n't* itch, but she said, "It keeps spreading!" She also mentioned that she has had problems with acne in the past. This is really a strange case. Please offer your advice and guidance.

A: Oh…This case is not strange at all! It is obviously postinflammatory hyperpigmentation (PIH) left behind after the folliculitis resolved. PIH is an acquired hypermelanosis that can occur after cutaneous inflammation in people of all skin types, especially those with darker skin.

Brown or *dark brown* appearance suggests that the hyperpigmentation is closer to the surface (epidermis) and thus will eventually resolve over time (faster with treatment!), whereas *bluish-grey* appearance suggests that the hyperpigmentation is at a deeper level (dermis) and thus may take a longer time to resolve or may even be permanent. The hyperpigmentation may get worse with ultraviolet (UV) radiation (e.g., sunlight) exposure and recurrent inflammation.

If the patient still presents with folliculitis, then first prescribe Xian Fang Huo Ming Yin adding Huang Qin, Ma Huang, Xing Ren, and Yi Yi Ren. Once the folliculitis (inflammation) has resolved, then you can change to either Ma Xing Yi Gan Tang (for *brown* or *dark brown* appearance) or Gui Qi Jian Zhong Tang (for *bluish-grey* appearance).

Unless the patient specifically requests that you prescribe decocting pieces (more expensive!), I would just consider prescribing commercial extract powder (granules), which may be more practical for treating this type of benign condition that may eventually resolve one day on its own anyways. TCM will accelerate the process of resolving the hyperpigmentation and reinstituting the "natural" coloration of the skin.

Section 6: Pigmentation Disorders

Case Study #1: Tinea Versicolor – Lingering White Macules

Q: A 35 y/o female explained that 7 years ago she began noticing an itchy, small, white macule on the left side of her neck. After receiving treatment from a dermatologist, the itch soon resolved, but the small white macules remain to this day.

The patient finds these spots unattractive and hopes that TCM can provide effective treatment to make the spots disappear. She currently has no other symptoms other than the white macules. I am not sure if there is anything I can do for this patient. Please offer your advice and guidance.

A: This sounds like a case of *tinea versicolor* (*pityriasis versicolor*), a common superficial skin infection caused by malassezia fungi (e.g., *Malassezia furfur*, *Malassezia globosa*). It can be triggered by factors, such as hot, humid weather, oily skin, hormonal changes, and weakened immune system, and presents with round macules that may manifest as hypopigmentation or hyperpigmentation.

The classical TCM pathological term for this condition is sweat macule (汗斑 hàn b□n) or purple and white patch wind (紫白癜風 zi bái diàn f□ng), which results from summer-heat damp settling in the exterior, opening and discharging of the interstices (腠裡開泄 còu li k□i xiè), and repeated contraction of wind toxin.

Usually, these macules will fade away in time, but it is possible that the infection has either never been completely eradicated or has recurred. In the acute stage, I would prescribe an exterior-resolving dampness-eliminating and lung qi-diffusing and -disinhibiting formula such as Ma Xing Yi Gan Tang. If itch presents, then also prescribe a topically applied formula such as Body Soothing Powder (resolves toxin and itch with clearing coolness, dissipates wind and dispels dampness, closes sores and engenders flesh, and clears heat and kills worms).

If this approach is *not* effective, then I would go ahead and treat this as if it were a case of *vitiligo*, which can be identified as kidney yang vacuity, liver blood vacuity, or spleen qi vacuity pattern. You could consider prescribing formulas that correspond with these patterns such as You Gui Yin, Sheng Yu Tang, Blood Desiccation Formula, or Bu Zhong Yi Qi Tang. Just make sure to include Bu Gu Zhi (supplements the kidney, assists yang, and secures essence), He Shou Wu (supplements and boosts essence-blood and secures the kidney and blackens the beard and hair), and Ci Ji Li (calms and courses the liver and dispels wind and serves as a pore conductor with the capacity to regulate opening and closing (開闔 k□i hé) of the pores and promote dermal circulation) in your formula.

Note: The classical TCM pathological terminology for *tinea versicolor* (*pityriasis versicolor*)—sweat macule (汗斑 hàn b□n) or purple and white patch wind (紫白癜風 zi bái diàn f□ng)—and *vitiligo*—white macules (白斑 bái b□n or 白瘢 bái b□n), white patch (白癜 bái diàn), and white patch wind (白癜風 bái diàn f□ng or 白駁風 bái bó f□ng)—just to name a few, simply describe the physical appearance of skin lesions.

In this case, both of the pathoconditions may present with the appearance of white macules (斑 b□n) or patches (癜 diàn) on the skin, and thus both may have macules or patches in the various forms of the nomenclature used to describe them throughout history. This is a prime example of similar or even identical terms being mutually applied to pathoconditions with very different etiologies and pathomechanisms.

Case Study #2: Vitiligo – Three Pattern Types

Q: Recently, I have been reaching out to other TCM physicians trying to get a better idea of how to treat vitiligo. A couple of them shared the following clinical experiences with me:

The first is a 23 y/o male patient who was diagnosed with vitiligo when he was 13. At that time, the white macules and patches started appearing on his face, abdomen, and back. Since then, the size and distribution of the skin depigmentation has enlarged and spread. He was administered TCM treatment for 6 months, which seemed to offer some moderate improvement, but the patient decided to discontinue treatment.

The other is a 4 y/o girl who was born with well-demarcated, white spots on her face, abdomen, and upper and lower extremities—basically dispersed over her entire body. The TCM physician tried prescribing medicinals at first, but the little girl hated the taste and adamantly refused to take the formula. Her parents did*n't* want to force the medicine on their daughter so they decided to have the physician perform acumoxatherapy (warm needling) instead. After administering this warm needling treatment for 6 months, the white macules and patches completely disappeared.

I have heard that vitiligo is difficult to treat, and especially, to completely cure. What has your experience been in treating vitiligo? Please offer your advice and guidance.

A: Vitiligo is a relatively rare skin condition that presents as well-demarcated, depigmented macules and patches. This depigmentation is thought to be caused by autoimmune destruction, oxidative stress, and/or intrinsic melanocyte defects in genetically predisposed individuals. It may also be triggered by physical and emotional stress and skin injury, and is commonly associated with other autoimmune diseases. Regardless of the treatment modality, many patients may continue to have episodes of skin depigmentation throughout their lives.

Indeed, vitiligo is difficult to definitively cure. A small percentage of these patients may spontaneously regain normal pigmentation, some may have varying degrees of therapeutic success, either *partially* or *completely* regaining their normal skin coloration, and in others the condition may persist indefinitely. Young patients whose depigmentation reaches its peak within 6 months tend to have a better chance of a complete cure than those who develop this condition later in life.

In classical TCM pathological terminology, vitiligo is commonly known as white macules (白斑 bái b□n) and white patch wind (白癜風 bái diàn f□ng or 白駁風 bái bó f□ng). This condition can be identified under the rubric of these three patterns and potential corresponding formulas:

- Kidney yang vacuity—You Gui Yin
- Liver blood vacuity—Sheng Yu Tang or Blood Desiccation Formula
- Spleen qi vacuity—Bu Zhong Yi Qi Tang

Regardless of the formula you choose, make sure to include Bu Gu Zhi, He Shou Wu, and Ci Ji Li (and/or Sha Yuan Ji Li). Depending on the presentation and pattern, you could also consider adding The Three Great Yang-Supplementers, Huang Bo, Ren Shen, and Lu Rong.

The administration of TCM medicinals usually can provide effective results, but it may take anywhere from 3 months to 1 year until noticeable improvements can be seen, and up to 2 to 3 years before repigmentation reaches the point where it is difficult to discern the boundaries of the affected areas and the normal skin. And even if results appear to be very good initially, the condition may exacerbate or recur again 3 to 5 years down the road. It is hard to say.

As for the little girl whom was administered acumoxatherapy (warm needling), it may be possible that warm needling qi- and blood-supplementing, blood-nourishing liver-emolliating, and kidney yang-supplementing acupoints could have had beneficial effects, but I doubt that it was the only factor involved. In my opinion, performing acumoxatherapy would only offer limited effects at best.

Case Study #3: Melasma

Q: I have noticed that many middle-aged women develop butterfly-shaped hyperpigmentation on their cheeks after giving birth. This hyperpigmentation is called melasma and the general medical consensus is that this condition is difficult to treat. What do you think?

A: Melasma is rather common, especially in women and people with naturally darker skin. This condition is known as dusty facial complexion (面塵 miàn chén) in classical TCM pathological terminology. There is a genetic predisposition for melasma and known triggers are pregnancy, oral contraceptive pills, certain medications, and sun exposure.

As for TCM treatment, it is not too difficult to achieve positive results. It just takes time and patience! You can plan on a minimum of 3 to 6 months, and possibly more, for the spots and patches to gradually fade away and become unnoticeable. However, even after the hyperpigmentation disappears, the patient will have to vigilantly avoid excessive sun exposure (ultraviolet radiation), which may activate melanocytes to produce more melanin and cause the melasma to reappear.

The traditional approach for the treatment of melasma usually revolves around formulas that treat liver depression and qi stagnation (e.g., Xiao Yao San), static blood (e.g., Tong Qiao Huo Xue Tang), spleen vacuity failing to transport (e.g., Gui Pi Tang), and kidney yin insufficiency patterns (e.g., Zhi Bo Di Huang Wan). These formulas may be effective, but if you prescribe them make sure to add Zi He Che (warms the kidney, supplements essence and boosts qi and nourishes blood, and contains proteins and steroid hormones that stimulate proliferation and reparative processes of the mucous membranes and skin) and Chuan Qi (quickens the blood and transforms stasis and improves tensility and promotes blood flow of the microvasculature).

However, I typically will prescribe either the yin and yang neutrally-supplementing, subduing and settling, and securing and astringing formula Gui Zhi Jia Long Gu Mu Li Tang adding Gan Jiang, Fu Zi, Huang Qin, and Zi He Che (powder); or the Shao Yang-harmonizing heat-clearing and fright-settling spirit-quieting formula Chai Hu Jia Long Gu Mu Li Tang adding Qing Hao, Zhi Mu, Di Gu Pi, and Zi He Che (powder).

Case Study #4: Acanthosis Nigricans and Melasma

Q: I have had a couple of cases involving hyperpigmentation of the skin.

One case was a 42 y/o female patient who explained that about 3 months ago, the skin on both wrists and ankles "began turning black" and "getting thicker," and it has continued to get worse since. There is no redness, heat, itchiness, or swelling.

The other was a 38 y/o woman who developed brown-colored hyperpigmentation around her mouth after giving birth to her second child, which almost looked like she was wearing a surgical mask, as well as a brown patch on the front of her neck. She explained that it started out as pimply pustules around her mouth, turned a purplish-red color and then evolved into a brownish-black color.

I am curious. How would you treat these types of cases?

A: The first case sounds like a classic case of benign *acanthosis nigricans* (aka *pseudoacanthosis nigricans*), which commonly presents on the wrists and ankles. Acanthosis nigricans can also be associated with obesity, certain syndromes (e.g., polycystic ovarian disease), drugs (e.g., nicotinic acid, insulin, systemic corticosteroids, hormone therapy), heredity, and malignancy (e.g., gastrointestinal cancers).

As for treatment, as long as there is no itchiness, redness, or swelling (i.e., heat pattern), then I would consider prescribing a blood-quickening qi-supplementing formula such as Bu Yang Huan Wu Tang variant. This approach will promote circulation and blood flow to the peripheries, gradually allowing the darkness to fade and the natural skin pigmentation to return.

The second case sounds like a classic case of *melasma* (aka *chloasma*). Melasma is caused by the overproduction of melanin by the melanocytes (pigment cells) and there seems to be a genetic predisposition to this condition. Some common triggers appear to be sun exposure, pregnancy, hormone treatments (e.g., oral contraceptive pills), and other drugs (e.g., targeted therapy for cancer). I would prescribe either the yin and yang neutrally-supplementing, subduing and settling, and securing and astringing formula Gui Zhi Jia Long Gu Mu Li Tang adding Gan Jiang, Fu Zi, Huang Qin, and Zi He Che (powder); or the Shao Yang-harmonizing heat-clearing and fright-settling spirit-quieting formula Chai Hu Jia Long Gu Mu Li Tang adding Qing Hao, Zhi Mu, Di Gu Pi, and Zi He Che (powder).

Section 7: Hyperhidrosis

Case Study #1: Palmer Hyperhidrosis – Therapeutic Options

Q: Recently, I have had quite a few patients visit me with the chief complaint of sweaty palms (palmer hyperhidrosis). The junior and senior high school-aged students say that when they feel nervous (such as during exams!) the sweating can be so profuse it makes the process of completing the task even more difficult. And adults say they feel awkward, embarrassed, and socially inhibited because they can't even shake hands with others.

Have you had any success treating hyperhidrosis? Can TCM effectively treat this condition?

A: At present, Western medicine offers various topical and oral medications, iontophoresis, botulinum toxin injections, surgical removal of sweat glands in the armpits, and sympathectomy.

The most effective treatment option for the face, armpits and hands is sympathectomy. However, this invasive treatment comes with potential risks and complications, such as a feeling of heat and dryness at the affected site and new-onset hyperhidrosis at other sites (e.g., torso, feet, buttocks) that functions as a kind of compensatory sweating mechanism (compensatory hyperhydrosis). Plus, even after undergoing sympathectomy, the hyperhidrosis may recur in a considerable number of patients.

Chinese medicine provides another therapeutic option for hyperhidrosis patients. The following are some basic guidelines:

(1) For patients who have *not* undergone sympathectomy, I would recommend prescribing a liver-settling wind-extinguishing and yin-enriching yang-subduing formula such as Jian Ling Tang adding Huang Bo, and Qing Hao, Zhi Mu, and Di Gu Pi (enrich yin and downbear fire, cool the blood and clear vacuity heat, and eliminate steaming bone).

(2) For patients who *have* undergone sympathectomy and are experiencing the *complications* of heat and dryness at the affected site(s) and/or compensatory hyperhidrosis, I would prescribe an yin-enriching fire-downbearing and steaming bone-eliminating formula such as Zhi Bo Di Huang Tang

adding Long Gu, Mu Li, and possibly Dai Zhe Shi. After about 1 month of administration, the patient should begin to notice gradual improvement, and in about 3 months these symptoms should completely resolve. If the patient is administered treatment for 6 months up to 1 year, then the probability of recurrence will be greatly reduced.

(3) For patients who have *not* undergone sympathectomy, but have received other *less invasive* procedures, such as botulinum toxin injections or iontophoresis, you can prescribe an yin-nourishing heat-clearing formula such as Tian Wang Bu Xin Dan, Bai He Gu Jin Tang, and Sha Shen Mai Men Dong Tang adding Ma Huang Gen, Fang Feng, Huang Qi, Mu Li, and Long Gu. Just make sure your formula includes yin-nourishing (e.g., Bai He, Yuan Shen, Mai Men Dong, Tian Men Dong, Sheng Di Huang, Dang Gui) and heart-quieting spirit-calming (e.g., Yuan Zhi, Suan Zao Ren, Bo Zi Ren) medicinals.

Additionally, you might also consider performing cupping on Hua Tuo's Paravertebral Points (EX-B2), and needle acupoints such as Feng Chi (GB20), Tian Zhu (UB10), Shen Men (HT7), Wai Guan (SJ5), San Yin Jiao (SP6), and Tai Chong (LV3).

Case Study #2: Complications of Axillary Sympathectomy

Q: A 31 y/o female patient of mine with palmer hyperhidrosis decided to undergo an axillary sympathectomy procedure. The procedure has proven successful in remedying her once sweaty hands, but now she has profuse sweating from her chest all the way down to her knees, and she says her legs "feel" swollen and tingly. How would you treat this patient?

A: Although undergoing an axillary sympathectomy procedure can indeed improve and sometimes even completely resolve palmar hyperhidrosis, these patients commonly experience the complications of heat in the palms of the hands, dry hands that crack easily and develop wrinkles, and compensatory sweating of the torso.

This condition can be identified as hyperactivity of yang due to yin vacuity pattern, requiring the administration of Zhi Bo Di Huang Tang adding Long Gu, Mu Li, Qing Hao, and Di Gu Pi. If necessary, you can also consider adding Ma Huang Gen (enters the lung channel and astringes and checks sweating), Fu Xiao Mai (enters the heart channel and constrains sweat), Gan Cao (boosts qi and supplements the center, clears heat and resolves toxin, and relaxes tension), and Long Yan Rou (supplements and boosts the heart and spleen and nourishes blood and quiets the spirit).

Case Study #3: Plantar Hyperhidrosis

Q: Recently, a patient with plantar hyperhidrosis visited me explaining that he has to change his socks (and shoes if available) 2 to 3 times a day. This is really a major inconvenience that can also cause embarrassment. Do you think Zhi Bo Di Huang Tang (including a large dose of Huang Bo) adding Bai Zhu (large dose) will be effective?

A: Yes, the yin-enriching fire-downbearing and steaming bone-eliminating formula Zhi Bo Di Huang Tang should be effective for treating plantar hyperhidrosis. However, for severe cases like this, you definitely need to include Sheng Long Gu and Sheng Mu Li (secure the essence and subdue yang) and Dai Zhe Shi (calms the liver and subdues yang).

These are among the essential medicinals of the liver-settling wind-extinguishing and yin-enriching yang-subduing formula Jian Ling Tang and will produce effective results much more quickly!

Case Study #4: Anxiety-Triggered Hyperhidrosis

Q: Over the past year, I have treated nearly twenty hyperhidrosis patients. My go-to formula is Jian Ling Tang adding The Three Yellows, Qing Hao, Zhi Mu, Di Gu Pi, and Ma Huang Gen (1 liang each). In most cases this formula has been effective. There are still some patients whom even after 2 months of administering this formula have had no improvements whatsoever.

Have you experienced these types of recalcitrant cases? Can you recommend any other approach that I could take?

A: Sure! You can also perform cupping on Hua Tuo's Paravertebral Points (EX-B2); needle (obliquely needling downwards) approximately 0.8 cun lateral to the lower border of the spinous processes (between EX-B2 acupoints and the urinary bladder channel back transport points (背俞穴 bèi shù xué)) from T1 down to T7; needle the body acupoints Feng Chi (GB20), Tian Zhu (UB10), Shen Men (HT7), Nei Guan (P6), Wai Guan (SJ5), Tai Chong (LV3), Di Wu Hui (GB 42), San Yin Jiao (SP6), and Yin Ling Quan (SP9); and needle auricular acupoints such as Shen Men, Jiao Gan (sympathetic), and Xin (heart).

If performing acupuncture is not convenient or suitable for the patient, then you can simply perform acupressure (massage the acupoints) and administer medicinals. Plus, you can prescribe a topical medicinal powder such as Body Soothing Powder (resolves toxin and itch with clearing coolness, dissipates wind and dispels dampness, closes sores and engenders flesh, clears heat and kills worms, and checks sweating) for application on the feet.

For patients whose hyperhidrosis is triggered by anxiety, aside from Zhi Bo Di Huang Tang and Jian Ling Tang, I would also consider prescribing Chai Hu Jia Long Gu Mu Li Tang (harmonizes Shao Yang and clears heat and settles fright and quiets the spirit), Wen Dan Tang (harmonizes the gallbladder and stomach, clears Shao Yang depressed heat, and dispels phlegm turbidity harassing the inner body), or Gan Mai Da Zao Tang Combining Ban Xia Hou Po Tang (harmonizes the center and releases tension and quiets the spirit and calms agitation). Just make sure to include Zhi Mu, Huang Bo, Qing Hao, Di Gu Pi, Long Gu, Mu Li, Dai Zhe Shi, and Long Yan Rou.

Case Study #5: Acrocyanosis with Coexisting Raynaud Phenomenon

Q: I have an interesting case involving a 17 y/o male patient with a history of sweaty hands and feet and a cutaneous tingling sensation. During the winter months, he has noticeably cold hands and feet that turn a bluish-purple color like the cyanotic discoloration of livedo reticularis, but when he warms them up they return to normal. He said that this condition runs in the family with varying manifestations and degrees of severity.

During his initial clinical visit, the chief complaint was hyperhidrosis, so I decided to prescribe Jian Ling Tang adding The Three Yellows, but this formula was not at all effective. Do you have any advice or suggestions on how to treat this patient?

A: This sounds like it could be a case of acrocyanosis, a hereditary condition caused by chronic vasospasm of cutaneous arterioles and venules, which includes symptoms of palmar and plantar hyperhidrosis and coldness of the extremities, and may coexist with chilblains, erythromelalgia, and *secondary* Raynaud phenomenon (aka Raynaud syndrome). However, in cases of *secondary* Raynaud phenomenon the blue discoloration of the fingers and toes is usually *persistent*, whereas *primary* Raynaud phenomenon (aka Raynaud disease) is an *episodic* exaggerated vasoconstrictive response of the digital arteries and arterioles to cold or emotional stress.

Depending on the extent of blood supply reduction, Raynaud phenomenon typically presents with a sequential discoloration of the extremities—fingers and/or toes and occasionally the tip of the nose and earlobes—white (ischemia)□ purplish-blue (hypoxia)□ red (reactive hyperemia).

Regardless of the pathological terminology, we can determine our treatment based on the following pattern identification:

- Profuse sweating of the hands and feet (hyperhidrosis) can be identified as yin vacuity with yang hyperactivity pattern. For this condition, I would consider prescribing a liver-settling wind-extinguishing and yin-enriching yang-subduing formula such as Jian Ling Tang adding Huang Bo, Qing Hao, Zhi Mu, Di Gu Pi, and Ma Huang Gen; or Zhi Bo Di Huang Tang adding Qing Hao, Di Gu Pi, Long Gu, Mu Li, and Dai Zhe Shi.
- Cold hands and feet that turn a bluish-purple color during the winter months can be identified as qi and yang vacuity with cold stasis pattern manifesting as reversal cold (Raynaud phenomenon). I would consider prescribing Gui Qi Jian Zhong Tang, Dang Gui Si Ni Jia Wu Zhu Yu Sheng Jiang Tang (substituting Sheng Jiang with Gan Jiang), Ren Shen Yang Rong Tang, or Bu Zhong Yi Qi Tang.
- Since this patient has a history of presenting with symptoms that involve both patterns concomitantly, this condition can be identified as heat-cold complex (寒熱夾雜 hán rè jiá zá).

Thus, you must determine the optimal balance of medicinals depending on whether the hyperhidrosis or Raynaud phenomenon is more pronounced. If the hyperhidrosis is more pronounced, your main formula can focus on treating this pattern, but you must also include the essential medicinals that treat Raynaud phenomenon (e.g., Huang Qi, Dang Gui, Wu Zhu Yu, The Three Great Yang-Supplementers, Ren Shen/Chuang Qi Powder). If Raynaud phenomenon is more pronounced, your main formula can focus on treating this pattern, but you must also include the essential medicinals that treat hyperhidrosis (e.g., Ma Huang Gen, Mu Li, Long Gu, Dai Zhe Shi, Qing Hao, Zhi Mu, Di Gu Pi, Sheng Di Huang).

As long as you accurately apply the eight principles—cold and heat, vacuity and repletion, exterior and interior, and yin and yang—to identify the pattern, it will be possible to effectively mitigate symptoms, improve the condition, and cure virtually any disease!

Section 8: Hair Loss

Case Study #1: First Alopecia Patient (My Wife) A Success!

Q: Originally, I had never thought much about the treatment of hair loss (alopecia). The reason why I began to look into this condition is because of my wife—she was my first alopecia patient!

It all started about 2 1/2 years ago. My wife had a cystectomy performed to remove a large ovarian teratoma. The surgery went fine, but soon after small patches of her hair began falling out (increased shedding) in a diffuse pattern, *not* in patches (areata). At that time, I tried prescribing regimens of Gui Zhi Jia Long Gu Mu Li Tang, Shi Quan Da Bu Tang, and You Gui Yin, but *none* of these approaches was effective. Fortunately, 7 months later she became pregnant (we were concerned that the cystectomy may have caused infertility!); the problem with hair loss gradually improved and she went on to give birth to our first son.

To our chagrin, her hair began to fall out again after giving birth. She would lose from 150 to 200 hairs a day, which she collected after combing or washing her hair. I continued to try the above approaches, but still no positive results. She was super stressed out about it. I found out that she had tried treatment from other TCM and Western medicine doctors as well, but *nothing* was effective. For about 1 1/2 years, she would have bouts of crying and depression. By that time, I also became really stressed out and was in a bad place mentally—then, my hair began to fall out too! That's when I realized firsthand that stress is indeed one of the reasons for hair loss.

From my research on hair loss, I know that there are different types of hair loss (i.e., anagen, telogen, and pattern) with different etiologies (e.g., genetic susceptibility, physical and psychological stress, drugs, associated autoimmune disease) and presentations (i.e., localized, diffuse, and generalized). I discovered that my wife has a family history of hair loss. That's what got me thinking about the possibility of prescribing medicinals that would suppress or inhibit the expression of these genes and effectively delay or mitigate the manifestation of hair loss.

Based on this logic, I prescribed Jian Ling Tang (including large doses of Huang Bo (1 liang) and Fu Ling (5 qian)). My wife began noticing positive results and has gone from losing approx. 180 strands down to approx. 30 strands. We are both very happy with the "hair-raising" results. I even wrote up a paper to document the results of this case.

A: Congratulations on finding an effective formula for hair loss! As a general rule for doctors, the most difficult patients to treat are your immediate family members, due to all of the emotional factors and expectations involved. To be able to effectively remedy your wife's hair loss (increased shedding) can be viewed as among the most "beautiful" achievements in the world. I often say that a person's greatest achievement is to make your parents proud, elevate the virtues of his/her spouse, and gain the trust of his/her spouse. You have done all of these. Congratulations!

Case Study #2: Hair Loss – A "Hair-Raising" Endeavor

Q: Recently, a 23 y/o female visited my clinic explaining that 4 years ago she began having hair loss (increased shedding) and has tried all types of different treatments, but nothing has been effective. The symptoms are almost the same as those of my wife: she feels a burning, prickly sensation (trichodynia) in her scalp at the top of her head (vertex), mild redness at the site of hair roots, and very emotionally sensitive.

I have tried prescribing various formulas for this patient over the past 3 months, such as Shi Quan Da Bu Tang, Gui Zhi Jia Long Gu Mu Li Tang, Wen Dan Tang, and Zhi Bo Di Huang Tang, but nothing has worked. I am not sure what I can do, if anything, for this patient. Please offer your advice and guidance.

A: Since antiquity hair has been known as "the silk of three thousand vexations." From this ominous description you can tell that hair has been giving people trouble for a long time. So pardon the pun, but the treatment of hair loss is a "hair-raising" endeavor.

Young people, especially females, tend to be more self-conscious of how their hair looks, putting lots of time and effort into haircare and experimenting with different styles. Hair loss can be a traumatic experience for these patients, causing anxiety, insecurity, reclusiveness, and even suicidal thoughts. There are a lot of potential causes of hair loss, including physical and emotional stress (e.g., child-bearing, hormonal changes, weight loss), viral infection, autoimmune response, medications (e.g., contraceptives), systemic disease (e.g., iron deficiency, hypothyroidism, systemic lupus erythematosus), and inflammatory skin conditions (e.g., tinea capitus, psoriasis, seborrheic dermatitis).

Based on my many years of clinical experience, aside from hair loss induced by *seborrheic dermatitis*, *folliculitis*, and *alopecia areata*—aka demon-licked head (鬼剃頭 gui shì tóu), patch balding (班禿 b□n t□), and glossy scalp wind (油風 yóu f□ng)—I have not found any "definitively" effective approaches for treating hair loss. If I have a patient who really wants to give treatment a try, I will usually prescribe a blood-quickening qi-supplementing formula such as Bu Yang Huan Wu Tang adding The Three Great Yang-Supplementers, Huang Qin, and Chuan Qi.

For patients with *seborrheic dermatitis*—aka wandering wind of the face (面游風 miàn yóu f□ng)—I would prescribe an exterior-resolving dampness-eliminating, lung qi-diffusing and -disinhibiting, heat-clearing toxin-resolving, and wind-dispelling formula such as Seborrheic Dermatitis Formula adding Pu Gong Ying. And in the acute stage or during flare-ups when exterior wind-heat or repletion heat is pronounced, bleed Da Zhui (GV14) (above, on, and below), and needle Feng Chi (GB20), Tian Zhu (UB10), Chi Ze (LU5), He Gu (LI4), and Zu San Li (ST36).

For patients with *folliculitis*—aka chicken's-droppings welling-abscess (雞屎癰 j□ shi y□ng)—I would prescribe a heat-clearing toxin-resolving, swelling-dispersing hardness-breaking, and blood-quickening pain-relieving formula such as Xian Fang Huo Ming Yin adding Huang Qin and Pu Gong Ying. You can also perform acupuncture on the acupoints Feng Chi (GB20), Tian Zhu (UB10), He Gu (LI4), and Zu San Li (ST36). This type of folliculitis that manifests on the scalp will continuously secrete purulent exudate, burrowing into the scalp and boiling upwards to form a mound, much like a cricket does when it burrows into the earth and forms a mound around the entrance of its dwelling.

For patients with *alopecia areata* (aka *autoimmune alopecia*), I would prescribe an yin and yang neutrally-supplementing, subduing and settling, and securing and astringing formula such as Gui Zhi Jia Long Gu Mu Li Tang. In the acute stage, make sure to add Huang Qin, Ma

Huang, Yi Yi Ren, Xing Ren, and Sheng Shi Gao, and perform acupuncture just as you would for seborrheic dermatitis above. If the patient has been administered corticosteroids (either intralesional or systemic) or the condition has evolved into the chronic stage, then I would add Gan Jiang, Fu Zi, Huang Qin, and possibly Huang Qi (supplements qi and upbears yang, boosts defense and secures the exterior, disinhibits water and disperses swelling, and expresses sores and engenders flesh). Or you could consider changing to Chao Mu Li and Chao Long Gu* and add Wu Zhu Yu (dissipates cold, warms the center, and assists yang). Additionally, you can topically apply Mugwort Ointment directly on the scalp patch and shine an infrared lamp on it for about 20–30 minutes each session.

For patients with *pattern hair loss* (*androgenetic alopecia*), I would consider prescribing either an yin-enriching fire-downbearing and steaming-eliminating formula, such as Zhi Bo Di Huang Tang, or a heat-clearing toxin-resolving formula, such as Huang Lian Jie Du Tang (if heat pattern is pronounced!). I can't guarantee anything, but you can give it a try.

*Note: Dr. Lee explains that the use of Sheng (生 sh□ng = raw—minimally processed, but not submitted to heat!) Long Gu and Mu Li preserves the full potency and actions of the calcium (Ca) constituents (e.g., subdues yang and quiets the spirit), whereas the Chao (炒 chao = stir-fried) processing method magnifies the actions of the magnesium (Mg) constituents (e.g., astringes and secures) in these medicinals.

Case Study #3: Alopecia Areata – Don't Take Corticosteroids or Cyclosporin!

Q: Recently, I have had a number of patients with hair loss visit me, including alopecia areata, male pattern hair loss, and female pattern hair loss. Even myself! I have been losing hair recently and it is becoming a concern. Many patients have tried Western medicine drugs and most say that initially the results were good, with their hair gradually growing back and the bald spots filling in, but after a period of time their hair started falling out again.

One woman with alopecia areata had taken methylprednisone orally daily for about 1 month, and was happy to see that her hair was growing back and the bald spot disappearing. But unfortunately, her hair began falling out again about two months later. Determined, she continued taking the corticosteroids up until the tell-tale side effects of "moon face" and weight gain appeared. That's when her doctor suggested she change her medication to cyclosporin, but she wasn't in to that idea so she decided to come see me for TCM treatment.

Since she has already taken corticosteroids for a period of time, how does that affect my pattern identification as the basis of treatment considerations? Please offer your advice and suggestions.

A: For most patients with alopecia areata (an autoimmune disorder in which T cell lymphocytes attack anagen hair follicles, suppressing hair growth and causing the hair to fall out in patches), my first-line formula is Chai Hu Long Gu Mu Li Tang (harmonizes Shao Yang and settles fright and quiets the spirit) or Gui Zhi Jia Long Gu Mu Li Tang (neutrally supplements yin and yang and subdues and settles and secures and astringes).

If the patient has been administered corticosteroids, then add Gan Jiang and Fu Zi (warm the center and expel cold, return yang and free the channels, and bolster right qi). If this is *not* effective, then add Wu Zhu Yu (dissipates cold, warms the center, and assists yang); and if this is *not* effective, then you can change to Chao Long Gu and Chao Mu Li*. Or, you could consider changing to a qi- and blood-supplementing and blood-quickening stasis-transforming formula, such as Bu Yang Huan Wu Tang, Xue Fu Zhu Yu Tang, Shao Fu Zhu Yu Tang, or Sheng Yu Tang; or a blood-nourishing yin-enriching and liver- and kidney-supplementing formula, such as Qi Bao Mei Ran Dan, Blood Desiccation Formula, or Dang Gui Yin Zi.

Both corticosteroids and cyclosporin come with the ever-present risk of unpleasant side effects, so it would be best for patients to avoid taking these drugs for such a benign condition like hair loss. I suggest that you proceed as mentioned above, prescribing Gui Zhi Jia Long Gu Mu Li Tang adding Gan Jiang, Fu Zi, and Huang Qin. And after a period of time, once most of the hair has grown back, you can change your formula to Gui Qi Jian Zhong Tang (supplements qi, blood, and kidney yang) or Bu Yang Huan Wu Tang (quickens the blood, transforms stasis, and supplements qi) adding Gan Jiang, Fu Zi, and

Huang Qin. Administer this formula up until the patient has a healthy head of flowing, radiant hair.

*Note: Dr. Lee explains that the use of Sheng (生 sh□ng = raw—minimally processed, but not submitted to heat!) Long Gu and Mu Li preserves the full potency and actions of the calcium (Ca) constituents (e.g., subdues yang and quiets the spirit), whereas the Chao (炒 chao = stir-fried) processing method magnifies the actions of the magnesium (Mg) constituents (e.g., astringes and secures) in these medicinals.

Case Study #4: Hair Loss Could Be "In the Head"

Q: A 44 y/o female patient explained that over the past three years she has been losing noticeable amounts of hair (shedding anywhere between 30 up to 200 hairs every day when she brushes her hair). She also sweats a lot on the head, has hot flashes (flushing), profuse dreaming, and poor sleep quality (awakens easily).

I prescribed Xiao Chai Hu Tang adding Qing Hao, Zhi Mu, Di Gu Pi, Long Gu, and Mu Li. Do you think this is a good approach?

A: Uhm…This hair loss (alopecia) sounds like it could be "in the head" instead of on the head, a psychosomatic symptom of menopausal transition. During this period of the woman's life, it is natural to shed relatively more hair than usual. Remember! The average human head has about 100,000 hair follicles. It is normal for her to shed 100 to 200 hairs every day. As long as she does *not* lose it in patches (alopecia areata) this shedding will *not* cause bald spots.

Thus, I would explain to the patient that there is no need to worry about this kind of "normal" hair loss. If she insists on treatment, then you could prescribe a formula that remedies the menopausal transition symptoms as well as nourishes the scalp and hair follicles.

In this case, I would consider prescribing an yin-enriching fire-downbearing and steaming bone-eliminating formula such as Zhi Bo Di Huang Tang adding He Shou Wu, Dang Gui, Tu Si Zi, and Gou Qi Zi (nourish the blood and replenish essence). Or, you could prescribe an yin-enriching essence-replenishing formula such as Qi Bao Mei Ran Tang or Blood Desiccation Formula adding Qing Hao,

Zhi Mu, and Di Gu Pi (enrich yin and downbear fire, cool the blood and clear vacuity heat, and eliminate steaming bone) and Huang Bo.

Case Study #5: Alopecia Totalis – Bald as an Egg and Soft as a Baby's Bottom

Q: About 4 years ago, a 23 y/o female patient began losing hair on the top of her head (*not* a bald patch like in alopecia areata, but just thinning) and the hairs on other parts of her head have gradually become softer, finer, and shorter in length (vellus hair).

She has tried all types of treatment, including TCM, Western medicine, and folk remedies, but nothing has been effective. What would you do for this patient?

A: This hair loss case reminds me of a young boy whom I treated a few years back. At the time, his grandmother brought him in saying that about 2 weeks ago the boy's hair started to "just fall out all over his head." When I saw him first, he was bald as an egg and it felt as smooth as a baby's bottom.

This type of sudden onset hair loss over the entire head (alopecia totalis) is thought to be caused by a hyperactive autoimmune response that can be triggered by viral infection, trauma, hormonal changes, and emotional and physical stress. At the onset, I identified this patient's condition as a mix between Shao Yang vacuity heat with hyperactivity of liver yang pattern and vacuity taxation with dual vacuity of yin and yang pattern, and thus prescribed Chai Hu Jia Long Gu Mu Li Tang (harmonizes Shao Yang and clears heat and settles fright and quiets the spirit) and Gui Zhi Jia Long Gu Mu Li Tang (neutrally supplements yin and yang, subdues and settles, and secures and astringes) for alternating periods as a means of subduing yang hyperactivity (autoimmune reaction) and promoting growth by mild supplementation. Gradually, over about a 6-month period, the boy's hair (vellus hair) filled back in, and within 1 year, the boy had a flowing head of healthy hair. We were all thrilled by the results!

Well, about 3 years later, this boy incurred the same type of hair loss once again. Based on my observations, I attributed this recurrence to being triggered by emotional stress and hormonal changes. Thus, over an approximately 8-month period, I prescribed a variety of formulas: Wen Dan Tang, Ban Xia Tian Ma Bai Zhu Tang, Chai Hu Jia Long Gu Mu Li Tang, and Gui Zhi Jia Long Gu Mu Li Tang. This therapeutic regimen produced effective results. His hair grew back again and his grandmother has kept in touch with me over the years, always mentioning her grandson's wonderful head of hair!

In addition to the above formulas, for some hair loss patients, you could also consider prescribing a center-harmonizing agitation-calming and stagnation-dissipating phlegm-transforming formula such as Gan Mai Da Zao Combining Ban Xia Hou Po Tang adding Yu Sheng Wan.

Case Study #6: Hair Loss in Adolescents and Young Adults

Q: Recently, I have had several young people, both male and female, come in for treatment of hair loss. The general clinical picture is noticeable anxiety and obvious concern over what they describe as a sudden onset of hair loss (general shedding and some in patches), and wonder how this could happen since no one else in their family has hair loss problems or baldness.

After conducting the patient interviews, the common thread that links these patients is stress and anxiety, whether it be facing pressure at school, on the job, conscription (compulsory military service), at home, or in a relationship. In attempts to subdue this anxiety and stress, I have tried administering Jian Ling Tang (even adding Zi He Che), but this approach has not provided noticeable improvement. Please offer your advice and guidance.

A: Hair loss is common in young people all over the world, regardless of gender or ethnicity. There are many potential factors (or combinations thereof) involved, including genetics, infection, hormonal changes, emotional and physical stress, and drugs.

There are likely multiple factors at play (e.g., infection, stress, hormones, genetics), which may result in various manifestations of hair loss. Inflammation may damage the hair follicle from external (e.g., tinea capitus, folliculitis, seborrheic dermatitis) or internal (e.g., autoimmune diseases) causes, while insufficient blood supply (capillary□ hair papilla□ hair bulb□ hair follicle□ hair shaft) may arise from any number of factors, thus resulting in hair loss.

The most common examples are *androgenetic alopecia* (pattern hair loss), *alopecia areata* (hair loss in patches), and *telogen effluvium* (shedding). *Androgenetic alopecia* may become apparent in men during their late 20s, and in women during their 40s or 50s. The common hypothesis for *alopecia areata* is that it involves autoimmunity in the form of a T-cell-mediated pathway. In *telogen effluvium*, hair continues to grow but at shorter lengths and has a bulb at the end (club hair), with shedding also possibly occurring.

I typically reserve the liver-settling wind-extinguishing and yin-enriching yang-subduing formula Jian Ling Tang for extreme cases of stress or yang-hyperactivity. In most cases, I would first consider prescribing an yin-enriching fire-downbearing and steaming bone-eliminating formula such as Zhi Bo Di Huang Tang or Tong Guan Wan; a qi- and blood-supplementing formula such as Sheng Yu Tang or Bu Yang Huan Wu Tang; a blood-nourishing yin-enriching and dryness-moistening formula such as Blood Desiccation Formula; an yin and yang neutrally-supplementing, subduing and settling, and securing and astringing formula such as Gui Zhi Jia Long Gu Mu Li Tang; or a Shao Yang-harmonizing heat-clearing and fright-settling spirit-quieting formula such as Chai Hu Jia Long Gu Mu Li Tang.

If there is pronounced inflammation, presenting with redness, heat, swelling, and serous or purulent exudate, then this can be identified as exterior wind-heat (damp) pattern, for which you could prescribe a formula such as Ma Xing Yi Gan Tang adding Sheng Shi Gao and Huang Qin.

Case Study #7: Hair Loss After Taking Antibiotics

Q: This 41 y/o male patient suffers from chronic purulent sinusitis. Back when he was 26 y/o, following administration of antibiotics by an otorhinolaryngolist to treat this condition, the patient began noticing hair loss that has gradually worsened over the years. He has tried taking medication to promote hair growth, but it has not been effective. The hair that remains has turned fine-textured, lighter in color, and shorter in length, and it looks like he is about to turn completely bald.

The patient emphasized that he has asked all of his relatives on both sides of the family about a history of baldness, and everyone he talked to said “absolutely *not*.” The scalp and follicles appear normal without any redness or signs of inflammation. How would you treat this patient?

A: It is possible that the antibiotic medication could have caused hair loss (thinning), but typically the hair would grow back over time. If the patient still has chronic purulent sinusitis symptoms, then you can prescribe Wen Dan Tang adding Lai Fu Zi, Ma Huang, Bai Zhi, Xin Yi, and Pu Gong Ying (or other heat-clearing toxin-resolving medicinals depending on the extent of heat).

If the chronic purulent sinusitis has already been resolved, then you can prescribe a qi- and blood-supplementing formula such as Dang Gui Bu Xue Tang or Bu Zhong Yi Qi Tang, or a qi-, blood-, and kidney yang-supplementing formula such as Gui Qi Jian Zhong Tang. These formulas will promote blood flow and provide nourishment to the scalp and hair follicles.

Additionally, you can perform acupuncture (warm needle) on acupoints such as Feng Chi (GB20), Tian Zhu (UB10), Shou San Li (LI10), Zu San Li (ST36), He Ge (LI4), and Chi Ze (LU5). And if the patient has bald patches, as opposed to diffuse thinning, then you could also topically apply Mugwort Ointment directly on the scalp at those sites and shine an infrared lamp on it for about 20–30 minutes each session.

I cannot guarantee this approach will work for all patients, but I have had phenomenal results with some patients, whereas others only marginal effects or none at all. It really depends on the individual patient and their specific condition.

Remember! Just because the patient doesn't have a known family history of androgenetic alopecia (male pattern hair loss) doesn't mean that he isn't the "progenitor" for his offspring. The chromosome mutation has to start somewhere, and maybe it's in his "own" genes!

Case Study #8: Hair Transplantation Ineffective? – Try TCM!

Q: A 24 y/o male patient suffers from severe hair loss. He underwent a hair transplantation procedure when he was 21 y/o, but now the only transplanted hair that remains is on the front of his head (the transplants on the top and sides of his head failed to grow), and he still has his natural hair on the back of his head. He feels that it looks ridiculous, and though I didn't tell him so, it really is a sore sight to behold!

You often say that male pattern hair loss (androgenetic alopecia) is normal and just a part of the person's genetic makeup, but I still want to conduct an experiment using TCM to treat this type of hair loss. Actually, I have already talked to a few patients about this and plan on carrying out a 1-year study. What do you think? Please offer your advice and suggestions.

A: As I have mentioned before, the type of hair loss I have had the best results treating is alopecia areata and shedding. However, if you are up for the challenge of conducting an experiment treating male pattern hair loss, more power to you! That sounds great!

Androgenetic alopecia can be identified as kidney yin vacuity with yang hyperactivity pattern. Thus, I suggest you prescribe a formula such as Zhi Bo Di Huang Tang adding Sheng Long Gu and Sheng Mu Li, or simpler yet, Tong Guan Wan (with Huang Bo as the sovereign medicinal). For some patients, you may also consider prescribing a Shao Yang-harmonizing heat-clearing and fright-settling spirit-quieting formula such as Chai Hu Jia Long Gu Mu Li Tang (including a large dose of Huang Qin).

You can give these a try!

Case Study #9: Stress-Induced Hair Loss – Prescribe Jian Ling Tang

Q: A 35 y/o male car salesman explained that he has been under a lot of pressure on the job and at home over the past year. He has tried oral and topical Western medicine medication and "hair growth" shampoos, but nothing has been effective. I know of other patients who have had success with various shampoos, unfortunately this patient has not.

Upon examination, I noticed that he had lots of dandruff and there was redness around the follicles, and he said that his scalp felt hot. I prescribed Jian Ling Tang adding Huang Bo (a large dose of 1.5 liang). Do you think this was a good approach?

A: For hair loss triggered by stress and anxiety, Jian Ling Tang (settles the liver and extinguishes wind and enriches yin and subdues yang) is a good choice, but you could also consider Chai Hu Jia Long Gu Mu Li Tang (harmonizes Shao Yang and clears heat and settles fright and quiets the spirit). However, redness around the hair follicles and a feeling of heat also suggests inflammation, so make sure to add Huang Bo (clears heat and resolves toxin) along with Qing Hao, Zhi Mu, and Di Gu Pi (enrich yin and downbear fire, cool the blood and clear vacuity heat, and eliminate steaming bone), and Gan Cao, Da Zao, and Long Yan Rou (harmonize (moderate) the nature of medicinals, boost qi and supplement the spleen and heart, and nourish the blood and calm the spirit) in your formula.

Section 9: Other Skin Disorders

Case Study #1: Chronic Cheilitis

Q: Two years ago, a female patient (now 21 y/o) developed red, swollen, and itchy lips with weeping (exudate) and scaling. She explained that every time her lips appear to improve a bit another flare-up occurs with the same pattern of presentation. She has received both TCM and Western medicine treatment, but nothing has provided a definitive cure.

I prescribed a 2-week regimen of Qing Wei San combining Huang Lian Jie Du Tang, but this didn't seem to help very much. What would you do for this patient?

A: There are many potential causes of chronic inflamed lips (cheilitis) with exudate. Qing Wei San (clears the stomach, drains fire, and cools the blood) is a good formula for this condition. However, due to the pronounced heat and dampness (weeping), I would consider adding Pu Gong Ying (clears heat and resolves toxin, disperses welling-abscesses, and disinhibits dampness), Sheng Shi Gao (clears heat and drains fire and astringes and engenders flesh), and Wan Ling Dan (resolves toxin and disperses welling-abscesses, quickens the blood, and dispels wind).

Plus, I would also perform bleeding on the four corners of the mouth (Di Cang (ST4), Ren Zhong (DU26), and Cheng Jiang (CV24)), Da Zhui (GV14) (above, on, and below), Cun Kou (Tai Yuan) (LU9), and the stomach channel well point (Li Dui (ST45)); and needle the acupoints He Gu (LI4), Chi Ze (LU5), and Zu San Li (ST40).

If this approach is still unable to achieve anticipated results, then you can add Huang Qin, Huang Bo, Ru Xiang, Mo Yao, Hua Shi, Lu Gan Shi, and Xiong Huang, or change the formula to Xian Fang Huo Ming Yin adding The Three Yellows, Pu Gong Ying, and Wan Ling Dan. And you could also consider prescribing the topical immersion and wash therapy Antimicrobial Wash, instructing the patient to soak her lips in this decoction (3x/day/20min/x) once it has cooled down to room temperature. This multifaceted therapeutic approach should provide effective results!

Case Study #2: Scrotal Dermatitis

Q: Recently, I have had several patients visit me with scrotal dermatitis (eczema), accompanied by other symptoms such as difficulty achieving erection, premature ejaculation, malaise, and hyperhidrosis.

I identified the chief complaint (scrotal dermatitis) as liver channel damp-heat pattern, and proceeded to prescribe Long Dan Xie Gan Tang variant. Unfortunately, this approach has *not* provided good results. How would you treat this condition?

A: Scrotal dermatitis is an umbrella term with variable etiology, including allergic reaction (e.g., clothing dye), infestations (e.g., scabies), chronic dermatological disease (e.g., psoriasis, atopic dermatitis, seborrheic dermatitis), systemic disease (e.g., diabetes, chronic renal failure), infections (e.g., syphilis), and nutritional deficiency (e.g., riboflavin, nicotinic acid, zinc).

In my clinical practice, the most common types of scrotal dermatitis can be distinguished as follows: scrotal wind-damp, bobble wind (scrotal folliculitis) (繡球風 xiù qiú f□ ng), and tinea cruris.

- Scrotal dampness can be classified as a type of water-damp and identified as exterior (defense aspect) vacuity pattern, exterior wind-damp pattern, or qi vacuity pattern. For exterior (defense aspect) vacuity pattern, you can consider prescribing Yu Ping Feng San adding Cang Zhu, or even the classic *Treatise on Cold Damage and Miscellaneous Diseases* formula Fu Ling Ze Xie Tang adding Huang Qi and Cang Zhu. For exterior wind-damp pattern, you can prescribe Ma Xing Yi Gan Tang (substituting Ma Huang with Gui Zhi (or Rou Gui)), Qiang Huo Sheng Shi Tang, or Qiang Huo Chu Shi Tang. If there is oozing (clear exudate almost like "perspiration") with a swollen scrotum, then this can be identified as qi vacuity pattern, for which you can prescribe Bu Zhong Yi Qi Tang adding Fu Ling, Ze Xie, and Di Long.
- For bobble wind (scrotal folliculitis), you can prescribe Long Dan Xie Gan Tang variant.
- For tinea cruris, you can prescribe Ma Xing Yi Gan Tang or Blood Desiccation Formula variants.

Regardless of the pattern, make sure to also prescribe Body Soothing Powder (resolves toxin and itch with clearing coolness, dissipates wind and dispels dampness, closes sores and engenders flesh, clears heat and kills worms, and checks sweating) for topical application and advise the patient to wear loose-fitting clothing.

Case Study #3: Post-Traumatic Hematoma – Yang Vacuity Pattern

Q: Two months ago, a 13 y/o boy was punched in the head during a fight with a classmate. Three weeks later, the bruising and swelling resolved, but he has continued to have an approx. 2 x 2 cm hard nodule right below the left zygomatic bone.

His mother brought him in last week for consultation and treatment. I have tried warm needling, but this has not been very effective. Do you have any advice or suggestions on how to treat this?

A: Post-traumatic hematoma results from blood extravasation into the muscle at the affected site and the swelling results from an increase in osmotic gradient that causes passage of the interstitial fluid through the muscle fascia. Most cases will spontaneously resolve in time, however, some cases may evolve into the complications of fibrosis or even myositis ossificans.

Since the acute phase with heat, bruising, and swelling have already resolved, this can be identified as yang vacuity pattern. First, if possible (may be difficult on the face, but on the body I definitely would) you should consider warm needling, inserting the needles in a radial pattern directly into the hematoma. Then, since the patient has already entered the post-acute/chronic stage, I would consider prescribing a qi-, blood-, and yang-supplementing such as Shi Quan Da Bu Tang, Gui Qi Jian Zhong Tang, or simply Yang Dan Tang adding Gan Jiang, Fu Zi, and Cang Zhu.

For patients in the acute stage, I would prescribe a blood-nourishing and -quickening, stasis-dispelling pain-relieving, network vessel-freeing channel-regulating, and swelling-dispersing flesh-engendering formula such as Ru Mo Si Wu Tang adding The Three Great Yang-Supplementers and Huang Qin. Or, if swelling is pronounced, then I would consider prescribing a kidney yang-warming qi transformation-promoting and bland-percolating dampness- and water-disinhibiting formula such as (Yu Sheng) Wu Ling San (Nephritis Formula) instead.

These approaches will expedite reabsorption and complete resolution of the hematoma.

Case Study #4: Garlic Paste on Steamed Buns – Gets Rid of "Foxy Smell"

Q: I have a 29 y/o female patient with a "knock out" physical appearance. She is very beautiful, but has long had a body odor (bromhidrosis) problem that makes her too self-conscious and apprehensive to go out and meet people.

She has tried the gamut of Western medicine treatment options from hygienic (e.g., germicidal soup, shaving, various deodorants and antiperspirants, staying dry) to various drugs and surgical procedures. Nothing has been ultimately effective.

Do you have experience at treating this type of patient with chronic body odor?

A: I most certainly do! I recommend trying Li Shi-Zhen's approach recorded in *Bin Hu's Simple Collection of Formulas* (瀕湖集簡方 *Bin Hu Ji Jian Fang*) (Ming dynasty). Crush up Da Suan (Garlic) into a paste and mix it together with Mi Tuo Seng (Lithargite), spread this paste on a warm steamed bun or cosmetic sponge, and apply it under the armpit. In the morning before going out, the patient can leave this application on for 15 to 30 minutes, and then wash off the residual paste about 30 minutes to 1 hour later. If the paste is applied prior to going to bed, then do the same procedure, but leave the residual paste on during sleep and wash it off the next morning after getting up.

The baseline recommended regimen is application of this paste everyday for 2 weeks straight. Some patients may be able to notice some positive results even after the first couple of days, but for others it may take longer. If necessary, the patient can continue applying this paste for a longer course of treatment up until she can work up a sweat without any offensive body odor. Just remember! Garlic may irritate some people's skin, causing a burning sensation or even a rash, so make sure to remind the patient that a very thin, fine layer of paste spread on the steamed bun or cosmetic sponge is all that is needed.

As a part of the therapeutic regimen, you can also prescribe a liver-settling wind-extinguishing and yin-enriching yang-subduing formula such as Jian Ling Tang adding Qing Hao, Zhi Mu, Di Gu Pi, Chai Hu, and Huang Bo.

The classical TCM pathological term for body odor is foxy smell (狐臭 hú chòu). By applying this dual—topical application and oral administration—approach, your patient will be well on her way to getting rid of that "foxy smell."

A bit of body odor is quite normal. *Homo sapiens* used to rely more heavily on "body odor" (just like many other mammals still do!) as a means of identification and attracting mates. It has become the norm for many humans today (but not all!) to rely on their sense of touch, sight, and hearing as a means of identification and attraction at the detriment of their olfactory sense. You should encourage your patient to overcome her self-consciousness and enjoy a healthy social life. Chances are, along the way, she will meet someone whose olfactory sense is stimulated and attracted to her scent. That person may very well be her true soulmate!

Case Study #5: Keratosis Pilaris – It's Common in Adolescents!

Q: A 16 y/o female patient has tiny bumps on her wrists, ankles, and chest. The bumps are colorless, translucent, painless, and do *not* itch, but she said that the tissue surrounding them feels a bit tight. She said that some of the furuncles produce clear, blood-tinged fluid (serosanguinous exudate) upon squeezing.

After prescribing Xian Fang Huo Ming Yin for 1 week, the bumps on her wrist appeared red colored and the skin around the affected areas felt less taut than before. Do you think this is a sign of efficacy?

A: Ahh!...That sounds like keratosis pilaris. It's very common in adolescence. It typically presents as skin-colored, red, or brownish scaly bumps at the sites of hair follicles (on some patients it looks just like "chicken skin"). It is *not* itchy or painful, and is more prominent at times of low humidity, such as during the cold winter months. In most people, it will usually resolve spontaneously in adulthood. However, tell the patient to stop picking and squeezing them, it only makes it worse!

Actually, it is not imperative that you treat this condition, but if the patient really wants you to administer treatment, then go ahead. If you have had success with Xian Fang Huo Ming Yin, then by all means continue with it. Typically, if the affected site appears red (indicating inflammation), then I would prescribe Xian Fang Huo Ming Yin variant; if skin-colored or brownish, then I would prescribe Blood Desiccation Formula; and if skin-colored with pustules at the surface, then I would prescribe Ma Xing Yi Gan Tang.

VIII. GYNECOLOGY & OBSTETRICS

This chapter covers a diverse scope of gynecological and obstetric pathologies and topics, including those involving menses (from menarche to menopause), gestation, parturition, and postpartum care. Disorders of the vagina, uterus, ovaries, and fallopian tubes will be presented and therapeutic protocols provided.

Section 1: Menstruation

Case Study #1: Oligomenorrhea – Delayed Menstruation

Q: A 26 y/o female visited me explaining that her period has *not* come in 3 months. She underwent a thorough examination, including transabdominal and transvaginal ultrasound, revealing *no* abnormalities of the uterus or ovaries. A gynecologist diagnosed her with oligomenorrhea (ovulatory dysfunction). How would you treat this patient?

A: Oligomenorrhea directly correlates with delayed menstruation (經遲 j□ng chí) in TCM classical pathological terminology. Gynecologists typically prescribe hormonal contraceptives (e.g., oral contraceptive pill (OCP) containing estrogen and progesterone), which is effective during administration, but once discontinued the problem will likely resume.

Hormonal therapy acts on the pituitary gland to regulate the secretion of FSH and LH, with the function of recalibrating the menstrual cycle. However, the downside of OCPs is that long-term administration will further suppress the body's natural capacity to generate hormones and regulate the menstrual cycle, thus resulting in further compromising ovarian function.

Typically, for these types of cases, I would consider prescribing either a blood-quickening blood-supplementing, qi-boosting spleen-fortifying, and kidney yang-supplementing formula, such as Shi Quan Da Bu Tang (including large doses of the blood-quickening stasis-resolving medicinals), or a blood-breaking, channel-freeing, and liver- and kidney-supplementing formula, such as Tong Jing Fang (includes Qian Cao) adding Chuan Qi and Hai Piao Xiao*.

*Note: The combination of Qian Cao and Hai Piao Xiao is taken from the formula Four Wu Zei Gu One Lu Ru Wan (四烏賊骨一藘茹丸) recorded in *The Yellow Emperor's Inner Canon*, which was prescribed for the treatment of blood desiccation (liver and kidney essence-blood depletion) menstrual block. This formula is comprised of the medicinal pair Wu Zei Gu (aka Hai Piao Xiao) and Lu Ru (aka Qian Cao).

Hai Piao Xiao supplements the kidney, boosts essence, and frees the blood vessels for the treatment of blood block (stasis obstructing the uterus), and Qian Cao quickens the blood and frees the channels (menstruation) for the treatment of inhibited menstrual flow (經水不通 j□ng shui bù t□ng).

The pill of this original formula also included Ma Que Luan (Sparrow Egg) (supplements essence-blood and regulates the thoroughfare and controlling vessels), and the pill was swallowed with a drink of Bao Yu Zhi (Abalone Juice) (nourishes the liver and transforms stasis).

Case Study #2: Menstrual Block – But She Is Still Lactating!

Q: A 45 y/o female made a clinical visit with a history as follows:

Approximately 5 years ago (when she was 40 y/o), she became pregnant for the first time (primagravida) and was also having difficulty sleeping, so her obstetrician/gynecologist (OB/GYN) prescribed sleeping pills (benzodiazepines). After taking these pills, she suffered from severe nausea and vomiting. She went on to conceive a healthy baby via cesarean section, but the entire process, especially the prenatal stage, was so grueling that she swore never to have another one.

She has *not* had a menstrual period since prior to her pregnancy 5 years ago and can still express breast milk by hand. An OB/GYN physician diagnosed her with hyperactivity of the pituitary gland resulting in hyperprolactinemia. She wants to know if TCM treatment would be effective for remedying this condition.

I am curious. Why would this patient still be lactating if she has already entered menopause and *no* longer menstruates (aka cessation of menstruation (停經 ting j□ng))? The patient has a good appetite, normal urine and stool, and *no* other remarkable signs, symptoms or concomitant pathoconditions. Please offer your advice and guidance on this case. Thank you!

A: She likely has *not* already entered menopause! The hormonal imbalance (i.e., hyperprolactinemia) is the culprit behind her lack of menstruation and breast milk expression.

Hyperprolactinemia can be identified as yang straying outward pattern. Prolactin (PRL) suppresses FSH and LH and thus inhibits follicle growth, resulting in galactorrhea (flow of milk from the breast not related to pregnancy) and lactational amennorhea. In this patient's case, this would be a "prolonged" galactorrhea and lactational amennorhea in which the higher brain centers become fooled into misperceiving the body is still in pregnancy and thus continues to secrete milk for the nursing mother and baby.

For this type of menstrual block (經閉 j□ng bì) with lactation, I would prescribe Jian Ling Tang (including Gan Cao) adding scorch-fried Ma Ya. Administration of this formula will gradually reduce the secretion of PRL and stop lactation. In patients presenting with anxiety, you can also consider adding medicinals such as Long Yan Rou, Chai Hu, Xiang Fu, Hou Po, Ban Xia, Lai Fu Zi, Zi Su, and Yu Sheng Wan.

Remember! Natural childbirth (vaginal delivery) offers a much better outcome for both the mother and the infant, especially for relatively younger women who still want to have more kids and are *not* at risk of other maternal or fetal complications. The mother will be able to breastfeed and the regulatory functions of the pituitary gland will naturally return to homeostasis.

Case Study #3: TCM Vaginal Suppository – Safe and Effective

Q: Societal norms continue to open up in regards to women's rights, and more young people are putting off marriage until later in life and engaging in sexual activity out of wedlock. It seems that despite modern advancements in sanitation, contraception, and healthcare, complications of induced surgical abortion (e.g., abrasions, scarring, infections of the cervix and uterine cavity) still arise and the prevalence of vulvovaginitis seems to be as high as ever.

That's why I think there is a definite demand for economical, easy to produce, and convenient to use TCM medicinal vaginal suppositories like the one you make and prescribe for your patients. Is there any potential for side effects and/or damage to the vaginal, cervical, or uterine lining (endometrium) that may result from the insertion of this type of medicinal suppository into the vagina?

A: (Yu Sheng) Vaginal Suppository (clears heat and resolves toxin, kills worms and relieves itch, and dispels wind and eliminates dampness) is inserted into the vaginal cavity and will *not* come into contact with the endometrium. And as long as it is used as directed, there will *not* be any iatrogenic effects on the vaginal and cervical mucosa. This suppository will provide therapeutic efficacy for pathologies of the vaginal and cervical lining that present with itching, irritation, and watery or viscous vaginal discharge such as vulvovaginitis (i.e., bacterial vaginosis, vulvovaginal candidiasis (vaginal yeast infection), trichomoniasis (parasites)), genital herpes, and gonorrhea.

The formula is composed of warm acrid medicinals (She Chuang Zi, Xiong Huang, and Liu Huang) and a cold bitter medicinal (Da Huang), all of which have potent toxin-resolving (antimicrobial) actions. She Chuang Zi functions as an excipient (bulking agent) facilitating drug absorption, reducing viscosity, and enhancing solubility, as well as having the action of promoting epithelial cell regeneration. Due to the potency of this formula, I only prescribe it for short durations. The infection usually resolves after only 1 week of administration, and if the condition has *not* resolved by then, I will go ahead and prescribe it for 2 weeks (the longest continuous regimen I have had to prescribe is 3 weeks).

Remember! For the treatment of vaginal infections and sexually transmitted diseases (STDs), I will apply a multifaceted therapeutic approach that also includes an orally administered formula decoction and possibly acupuncture. Typically, I will prescribe a formula such as Long Dan Xie Gan Tang (drains liver-gallbladder repletion fire and clears damp-heat in the lower burner), Jin Suo Gu Jing Wan (supplements the kidney and astringes essence), or Bu Zhong Yi Qi Tang (fortifies the spleen and supplements qi, upbears yang and raises the fall, and supplements and quickens the blood). And for acupuncture, I will needle acupoints such as Tai Chong (LV3), Zhong Feng (LV5), San Yin Jiao (SP6), Yin Ling Quan (SP9), and Zu San Li (ST36).

Case Study #4: Dizziness, Shortage of Qi, Profuse Menstruation – Look Out for Anemia!

Q: Today, a female patient presented with a chief complaint of dizziness, shortage of qi, and profuse menstruation resulting in anemia. She mentioned that during day 2 of her last menstrual cycle bleeding was so profuse that blood soaked completely through her sanitary pads, and she had to change underpants 4 times.

The initial lab work up she brought was as follows: Hb 9.5 (12.0–15.5), Hct 31.4% (32.4%–44%), red cell distribution width (RDW) 18.2 (11.5–14.5), Ferritin 3.27 (20–200), and Iron 4 (10–30). Her gynecologist diagnosed her with iron-deficiency anemia and she is currently taking iron supplements, but the most recent lab tests showed only a minor increase in iron levels (now 5). How would you treat this patient?

A: Yes, this can technically be diagnosed as *iron-deficiency anemia*, but the key here is that the patient obviously has enough iron and ferritin in her blood; it's just that she is losing too much blood during menstruation.

For patients such as this who present with severely profuse menstruation (*hypermenorrhea*) to the point of causing *anemia*, as well as those in which flooding (崩 b□ng) (roughly correlates with menometrorraghia) and recalcitrant profuse menstruation (*menorrhagia* or *hypermenorrhea*) present as a result of *endometrial hyperplasia*, you can consider prescribing Ru Mo Si Wu Tang adding Huang Qin, Ce Bo Ye, Ou Jie, Ai Ye, Chuan Qi, and Zhu Sha. Plus, advise the patient to eat a well-rounded diet that includes iron-supplementing foods (e.g., raisins, spinach, kale, collard greens, meat (especially liver!), poultry, and seafood).

If your formula is successful in reducing the volume of blood during menstruation, but signs and symptoms of anemia still present, then you can add Si Ni Tang (warms the channels and expels cold and returns yang and stems counterflow) to your original formula. And if this approach still does*n't* reduce the amount of bleeding and improve the anemia, then change your formula to either Sheng Yu Tang or You Gui Yin adding Si Ni Tang and Xi Lu Rong.

For women, especially older women, who do *not* want to have children, they could also consider the more invasive, but sometimes necessary, alternative of hysterectomy. This will resolve the problem once and for all!

Case Study #5: Menstrual Vomiting – Quicken the Blood, Transform Stasis, and Dispel Phlegm

Q: This 31 y/o female patient visited me explaining that ever since the onset of menarche in elementary school she has suffered from nausea and vomiting during menstruation. Sometimes she can't even keep liquids down and it has gotten so bad that she has had to go to the hospital to receive intravenous infusions. She has received both TCM and Western medicine treatment, but nothing has been effective in remedying the condition.

I decided to administer Jian Ling Tang adding Ban Xia and Fu Ling for 1 month, which unfortunately has not been effective either. Other than this problem, she appears to be both physically and mentally healthy and said she eats a well-balanced diet, gets enough sleep, and exercises regularly. Please offer your advice and guidance.

A: Menstrual vomiting starting as far back as menarche…hmm…this sounds like a classic case of endometriosis to me. If so, then I would prescribe a blood-quickening stasis-transforming formula such as Ru Mo Si Wu Tang adding Huang Qin (large dose), Gu Sui Bu and Xu Duan (enter the kidney channel, quicken the blood and transform stasis, and break blood), and Ban Xia, Fu Ling, and Sheng Jiang (dispel phlegm and move water and dissipate qi and disperse glomus).

Actually, what I like to do is administer the Ban Xia, Sheng Jiang, and Fu Ling (aka Xiao Ban Xia Jia Fu Ling Tang) *only* during menstruation. At that time, I will instruct the patient to take these medicinals in either extract powder or raw pulverized powder form. The key here is to let the powder mix in with just enough saliva (or water if necessary) so it moistens and can be swallowed.

The following TCM classical pathophysiological terms describe symptoms that may accompany endometriosis during menstruation: pain, frequent urination, urinary incontinence, constipation, abdominal urgency and rectal heaviness (tenesmus), diarrhea, abdominal distention, distending pain in the breasts, axillary swelling (suppuration, yellow sweat, or perspiration), headache, nausea and vomiting, nosebleed, coughing of blood, and bleeding gums.

The terminology may not be exactly the same as today but the etiology and pathomechanisms all involve stasis obstructing the uterus with heat pattern. That's why I would prescribe the Ru Mo Si Wu

Tang variant for this patient and *not* Jian Ling Tang (settles the liver and extinguishes wind and enriches yin and subdues yang)!

Note: Ban Xia (an essential medicinal for drying dampness and transforming phlegm, warming and transforming cold phlegm, and checking vomiting), Sheng Jiang (a sage medicinal for people suffering from retching and vomiting), and Fu Ling (an essential medicinal for disinhibiting water and percolating dampness) provide effective relief for patients with vomiting during pregnancy, especially those who incur episodes of stomach reflux vomiting in response to rancid odors (e.g., the smell of vomit).

Zhang Zhong-jing utilized this therapeutic approach very effectively with Xiao Ban Xia Jia Fu Ling Tang in his *Treatise on Cold Damage and Miscellaneous Diseases* (subsequently presented in the *Essential Prescriptions of the Golden Coffer*).

Case Study #6: Menstrual Aversion to Cold and Vomiting – For the Past 20 Years

Q: A 47 y/o female patient has incurred aversion to cold and nausea and vomiting on the first day of menstruation for the past 20 years. She has undergone thorough examinations and testing, but nothing abnormal has been revealed, and has tried taking various Western medicine drugs without any improvement. How would you explain this condition? How can I treat this patient?

A: Hmm…this is strongly suggestive of endometriosis that has invaded the stomach duct and affected the vagus nerve.

As for treatment, I would consider prescribing a blood-nourishing blood-quickening, stasis-dispelling pain-relieving, and network vessel-freeing channel-regulating formula such as Ru Mo Si Wu Tang adding Huang Qin, Ban Xia, Fu Ling, Ze Xie, Xu Duan, Gu Sui Bu, and Chuan Qi. Administer this formula up until the patient incurs 2 to 3 symptom-free menstrual cycles. That's when you know you can discontinue the therapeutic regimen.

If this approach is *not* effective, then you could consider changing the formula to a blood-nourishing network vessel-freeing and cold-dissipating counterflow-downbearing formula such as Dang Gui Si Ni Jia Wu Zhu Yu Gan Jiang Tang adding Huang Qin.

Endometriosis is a chronic disease in women of reproductive age characterized by the occurrence of endometrial tissue outside the uterus and reacts to the hormone cycle (e.g., estrogen) in much the same way as the endometrium. Once ovulation stops and the patient enters menopause, these symptoms will naturally resolve. So technically, at this woman's age in particular, it may *not* be imperative to aggressively treat this condition. You can discuss the options with her as well.

Remember! The physiological and psychological symptoms that commonly arise during menopause (e.g., hot flashes, mood swings, anxiety, vaginal dryness) can be identified as Shao Yang channel depressed heat pattern and yin vacuity pattern. Up until the 1970s and into the 1980s, it was common for the TCM community here in Taiwan (and China) to treat menopausal symptoms with kidney yang-supplementing medicinals (e.g., Yin Yang Huo, Rou Cong Rong, Suo Yang). But over the past 30 years or so nutritional intake and the administration of hormone replacement therapy has become widespread. Nowadays, TCM treatment of menopausal symptoms typically consists of yin-supplementing, heat-abating, and spirit-quieting medicinals.

Case Study #7: Menstrual Pain and Irregularities – Patterns Then and Treatment Now

Q: Menstrual pain is a very common condition, but not easy to treat. I know that some doctors will tell their patients: "This problem will improve dramatically or completely resolve once you marry and have children." But I have *not* consistently born witness to this in my own clinical experience. I am curious as to what your experience has been regarding this condition?

A: In TCM classical texts on gynecology some of the most common menstrual irregularities documented during times of antiquity were generally identified as the following patterns:

- Premenstrual abdominal pain (經前腹痛 j□ng qián fù tong) (dysmenorrhea)—qi stagnation and stasis obstruction
- Abdominal pain during menstruation (經期腹痛 j□ng qí fù tòng) (dysmenorrhea)—stasis heat or qi depression

- Profuse menstruation (月經過多 yuè j□ng guò du□) (menorrhagia, hypermenorrhea)—qi vacuity and blood heat
- Scant menstruation (月經過少 yuè j□ng guò shao) (hypomenorrhea)—constitutional vacuity or blood and qi vacuity
- Delayed menstruation (經行後期 j□ng xíng hòu qí) (oligomenorrhea)—blood cold
- Premature menstruation (經行期前 j□ng xíng qí qián)—blood heat, vacuity heat, or qi vacuity
- Flooding and spotting (崩漏 b□ng lòu)—blood heat and qi vacuity
- Menstrual block (經閉 j□ng bì) (amennorhea)—liver and kidney insufficiency or qi stagnation and blood stasis
- Cessation of menstruation (停經 ting j□ng) (amenorrhea in menopause)—blood and essence vacuity

Again, these are simply the conditions and patterns that were most commonly documented and reflect the way of life and environment during those times.

With advancements in modern medicine, we now have the capacity to access lab workups, imaging studies, and histological findings that oftentimes are capable of definitively revealing the presence of pathologies such as uterine fibroids, adenomyosis, endometriosis, endometrial hyperplasia, and thin endometrium among other conditions. In my clinical setting, these pathoconditions can most commonly be identified as the following patterns:

- Thin endometrium—cold or dual qi and blood vacuity
- Endometrial hyperplasia—stasis heat
- Leiomyomas (uterine fibroids) and adenomyosis—stasis heat with phlegm-rheum

Nowadays, in advanced industrialized societies the standard of living, lifestyle and nutritional intake has dramatically improved compared to times of antiquity. Thus, in my clinical setting most women with menstrual pain can be identified as stasis heat pattern. And as long as the patient completes the therapeutic regimen by taking the TCM medicinals up until 2 to 3 menstrual cycles have passed without pain, then the patient will likely remain menstrual pain-free in the future.

The treatment of endometrial hyperplasia will require administration of TCM medicinals for at least 6–10 months, adenomyosis approx. 1–3 months, and leiomyomas approx. 6–12 months. For these pathoconditions, I would typically prescribe Ru Mo Si Wu Tang (nourishes and quickens the blood, dispels stasis and relieves pain, and frees the network vessels and regulates the channels) or Tong Jing Fang (breaks blood, frees the channels, relieves pain, and supplements the liver and kidney) adding Huang Qin, Huang Lian, Fu Ling, and Ze Xie.

However, some patients may consider concomitant treatment with injections (or nasal spray) of GnRH agonists (e.g., buserelin, goserelin), which agonizes the gonadotropin-releasing hormone receptor (GnRHR) in the pituitary gland and leads to desensitization of the pituitary gland, which reduces the secretion of gonadotropins (LH and FSH) and thus lowers estrogen levels. This will expedite the therapeutic process, effectively reducing the thickness of the endometrium by 1/2 within 1 month, another 1/2 in 2 months, and after 6 months the thickness will be down to 1 cm–1.5 cm. Just continue prescribing your formula, treating the condition and gradually regulating the constitution up until the endometrial thickness is reduced back down to normal (< 5 mm).

As for doctors telling their nulliparous patients of childbearing age "This problem will improve dramatically or completely resolve once you marry and have children," yes, this has indeed "born out" in my clinical experience about 80 to 90% of the time.

Case Study #8: High FSH Levels – Further Testing and Follow-Up

Q: This 32 y/o female patient has had scant menstruation since her periods first started in her early teens. She has already given birth to two healthy children, but recent lab tests have indicated high levels of follicle-stimulating hormone (FSH) 35.97.

A woman of her age would not likely already be going through menopausal transition, would she? Do you think this condition can be identified as yang hyperactivity pattern?

A: It seems unlikely that the patient would be going through menopausal transition already. Hormone levels (e.g., FSH, LH) may fluctuate widely in response to variables such as stage of menstrual cycle, emotional stress, physical exhaustion, and sleep deprivation. In fact, traumatic stress and extreme exercise may even induce a period of *temporary menopause* (*amenorrhea*) that may subside once the causal factors have been removed and the body resumes normal functioning.

You should follow up on this to determine the nature of her periods (e.g., duration, blood loss volume, any changes in cycles) and make sure that she gets her FSH tested periodically over an extended period of time. That will provide you with a clearer clinical picture and allow you to make an accurate diagnosis.

Another possibility you must rule out is a *space-occupying brain lesion* that may be compressing the pituitary gland or hypothalamus. If imaging studies reveal the presence of a brain tumor (likely benign), then the best approach would be to undergo surgical resection and decompression followed by administration of either Ru Mo Si Wu Tang or Jian Ling Tang adding The Three Yellows and Lai Fu Zi and Zi Su Zi (downbear qi and transform phlegm).

If there is not a tumor, just elevated FSH levels and *endometrial hyperplasia*, then I would prescribe Ru Mo Si Wu Tang adding The Three Yellows, Zhi Zi, Mu Dan Pi, Chuan Qi, Fu Ling, Ze Xie, Long Gu, Mu Li, and Niu Xi. If further diagnostic tests and imaging reveal *endometrial cancer*, then I would consider prescribing either Ru Mo Si Wu Tang or possibly Xian Fang Huo Ming Yin adding The Three Yellows, Mu Dan Pi, Zhi Zi, Pu Gong Ying, Sheng Shi Gao, Chuan Qi, Long Dan Cao, and Wan Ling Dan.

Case Study #9: Early Menopause – To Each Her Own!

Q: A 40 y/o female is already experiencing menstrual block (amenorrhea), indicating that she may be in perimenopause, which is much earlier than her mother who began the menopausal transition at 50 y/o. This patient began having irregular menstruation about 3 years ago, with delayed menstruation (periods coming approx. every 2 months) (oligomenorrhea) and scant menstruation (hypomenorrhea).

She went in for a thorough gynecological examination and testing that revealed the following: T3 111.2 (normal range 58–159), TSH 1.50 (0.35–4.94), Free T4 0.95 (0.7–1.48), LH 39.36 (menopause 9.14–58.32), FSH 36.60 (postmenopause 13.5–87.2), and E2 $<$ 10.0 (30–400 pg/mL). The right ovary size was 2.85 cm × 1.68 cm and the left 2.35 cm × 1.71 cm (normal range 3.0–5.0 cm in length x 1.5–3.0

cm in width).

She recently took TCM medicinals prescribed by another physician for 3 months, without any noticeable effects. My idea is to prescribe Shi Quan Da Bu Tang adding Ai Ye, Shan Yao, and Xu Duan (I would consider prescribing Zi He Che (Dried Human Placenta), but we don't have access to this medicinal here in South Korea). Can TCM directly stimulate an increase in ovarian hormones?

A: Hmm! High levels of follicle-stimulating hormone (FSH) and luteinizing hormone (LH) and low levels of estradiol (E2), along with slightly atrophied ovaries. This *does* suggest the patient may have already entered perimenopause. Yes, I think a blood-quickening blood-supplementing, qi-boosting spleen-fortifying, and kidney yang-supplementing formula such as Shi Quan Da Bu Tang adding Ai Ye, Shan Yao, and Xu Duan is the right approach. However, I would make sure to include The Three Great Yang-Supplementers, Zi He Che, and Tu Si Zi.

If you don't have access to Zi He Che, then you can add large doses of other "seed (子 zi)" medicinals, such as Tu Si Zi, Sha Yuan Zi, and Ji Li Zi, instead. These types of medicinals will also promote partial restoration and revitalization of ovarian function and increase estrogen and progesterone levels.

Remember! The average age for menopause is 49 to 51, but it is *not* abnormal for some women to begin the menopausal transition and even complete cessation of menstruation (menopause) as young as 35 years old. If your patient *no* longer desires to become pregnant and is not experiencing any discomfort or problematic symptoms, then it really is*n't* imperative to administer any type of treatment.

Case Study #10: Bimonthly Menstruation – It May Be "Normal"!

Q: Recently, a 24 y/o nulliparous female patient visited me explaining that she has had irregular menstrual cycles for about 4 years now. The strange thing is that her menses comes "regularly" at about 50- to 60-day intervals with a normal volume of bleeding and no other symptoms or abnormalities. She has undergone thorough gynecological examinations and testing on several occasions, without any specific findings. Do you think I should try to regulate this patient's constitution and get her cycle back on track?

A: It sounds to me like this just may be a "normal" physiological menstrual cycle and *not* a pathological irregularity. Her menstrual cycle may simply come at different intervals than most other women.

For most women, menses usually comes "monthly" at 3- to 5-week intervals. However, in some women, menses may come every 45 days, 60 days—bimonthly menstruation (併月 bìng yuè), 3 months—residing (居經 j□ j□ ng) or quarterly (季經 jì j□ ng) menstruation, 6 months, 1 year—annual evasion (避年 bì nián), and bleeding may never appear—surreptitious menstruation (暗經 àn j□ ng), with lumbar pain being the only sign of ovulation.

Women with this type of "normal" physiological menstrual cycle are in fact ovulating and may conceive *in sync* with their individual menstrual cycles. Again, for these women it is *not* a problem of ovarian atrophy or uterine dysfunction, but involves a *glitch* in the hormonal regulation of the brain centers and the feedback mechanisms in the uterus and ovaries. This results in physiologically "normal" menstrual cycles that come at "regular" intervals, based on individual constitution.

Thus, I would simply advise the patient to chart her daily basal body temperature to verify whether or not ovulation is indeed occurring. Evaluate these results over a period of time until it can be determined if a definitive interval pattern between ovulation and menses appears. Then, you will know for sure if her condition is "regular" or "irregular." In the meantime, unless the patient presents with symptoms, technically, you really do*n't* need to provide any type of treatment. If she really wants to take TCM medicinals, then you could prescribe a blood-nourishing blood-quickening, stasis-dispelling pain-relieving, and network vessel-freeing channel-regulating formula such as Ru Mo Si Wu Tang or Tong Jing Fang until you are certain about the diagnosis and pattern identification of her condition.

Remember! Women with bimonthly menstruation, residing (or quarterly) menstruation, annual evasion, and surreptitious (or absent) menstruation continue to ovulate and are perfectly capable of being impregnated. Make sure your patient is aware of this and takes necessary precautions if she does *not* want to become pregnant, and if she does, then follow her daily basal body temperature chart accordingly. Typically, after childbirth the *glitch* in the hormonal regulation of the brain centers and the feedback mechanisms will gradually "awaken" autoregulation and recalibrate back to monthly menstrual cycles over time.

Case Study #11: Menopause – Nature's Course!

Q: A 49 y/o female patient has been having lighter (hypomenorrhea) and delayed menstruation (oligomenorrhea), with menses occurring in two-month intervals. She wants to take TCM medicinals to prolong her menopausal transition. Do you think this is necessary, or possible?

A: Ahh! Menopausal transition is a natural part of the aging process. Let it come, when it comes! Many people have the misconception that by prolonging menopausal transition they can somehow slow down the aging process. In fact, the longer menstruation occurs, the more likely it is for a woman to develop a genitourinary tract tumor.

This is a natural physiological process that has been programmed into the DNA of *Homo sapiens* since our inception on this planet at least 300,000 years ago. There is no need, nor healthy way, to alter this programmed sequence. It's just nature's course!

Section 2: Ovarian Disorders

Case Study #1: Ovarian Cysts – Phlegm-Rheum with Stasis Heat Pattern

Q: A 26 y/o unmarried, nulliparous woman presented as asymptomatic with menstrual cycles of about 35–40 days. Recently, she had a routine ultrasound which revealed an ovarian cyst 6.7 cm × 6.8 cm in size. Can TCM provide effective treatment for such a large ovarian cyst?

A: Ovarian cysts (i.e., follicular cysts and corpus luteum cysts) that fluctuate in size with the hormonal changes of the menstrual cycle can be identified as phlegm-rheum with stasis heat pattern. For these types of ovarian cysts, I would prescribe Ru Mo Si Wu Tang combining Wen Dan Tang (including a large dose of Huang Qin), adding either Yan Hu Suo and Mu Xiang (for gripping or colicky pain resulting from qi stagnation) or Wu Ling Zhi, Pu Huang, and Chuan Qi (for distention and oppressive pain resulting from static blood).

Make sure to have the patient get an ultrasound performed every 2 months so you both can see how things are progressing. During the first 2 weeks of administration, the size of the cyst may slightly enlarge in circumference appearing like a "halo" as the fluid (and possibly blood) inside begins to break down and dissipate. As you continue administering this formula, the cyst will shrink gradually up to a certain point until it will once again (due to hormonal fluctuations and subsequent break down and dissipation) appear like a "halo" image on ultrasound. Then, as before, the cyst will continue gradually shrinking in size up until it completely vanishes.

Remember! These slight "halo" perturbations may occur throughout the therapeutic process, but as long as you can see a definitive shrinking trend, then you know you are on the right track. You should inform your patient about this progressive process at the onset of treatment, that way everyone knows what to expect. It's ok to see the "halo."

Ovarian cysts that are *not* related to variations in normal hormonal fluctuations (i.e., endometriomas (chocolate cysts), dermoid cysts (cystic teratomas), and cystadenomas (serous cystadenomas)) tend to be more difficult to treat than those mentioned above. Typically, for these types of ovarian cysts I will prescribe a blood-breaking, channel-freeing, and pain-relieving formula such as Tong Jing Fang adding heat-clearing toxin-resolving and dampness-disinhibiting by bland percolation medicinals.

If this is *not* effective, then I will return to the *Treatise on Cold Damage and Miscellaneous Diseases* classical approach by prescribing (Yu Sheng) Gui Zhi Fu Ling Wan (including larger doses of medicinals than in the original version) adding Chuan Qi, Wan Ling Dan, and Yu Sheng Wan; or possibly Dang Gui Shao Yao San (including large doses of Fu Ling and Ze Xie) adding Gui Zhi, Bai Zhu, Chuan Qi, Wan Ling Dan, and Yu Sheng Wan.

Case Study #2: Large Follicular Cyst – Surgical Resection

Q: My wife has a follicular cyst (about 8 cm in diameter) on her left ovary. She had been experiencing distention in her lower abdomen and lower back (more pronounced a few days before and during menses) and irregular intervals, so she went in to get it checked out with her gynecologist. The gynecologist advised her to go ahead with surgery and she is scheduled for surgical resection next week. Since we still want to have children, we are worried that surgery may impact fertility.

Do you think it is really necessary to have surgery or could TCM provide effective treatment for a follicular cyst of this size? Also, what would be a good formula to regulate the constitution following surgery?

A: For a large ovarian cyst that does *not* resolve on its own or through other therapeutic means there is a definite risk of ovarian torsion or ruptured ovarian cyst (which is a bona fide medical emergency!). So yes, in order to eliminate this risk, I would say go ahead with surgical resection. With the modern surgical advancements of today, it may be possible to preserve the function of her left ovary, and even if it cannot be preserved, your wife still has a normal functioning right ovary for children in the future. Generally, for persistent ovarian cysts $\geq$ 8 cm it is advisable to undergo surgical resection. It's just *not* worth the risk!

Ovarian cysts can most often be identified as stasis heat with phlegm-rheum pattern. Thus, to regulate the constitution following surgery, I would prescribe a formula such as Ru Mo Si Wu Tang (nourishes and quickens the blood, dispels stasis and relieves pain, and frees the network vessels and regulates the channels) combining Wen Dan Tang (clears Shao Yang depressed heat and dispels phlegm turbidity harassing the inner body) adding Pu Gong Yin, Wu Ling Zhi, Xu Duan, Gu Sui Bu, Yan Hu Suo, Mu Xiang, and Chuan Qi.

Remember! A little extra love and understanding may be the best way to "regulate the constitution." Say hello to your wife for me…I look forward to visiting your family and kids soon.

Case Study #3: Can TCM Treat Polycystic Ovary Syndrome?

Q: A 30 y/o female patient explained that after getting married 5 years ago she rapidly gained 20 kg, her menstrual cycle became irregular (delayed menstruation), and attempts to get pregnant have been unsuccessful. Her gynecologist advised lifestyle changes (e.g., dietary modifications, exercise) and prescribed unspecified medication, which was not effective, so she decided to come see me.

I suspected immature ovarian follicles. Identifying this condition as qi and blood vacuity with insufficiency of kidney yang pattern, I prescribed Shi Quan Da Bu Tang variant to regulate the menses and promote the development of healthy follicles. After taking this formula for 1 week, the patient began to have irregular uterine bleeding (approx. 10 ml/day) every time she urinated. I advised her to go back for a thorough gynecological examination, upon which she was diagnosed with polycystic ovary syndrome (PCOS). How would how to treat this patient?

A: PCOS is a clinical syndrome that typically includes the presence of many tiny (occasionally larger ones) follicular cysts in the ovaries, involves anovulation or ovulatory dysfunction and androgen excess of unclear etiology, and carries an increased risk of developing metabolic syndrome (e.g., large waist circumference, hypertension, plasma glucose or insulin resistance, and dyslipidemia).

In TCM, this condition can be identified as *life gate stasis heat and static blood obstructing the uterus (ovaries) with phlegm-heat and yang hyperactivity* pattern.

If blood tests reveal elevated levels of LH, FSH, testosterone, DHEA-S, and postprandiol blood glucose (PPBG), along with signs and symptoms of *yang hyperactivity* pattern, then I would proceed by prescribing one of the following formula variations along with modifications based on specific signs, symptoms and pattern:

- Ru Mo Si Wu Tang (nourishes and quickens the blood, dispels stasis and relieves pain, and frees the network vessels and regulates the channels) adding Niu Xi (quickens the blood, frees the channels, and conducts medicinals downwards), Huang Qin and Zhi Zi (abate heat with cold and bitterness), Mu Dan Pi (cools the blood and clears heat and quickens the bloods and disperses stasis), and Long Gu, Mu Li, and Dai Zhe Shi (calm the liver and subdue yang).
- Jian Ling Tang (settles the liver and extinguishes wind and enriches yin and subdues yang) combining Huang Lian Jie Du Tang (clears heat and resolves toxin) adding Chuan Qi (transforms stasis and stanches bleeding and quickens the blood and settles pain), Xu Duan and Gu Sui Bu (enter the kidney channel, quicken the blood and transform stasis, and break blood), San Leng and E Zhu (break blood and move qi and disperse accumulations and relieve pain), and Yan Hu Suo (quickens the blood, moves qi, and relieves pain).
- In the absence of noticeable signs or symptoms of *yang hyperactivity*, then this pathocondition can be identified more at *phlegm-rheum heat* pattern, for which I would add Wen Dan Tang, Sang Bai Pi, and Sheng Shi Gao to the formula chosen from above.
- If *static blood and stasis heat* pattern is more pronounced, then you can consider changing your formula to Gui Zhi Fu Ling Wan adding The Three Yellows, Sang Bai Pi, and Sheng Shi Gao.
- And if *constipation* presents, make sure to add Da Huang; for *menstrual pain* (dysmenorrhea), add Yan Hu Suo and Mu Xiang (or Gu Sui Bu and Xu Duan); and for *uterine bleeding* involving heat pattern, add Chuan Qi and Zhu Sha.

Section 3: Uterine Disorders

Case Study #1: Aplastic Anemia and Endometrial Cancer – Therapeutic Approach

Q: A 73 y/o female patient began feeling dizziness, light-headedness, and a lack of energy about 6 months ago so she went to see her doctor to get it checked out. Blood tests confirmed low Hb, WBC, and PLT levels, and she was diagnosed with aplastic anemia, requiring administration of bimonthly blood transfusions.

Recently, she incurred episodes of profuse uterine bleeding whenever she engaged in slightly straining physical activity. This prompted a thorough gynecological examination, which revealed endometrial cancer (6 cm × 6 cm). After administration of progestins, the tumor has shrunk a little bit to 5 cm × 4 cm. Since she still needs to have bimonthly transfusions (whole blood and clotting factors) for the treatment of anemia, she said that she is unable to undergo immediate cancer treatment (i.e., surgery, chemotherapy, radiotherapy). That's why she wants to see if TCM can help resolve this problem.

Her most recent lab test results are as follows: Hb 8.7 (12–16 g/dl), WBC 2,300 (5,000–10,000/ul), PLT 60,000 (150–400 x10 ^{3}/ul), and Hct 25.3% (37–47%). The patient also said that her oncologist didn't think the aplastic anemia had anything to do with her endometrial cancer, but I want to try treating both at the same time. My idea for treatment is to prescribe kidney yang-supplementing medicinals, but I am concerned this approach might stimulate cancer growth and possibly metastasis. What is the best approach for treating this patient?

A: If there is *no* relationship between the aplastic anemia and the abnormal uterine bleeding resulting from endometrial cancer, then your treatment focus should be to first stanch bleeding and promote hematopoiesis, *not* on supplementing yang!

Endometrial cancer can be identified as frenetic movement of hot blood in the sea of blood (血海 xuè hai) and liver depression and blood stasis failing to contain the blood pattern. As for treatment, I would prescribe Ru Mo Si Wu Tang adding Huang Qin, Mu Dan Pi, Fu Ling, Ze Xie, Long Dan Cao, Ou Jie, Ce Bo Ye, Xu Duan, Gu Sui Bu, Chuan Qi (powder), Zhu Sha (powder)*, Yu Sheng Wan, and Wan

Ling Dan.

Regarding specific doses, for Huang Qin and Mu Dan Pi you can start out at 8 qian, and Chuan Qi (powder) 3 g and Zhu Sha 4 g (3x/day of each), gradually increasing the doses of each medicinal. A normal dose of Long Dan Cao would be from 5–8 qian, but if the patient has a poor appetite, then add only 3 qian along with Cang Zhu and Shan Zha to disperse food and promote digestion and fortify the spleen and open the stomach. Shan Zha also offers excellent blood-quickening, blood-stanching, heart-strengthening, and pain-relieving actions, especially for pathoconditions in the pelvic region.

As for Zhu Sha, if you are concerned about the possibility of toxicity, then the safest way is to advise the patient to separately decoct Tu Fu Ling, drinking the decoction like a tea (beverage) throughout the therapeutic regimen. And if you don't have access to Zhu Sha, then you can substitute it with Dai Zhe Shi (powder), which effectively cools the blood and stanches bleeding, quiets the spirit by heavy settling, and calms the liver and subdues yang (for hypertension and overactive endocrine disorders), but it cannot replace Zhu Sha's superior blood-stanching and antitumor actions.

*Note: The traditional method of processing Zhu Sha is to crush, grind in a mortar with water, place the contents in the mortar into a container adding more water, use a sieve to collect the fine powder in suspension (or floating on top), dry under the sun, and then repeat this process repeatedly until the mineral has been reduced to the finest particles. In this "purified" form, it can be considered free of toxicity and safe to ingest in small doses. Obviously, this is a time-consuming and arduous practice that nowadays has been supplanted by automated methods. Depending on the machines used and their operators, this may lead to the rapid induction of excessive temperatures that result in the transformation of cinnabar into high concentrations of mercury sulfide (HgS) and a host of other toxic mercurial compounds.

Case Study #2: Endometrial Cancer with Abdominal Metastasis

Q: This 42 y/o female began noticing an enlarged abdomen along with shortness of breath, prompting her to go in to get it checked out.

Thorough examination revealed endometrial carcinoma (type 1). While performing the hysterectomy surgeons discovered an 18 cm cancerous tumor in the abdominal cavity as well. She is currently receiving radiotherapy (no chemotherapy). How would you treat this patient?

A: For the treatment of endometrial carcinoma with abdominal metastases, I would prescribe a blood-breaking, channel-freeing, and pain-relieving formula such as Tong Jing Fang adding Bai Zhu, Fu Ling, and Ze Xie (dry dampness and disinhibit water by bland percolation); San Leng, E Zhu, Yan Hu Suo, and Yu Jin (break blood, disperse accumulations, and relieve pain); Ban Xia and Bai Jie Zi (transforms phlegm and disperse binds); Chuan Qi (transforms stasis and stanches bleeding and quickens the blood and settles pain); and Wan Ling Dan (resolves toxin and disperses welling-abscesses, soothes the sinews and quickens the blood, and dispels wind and relieves pain).

Remember! Add 2 tablespoons (approx. 30 ml) of vinegar and rice wine (approx. 150 cc) into water (approx. 1,200–1,400 cc) and steep (a minimum of 30 min. up to 12 hrs.) prior to decoction. This method will greatly enhance the overall blood-breaking accumulation-dispersing potency of these medicinals.

Case Study #3: Too Much and Too Little Is No Good

Q: I have a 44 y/o patient with endometrial hyperplasia and profuse menstruation. About 8 months ago, she began having monthly menses that lasted over 10 days, excessive bleeding (menorrhagia), and lower back pain (no radiating pain). She has already been administered nearly 6 months of Western medicine therapy (i.e., progestin), but this has *not* improved the condition. How would you treat this patient?

A: Hmm! This pathocondition can be identified as depressed blood with stasis heat pattern. I would consider prescribing either Ru Mo Si Wu Tang or Tong Jing Fang adding The Three Yellows, Mu Dan Pi, Zhi Zi, and Chuan Qi. If excessive bleeding remains a problem, then you could consider adding liver-calming yang-subduing, spirit-quieting by heavy settling, blood-cooling bleeding-stanching, and astringing and securing medicinals such as Sheng Mu Li, Dai Zhe Shi, and Zhu Sha into your formula.

Lumbar pain suggests that the patient may have concomitant endometriosis that has become implanted in the pelvic region and enlarges under the influence of estrogen during the menstrual cycle. For this condition, I would consider adding Du Zhong (or Gou Ji) and Di Long to the main formula; bleed the well points of the kidney (Yong Quan (KI 1)) and liver (Da Dun (LV1)) channels, along with Wei Zhong (UB40); and needle Nei Guan (PC6), Tai Chong (LV3), San Yin Jiao (SP6), and Zu San Li (ST36). If constipation presents, then add Da Huang.

Remember! Patients with endometrial hyperplasia (especially the type *with atypia*) are at greater risk of developing into endometrial cancer. Thus, make sure the patient goes back for periodic gynecologic follow-up examinations and be on the lookout for elevated ovarian cancer marker CA-125 levels. Typically, I would administer this therapeutic regimen for a period of 6–10 months. Once the ultrasound shows the endometrium has shrunk back down to its normal size, then you can begin to gradually discontinue administration. Naturally, it's *not* good to have too much menses with lots of clots, but it's also *not* good to have too little without any clots. The middle path is best!

Case Study #4: Endometriosis – Treatment Based on Pattern Identification

Q: I am currently treating a patient with endometriosis who initially presented with profuse menstruation (menorrhagia). After taking Ru Mo Si Wu Tang variant for about 1 month, she incurred episodes of intense cramping pain in the pelvis (dysmenorrhea) just before menses and even larger amounts of blood than before.

What do you make of this situation? Do you think this is a sign that the therapeutic process is taking effect or is her condition worsening? If there is no response to therapy, is it necessary to have surgery (e.g., laparoscopic excision and ablation of endometrial implants, hysterectomy)? Please offer your advice and guidance.

A: *Endometriosis* can be identified as static blood obstructing the uterus (or uterine vessels) pattern. In modern advanced societies with high nutritional intake and comfortable living environs, this pathocondition most commonly involves stasis heat pattern (e.g., presents with viscous, dark blood with clots) as opposed to cold stasis pattern (e.g., presents with watery, light-colored blood), which was prevalent in times of antiquity and still may be in disadvantaged populations with poor nutritional intake and living environs.

Stasis heat pattern requires the administration of formula variants such as Ru Mo Si Wu Tang or Tong Jing Fang, making sure to add Huang Qin (or Huang Lian), Mu Dan Pi, Zhi Zi, and Chuan Qi. If pain is pronounced, then add Yan Hu Suo and Mu Xiang; and if bleeding is profuse add Pu Huang, Ce Bo Ye, Ou Jie, Ai Ye, and Zhu Sha

For patients presenting with profuse (copious) menses you must consider the possibility of *endometrial hyperplasia*, *uterine fibroids* (*leiomyoma*), or *adenomyosis*. These pathoconditions will lead to excessive proliferation of the endometrium and profuse bleeding when the endometrium sloughs off (desquamation) during menses.

In the treatment of *endometriosis*, I administer TCM medicinals up until the patient has gone through 2–3 menstrual cycles without experiencing pain. That's when I consider the condition cured and can discontinue treatment. For *endometrial hyperplasia*, the patient will typically need to be administered TCM medicinals for 8–10 months in order to prevent abnormal uterine bleeding (e.g., constant, intermenstrual, postmenopausal), infertility, and the development of endometrial cancer.

For patients with *endometriosis*, hysterectomy is an option, but the best way is to conceive and have children. This gives the ectopic endometrial tissue a respite from the hormonal fluctuations of the menstrual cycle during the 9–10 months of gestation and allows these endometriotic implants to shrink and resolve. Women in our modern society are getting married later in life and having fewer children, if any at all, which sets the stage for the development of *endometriosis*, *uterine fibroids*, and *adenomyomas*. After undergoing hysterectomy, it is common for patients to experience posthysterectomy depression, anxiety (even acute psychosis), reduced sexual pleasure, dyspareunia, infection, excessive bleeding, vaginal vault prolapse, injury to the ureter, bladder and bowel, and pelvic adhesions. So if possible, by all means hold onto your reproductive organs!

If it is vital for the health of the patient to undergo hysterectomy, I would prescribe a formula variant such as Bu Zhong Yi Qi Tang or Shen Ling Bai Zhu San adding Du Zhong, Gan Jiang, Fu Zi, Huang Qin, Zi He Che, and Yu Sheng Wan to promote tissue healing and ameliorate the postsurgical menopausal symptoms. If dizziness presents, then add Tian Ma; and for dry mouth add Zhi Mu and Tian Hua.

Once the tissue damage from surgery has healed, if the patient still presents with noticeable autonomic symptoms (e.g., hot flashes), mood disorders (e.g., irritability, insomnia, loss of libido), and atrophic changes due to decreased estrogen production (e.g., vulvovaginal atrophy, decreased breast size), this can be identified as Shao Yang pattern or cold phlegm visceral agitation (aka Tai Yin-Jue Yin phlegm-rheum dizziness) pattern, requiring the administration of either Wen Dan Tang or Ban Xia Tian Ma Bai Zhu San adding Gan Cao, Da Zao, and Du Zhong.

In very rare cases, where the patient presents with insomnia due to yang hyperactivity, I have had to prescribe Jian Ling Tang (including Gan Cao) adding Long Yan Rou, Huang Bo, Huang Lian, Tian Ma, and Yu Sheng Wan. And for patients presenting with yin vacuity tidal heat and heart palpitations, I would prescribe Zhi Bo Di Huang Tang adding Gan Cao, Cang Zhu, and Yu Sheng Wan; for Shao Yang vacuity heat with hyperactivity of liver yang symptoms (e.g., vexation and susceptibility to fright), I would prescribe Chai Hu Jia Long Gu Mu Li Tang; and for vacuity taxation with dual vacuity of yin and yang symptoms (e.g., emotional depression), I would prescribe Gui Zhi Jia Long Gu Mu Li Tang, Shen Qi Wan, or You Gui Wan.

Pelvic adhesions can be identified as either stasis obstruction pattern or qi vacuity pattern, requiring administration of formulas such as Gui Zhi Fu Ling Wan, Dang Gui Shao Yao San, Bu Zhong Yi Qi Tang, or Tiao Zhong Yi Qi Tang. Just make sure to add Chuan Qi, Yan Hu Suo, Mu Xiang, and Yu Sheng Wan to your formula. If constipation presents, then add Da Huang; for lumbar pain add Du Zhong; and for urinary incontinence add Huang Qi, Bai Guo, and Long Yan He.

Case Study #5: Physical and Emotional Complications of Hysterectomy

Q: A 40 y/o patient with endometriosis decided to have a total hysterectomy with unilateral oophorectomy (right ovary resected) performed and has received two GnRH agonist injections to remedy the troubling chronic symptoms of pelvic pain, dysmenorrhea, and profuse uterine bleeding.

Unfortunately, following the surgical procedure and drug administration, she has experienced the following complications and side effects: rectal, urethral, and vaginal pain (especially after defecation); episodes of diarrhea during intense pain flare-ups; lower abdominal distention and pain in the anal region upon full bladder; episodes of left hip pain so severe that she can't even touch it; profuse sweating on the back of the neck; and profuse sweating on the upper chest and upper arms (sweat will even drip off at times). How would you treat this patient?

A: This patient is likely experiencing both the emotional and physical complications (e.g., pain resulting from ureter, bowel, and bladder injury) following the hysterectomy, as well as potential side effects of the GnRH injections (e.g., profuse spontaneous sweating). Lingering, persistent pain may result from damage to nerves and is an iatrogenic complication that I liken to "phantom pain."

For cases involving profuse spontaneous sweating, I typically prescribe Jian Ling Tang (including Gan Cao) adding Long Yan Rou, Qing Hao, Zhi Mu, Di Gu Pi, Huang Bo (large dose starting at 8 qian), Du Zhong, The Three Insects, Di Long, and Yu Sheng Wan (3 pills/1x/day). If sloppy stools present, then add Fu Ling and Ze Xie.

This therapeutic regimen will provide quick and effective relief of symptoms. You can continue administration up until the spontaneous sweating and phantom pain completely resolves.

Case Study #6: Hysterectomy – Emotional Complications Pattern Types

Q: What are the most common complications of hysterectomy? And what are the principles, methods, and medicinals you use to treat these complications?

A: The most common physical complications are infection, hemorrhage, vaginal vault prolapse, and injury to the ureter, bowel, or bladder. However, in my clinical practice I see many patients with psychological complications (e.g., fatigue, depression, anxiety, psychosexual dysfunction, and even psychosis) and menopausal symptoms (e.g., hot flashes, night sweats, vulvar and vaginal atrophy, vaginal dryness, and insomnia). Here are the pattern types I most commonly encounter:

1) Hyperactivity type (e.g., menopausal symptoms of agitation, anxiety, insomnia, tidal heat, palpitations, night sweats, vaginal dryness, psychosis)—Prescribe an yin-enriching fire-downbearing and liver-settling yang-subduing formula such as Zhi Bo Di Huang Tang, Dang Gui Liu Huang Tang, Tian Wang Bu Xin Dan, or Jian Ling Tang. Just make sure to include Qing Hao, Zhi Mu, Di Gu Pi, Long Yan Rou (or Da Zao), Zi He Che, and Yu Sheng Wan.
2) Depression type (e.g., menopausal symptoms of depression, sleeplessness)—For phlegm-heat pattern sleeplessness (insomnia) and profuse dreaming, prescribe Wen Dan Tang or Di Tan Tang adding Qing Hao, Zhi Mu, Di Gu Pi, Zi He Che, and Yu Sheng Wan. For cold rheum pattern, prescribe Ban Xia Tian Ma Bai Zhu San adding Gan Cao, Long Yan Rou, Du Zhong, Qing Hao, Zhi Mu, Di Gu Pi, Zi He Che, and Yu Sheng Wan.
3) Fatigue type (e.g., fatigue, general malaise, dizziness, blurred vision, headache)—Prescribe Ban Xia Tian Ma Bai Zhu San adding Gan Cao, Long Yan Rou, Da Zao, Ren Shen, Zi He Che, and Yu Sheng Wan.
4) Qi vacuity type (e.g., pelvic organ prolapse, lack of strength in the lumbus and knees, shortage of qi)—Prescribe a spleen-fortifying qi-supplementing formula such as Bu Zhong Yi Qi Tang adding Gan Jiang, Fu Zi, Du Zhong, Huang Qin, Da Zao, Long Yan Rou, Zi He Che, and Yu Sheng Wan.
5) Kidney yang vacuity type (e.g., limp wilt, cold aching lumbus and knees, vaginal atrophy)—Prescribe either a kidney yang-supplementing or essence-replenishing formula such as You Gui Yin, Shen Qi Wan, He Che Da Zao Wan, or Gui Lu Er Xian Jiao. Just make sure to include Da Zao, Long Yan Rou, Qing Hao, Zhi Mu, Di Gu Pi, Zi He Che, and Yu Sheng Wan.

However, in the clinical setting, patients often present with combinations of symptoms that overlap various pattern types. The majority of my patients present with a combination of depression, fatigue, and qi vacuity type symptoms, for which I most commonly prescribe Bu Zhong Yi Qi Tang variant. If lumbar pain presents, then add Du Zhong; for dizziness add Tian Ma; for severe headache add

Tian Ma and Wu Zhu Yu; and for tidal heat and night sweating add Qing Hao, Zhi Mu, and Di Gu Pi.

Some patients respond very well to acupuncture, so you can also consider needling acupoints that correspond with the presenting symptoms such as Feng Chi (GB20), Bai Hui (GV20), He Gu (LI4), Shen Men (HT7), Nei Guan (PC6), Guan Yuan Shu (UB26), Huan Tiao (GB30), Wei Zhong (UB40), Tai Chong (LV3), and San Yin Jiao (SP6).

Case Study #7: I Feel Pain All Over!

Q: A 44 y/o female patient had been having increasingly heavy menstruation (menorrhagia and hypermenorrhea) over a period of 6 months (6 relatively regular cycles), prompting her to get it checked out.

Following a thorough gynecological examination, she was diagnosed with adenomyosis and administered oral contraceptives that proved ineffective. Bleeding began occurring between periods (metrorrhagia) and then became heavy (menometrorrhagia), thus her gynecologist recommended hysterectomy. After this invasive surgical procedure, she has felt pain all over, shortage of qi (weakness), and heaviness.

She has taken Chinese medicine at another clinic, but the treatment was *not* effective in remedying symptoms. I decided on prescribing Bu Zhong Yi Qi Tang variant. Do you think this is a good approach?

A: Adenomyoma with irregular bleeding can be identified as static heat and frenetic movement of hot blood pattern, requiring the administration of Ru Mo Si Wu Tang adding Huang Qin, Huang Lian, Ce Bo Ye, Chuan Qi, Mu Dan Pi, and Zhi Zi.

However, your patient has already undergone a hysterectomy. Both the tissue healing process and most of the symptoms arising from posthysterectomy complications can be identified as qi vacuity pattern. So yes, Bu Zhong Yi Qi Tang variant is a good formula for this patient. Just make sure to include Yan Hu Suo, Mu Xiang, Huang Qin, Du Zhong, Zi He Che (powder), and Yu Sheng Wan.

Remember! Immediately following surgery, heat and swelling (serous and serosanguinous fluid) will be pronounced at and around the sites of resected tissue, so you should also add large doses of The Three Yellows (clear heat and resolve toxin) and Fu Ling and Ze Xie (disinhibit water and percolate dampness).

If these symptoms persist beyond the acute and postacute stages into the chronic stage, then this can be identified as qi vacuity with yang vacuity pattern, requiring the addition of The Three Great Yang-Supplementers. If lumbar pain presents, then add Du Zhong; for dizziness and neck tightness, add Tian Ma and Ge Gen; for palpitations, add large doses of Gan Cao, Da Zao, and Long Yan Rou; for tidal heat (hot flashes) and night sweating, add Qing Hao, Zhi Mu, and Di Gu Pi; and for insomnia, add Long Gu, Mu Li, Long Yan Rou, Gan Cao (large dose), Fu Shen, and Yu Sheng Wan.

Case Study #8: Vaginal Dryness Following Hysterectomy

Q: A 40 y/o female patient visited me with the chief complaint of vaginal dryness following hysterectomy. In the past, I had prescribed Gui Zhi Jia Long Gu Mi Li Tang variant for this type of condition, but results were *not* very satisfactory. How would you treat this condition?

A: Menopausal symptoms (e.g., hot flashes, emotional distress, vaginal dryness, night sweating) and psychosomatic disorders (i.e., either existing symptoms that are exacerbated by mental factors or mental factors causing the manifestation of perceived symptoms (aka somatization, somatic symptom disorder, somatoform disorder)) are common posthysterectomy complications.

Bu Zhong Yi Qi Tang variant is a good formula for treating a broad spectrum of the symptoms that may manifest following hysterectomy. I commonly prescribe this formula variant for both physical and psychological posthysterectomy complications, adding other medicinals depending on the specific presenting signs, symptoms, and pattern. For instance, for dizzy head (dizziness), add Tian Ma; for lumbar pain, add Du Zhong; for palpitations, add Da Zao and Long Yan Rou; for tidal heat (hot flashes), add Qing Hao, Zhi Mu, and Di Gu Pi; and for vaginal dryness, add medicinals such as Zi He Che, Yin Yang Huo, Tu Si Zi, Rou Cong Rong, and Lu Rong.

Remember! If these symptoms persist and become chronic, make sure to include adequate doses of The Three Great Yang-Supplementers and Huang Qin.

Case Study #9: Lower Extremity Lymphedema Following Hysterectomy

Q: A 43 y/o female patient incurred lower extremity lymphedema in her left leg following a hysterectomy.

Is this a common complication? What's the best approach for treating this condition?

A: It is a common complication, particularly so for patients with gynecologic cancer (e.g., cervical, endometrial, vulvar) who also undergo lymphadenectomy and/or radiotherapy. For your patient there are two likely scenarios:

1) Malignancy with lymph node metastases has occurred independent of the hysterectomy procedure, causing lymphatic obstruction and lower limb lymphedema.
2) Either damage to the tissue and nerves with subsequent swelling or direct damage to the lymph nodes occurred during the hysterectomy, causing lymphatic obstruction and lower limb lymphedema.

The key here for you is to determine whether or not *malignancy* is involved. If *so*, then I would consider prescribing Wu Ling San (Nephritis Formula) (including large doses of Fu Ling and Ze Xie) adding Huang Qin (large dose), Yin Xing Ye, Huang Qi, and Ren Shen/Chuan Qi Powder. If *not*, and the lower limb lymphedema results from a complication of the hysterectomy procedure, then I would consider prescribing Ru Mo Si Wu Tang adding The Three Yellows, Fu Ling, Ze Xie, and Qing Hao.

Case Study #10: Uterine Polyp

Q: A 25 y/o female patient recently incurred irregular menstrual bleeding (menorrhagia and occasional spotting), prompting her to undergo a thorough gynecological examination. A uterine (endometrial) polyp 1.3 cm in size was found, and her gynecologist decided to wait and see if the symptoms continued progressing before prescribing hormonal treatment (e.g., progestins, GnRH agonist).

I have been prescribing Ru Mo Si Wu Tang combining Wen Dan Tang and adding Wan Ling Dan for the past 2 months now, but the patient's symptoms have *not* improved. How would you proceed from here?

A: Uterine polyps can be identified as liver channel depressed heat, depressed accumulation of static blood, and stasis obstructing the uterus pattern. For uterine polyps with menorrhagia and occasional spotting, I would prescribe Ru Mo Si Wu Tang adding Huang Qin, Huang Lian, Mu Dan Pi, and Zhi Zi. If irregular menstrual bleeding persists, then add Chuan Qi (powder) (3 g/3x/day), Dai Zhe Shi (powder)* (4 g/3x/day), Fu Ling, and Ze Xie. Also, make sure to needle acupoints such as Tai Chong (LV3), Zhong Feng (LV4), San Yin Jiao (SP6), and Bai Hui (GV20).

*Note: Dai Zhe Shi calms the liver and subdues yang, downbears counterflow by heavy settling, cools the blood and stanches bleeding, and has the capacity to affect the hypothalamus-pituitary axis, which mediates the effects of ovarian hormones and regulates the menstrual cycle via follicle-stimulating hormone (FSH) and luteinizing hormone (LH).

Put simply, Dai Zhe Shi "tells the brain that the uterus already has enough blood flow," thus restoring autoregulation and recalibrating the errant feedback mechanism to resolve the menstrual bleeding.

Case Study #11: Malodorous Yellow Vaginal Discharge Indicates Infection

Q: A 51 y/o female patient of mine explained that about 6 months ago she began experiencing symptoms of pelvic pain, excessive menstrual flow (menorrhagia), and malodorous yellow vaginal discharge that occasionally stained her underwear and had such a fishy smell it was even noticeable upon changing pants.

The condition was not getting any better, so she decided to go in for a thorough gynecological examination, which revealed endometrial hyperplasia, an enlarged uterus, and 1 endometrial polyp (< 1 cm). Her period has not come over the past 3 months, and it appears that she may be either in the menopausal transition stage or has already entered menopause.

How would you treat this patient?

A: Endometrial hyperplasia, uterine polyps, leiomyomas (uterine fibroids), and endometrial cancer do *not* produce this type of malodorous yellow vaginal discharge. It is obvious that this patient has an infection. Malodorous yellow vaginal discharge is caused by an infection in the vaginal cavity that does *not* extend beyond the cervix. If an infection does extend beyond the cervix into the uterus or pelvis, then the patient would present with symptoms of fever and lower abdominal pain.

As for the treatment of malodorous yellow vaginal discharge, if heat is pronounced with viscous discharge, then I would recommend prescribing a liver and gallbladder repletion fire-draining and lower burner damp-heat-clearing formula such as Long Dan Xie Gan Tang adding Ru Xiang, Mo Yao, Lian Xu, Qian Shi, and Sheng Mu Li. If the discharge is watery with only mild heat, then I would prescribe a blood-nourishing blood-quickening, stasis-dispelling pain-relieving, and network vessel-freeing channel (menstruation)-regulating formula such as Ru Mo Si Wu Tang adding Long Dan Cao and Zhi Zi.

Case Study #12: HPV Increases Risk of Cervical Cancer

Q: Many women test positive for the human papillomavirus (HPV). How does TCM classify HPV? Can TCM play a role in effectively treating this infection?

A: Women who test HPV positive have a greater risk of developing cervical cancer, especially in the case of high-risk subtypes such as HPV 16, 18, 31, and 33. In TCM, HPV can be identified as either ascendant hyperactivity of liver yang, liver channel depressed heat, or Shao Yang exterior heat with static blood pattern.

I would consider prescribing a formula variant such as Long Dan Xie Gan Tang combining Huang Lian Jie Du Tang, Xiao Chai Hu Tang combining Gui Zhi Fu Ling Tang, Xiao Chai Hu Tang adding Qing Hao and Zhi Mu, or Xiao Chai Hu Tang combining Long Dan Xie Gan Tang.

Regardless of the formula you choose, make sure to add Wan Ling Dan for its antimicrobial actions and capacity to effectively lower the viral load in the blood.

Case Study #13: Headaches During Ovulation and Menses

Q: This 43 y/o female underwent bilateral tubal ligation about 4 months ago. Following the procedure, she began having headaches during ovulation and menses, lower abdominal pain that extends to the back and lumbar region, generalized aches, loss of appetite, yellow vaginal discharge, and difficult urination (dysuria).

Do you think it is possible for this patient to go back in for fallopian tube reconstruction? From what I have read, this procedure will *not* yield effective results. How would you treat this patient?

A: As far as the fallopian tube reconstruction is concerned, you will have to let the patient discuss those options with her gynecologist. However, I can tell you that headache during menstruation strongly suggests *endometriosis.*

In classical TCM texts, *endometriosis* correlates with headache, lumbar pain, abdominal pain, poor food intake, and vaginal discharge during menstruation. Most of the endometriosis patients I treat in my clinical practice can be identified as stasis obstructing the uterine vessels (瘀阻胞脈 y□ zu b□ o mài) with heat and liver wind pattern or thoroughfare and controlling vessel stasis obstruction (衝任瘀阻 ch□ ng rèn y□ zu) with heat and liver wind pattern.

For this pathocondition, I typically prescribe Ru Mo Si Wu Tang (including Chuan Xiong up to 8 qian) adding Tian Ma (at least 8 qian), sliced and crushed Sheng Du Zhong, Huang Lian, Huang Qin, Chuan Qi, and Yu Sheng Wan. You should prescribe this formula up until the patient has 2–3 menses and/or ovulations with*out* headache. That's when you can modify the dosage, instructing the patient to take 1 packet (typical daily dose) over a 2–3 day period, continuing an incremental reduction in dosage over time up until the formula has been completely discontinued.

If the headache does *not* resolve, then add combinations of the following medicinals: crushed Wu Zhu Yu (5 qian) (opens depression, transforms stagnation, and relieves Jue Yin phlegm drool headache),

Yan Hu Suo and Mu Xiang (quicken the blood, move qi, and relieve pain), and Gu Sui Bu and Xu Duan (quicken the blood and transform stasis, break blood, treat injury and mend breakages, and serve as hard tissue conductors). You could also consider changing the formula to Tong Jing Fang (breaks blood, frees the channels, and relieves pain) adding Huang Lian, Huang Qin, Sheng Du Zhong, Tian Ma, Wu Zhu Yu, Chuan Qi, and Yu Sheng Wan.

If headache is caused by blood desiccation during menstruation, then you can prescribe Blood Desiccation Formula adding Tian Ma, Wu Zhu Yu, and Chuan Qi. If headache is simply the result of premenstrual syndrome (PMS), then you can consider prescribing Wen Dan Tang (clears heat and transforms phlegm for disharmony of the gallbladder and stomach and phlegm turbidity harassing the inner body (痰濁内擾 tán zhuó nèi rao)) or Chai Hu Gui Zhi Tang (resolves both the exterior and interior and concurrently eliminates cold and heat) adding Tian Ma, Chuan Xiong, Wu Zhu Yu, and Chuan Qi.

Remember! You must also take into consideration environmental, social, and cultural factors—different ethnic groups, climates, lifestyles, and eating habits all impact the physical constitution and manifestation of pathological conditions. South Koreans are a strong-willed, hard-working and principled people who tend to enjoy eating spicy foods. Thus, I would anticipate that many endometriosis patients in South Korea would present with stasis obstructing the uterine vessels pattern. This would require administration of Ru Mo Si Wu Tang adding crushed Da Huang (drains and precipitates, attacks accumulations, clears heat and drains fire, quickens the blood and dispels stasis, and resolves toxin) or commercial granules of Di Dan Tang (attacks and expels static blood) combining Tao Ren Cheng Qi Tang (quickens the blood, transforms stasis, and precipitates stasis heat).

For Da Huang, start out at a dose of 5 fen, incrementally increasing the dose up until the patient maintains 2–3 stools per day, and then reduce the dose accordingly. For Di Dan Tang and Tao Ren Cheng Qi Tang, start out at a dose of 2 g each, incrementally increasing the dose by 0.5 g each up until the patient maintains 2–3 stools per day, and then reduce the dose accordingly (e.g., down to 1 g each□ 0.5 g each□ discontinue altogether).

For my *endometriosis* patients in Taiwan, most present with stasis obstructing the uterine vessels with phlegm turbidity harassing the inner body (or vacuity wind harassing the upper body) pattern. Thus, I will typically prescribe Ru Mo Si Wu Tang combining Wen Dan Tang (or Ban Xia Tian Ma Bai Zhu San) adding Gan Cao, Long Yan Rou, Tian Ma, Wu Zhu Yu, Chuan Xiong, and Chuan Qi.

Case Study #14: Asymptomatic Renal Cyst – Don't Worry About It!

Q: A 46 y/o female patient went in for an annual gynecological examination. A routine ultrasound revealed a leiomyoma (4 cm) and also a renal cyst on the left side (2 cm x 1 cm). The patient has *no* menstrual pain (dysmenorrhea), excessive menstrual bleeding (menorrhagia), or any other symptoms for that matter. What is your opinion about this case? Should I be concerned about the renal cyst or just ignore it?

A: A 4 cm uterine fibroid (leiomyoma) is *not* considered large, plus the patient is 46 y/o and will likely be going through menopausal transition on her way to menopause within the next few years. As long as she does *not* take any hormone supplements, usually, the fibroids will spontaneously resolve 2 to 3 years after the onset of menopause.

A renal cyst is a sac of fluid that forms in or on the surface of the kidneys. Simple cysts have a thin wall and clear, watery fluid inside. They are fairly common in the elderly and typically do not cause any symptoms or harm. As long as the cyst does *not* rapidly enlarge you do *not* need to worry about it!

If your patient is worried about the leiomyoma (uterine fibroid) and really wants treatment, then you can prescribe Ru Mo Si Wu Tang (nourishes and quickens the blood, dispels stasis and relieves pain, and frees the network vessels and regulates the channels) or Tong Jing Fang (breaks blood, frees the channels, and relieves pain) adding Huang Qin, Fu Ling, and Ze Xie. Over time, this formula will gradually shrink the fibroid and renal cyst.

Case Study #15: Adenomyosis – Optimal Therapeutic Approach

Q1: A 42 y/o female patient explained that she has always had a relatively large volume of bleeding during menses. But recently she has incurred intense aching pain in her lower abdomen, excessive menstrual bleeding (hypermenorrhea), and malodorous menstruation.

Gynecological examination revealed adenomyoma and concomitant infection with what is likely human papillomavirus (HPV) or Epstein-Barr virus (EBV). I prescribed Ru Mo Si Wu Tang adding Huang Qin, Chuan Qi, and Ce Bo Ye. Do you think this is a good approach?

A: Adenomyosis typically does *not* present with flooding. Flooding (血崩 xuè b□ng) (metrorrhagia or menometrorrhagia) and spotting (漏下 lòu xià) commonly present in patients with endometrial hyperplasia, leiomyomas, uterine polyps, endometrial cancer, and cervical cancer. The presentation of flooding and spotting (崩漏 b□ng lòu) in these pathoconditions can be identified as stasis obstructing uterine vessels with stasis heat, depressed blood with stasis heat, or stasis heat with phlegm-rheum pattern. Obviously, the heavy bleeding has *nothing* to do with the viral infection.

As for treatment, yes, for stasis heat with phlegm-rheum pattern, I would consider prescribing Ru Mo Si Wu Tang combining Wen Dan Tang (including a large dose of Huang Qin). For stasis obstructing uterine vessels, I would prescribe Ru Mo Si Wu Tang adding Bai Zhu, Fu Ling, Ze Xie, Gu Sui Bu, and Xu Duan. If a pungent, fishy odor presents during menstruation or as vaginal discharge, then this indicates that stasis heat and heat-toxin (infection) is pronounced, requiring a prescription of Ru Mo Si Wu Tang adding Mu Dan Pi, Zhi Zi, Long Dan Cao, and Huang Qin (large dose).

Q2: After 6 weeks of administering the Ru Mo Si Wu Tang variant you recommended, her first period since taking this formula was relatively normal, but during her second period, the patient incurred another cycle of extremely heavy menstruation (hypermenorrhea).

Do you think this could be a normal "therapeutic response" to the TCM formula? Or should I consider modifying the formula?

A: Adenomyosis is a benign pathocondition characterized by the occurrence of endometrial tissue (glands and stroma) within the uterine wall (myometrium). Leiomyomas (uterine fibroids) are benign tumors that may grow beneath the endometrium (submucosal), within the uterine wall (intramural), or beneath the peritoneum (subserosal). Both are hormone-sensitive, producing symptoms such as menstrual abnormalities (e.g., excessive bleeding during menses and between periods) and mass effects (e.g., lower abdominal, lumbar, and sacral pain) that wax and wane with the fluctuations of the menstrual cycle.

Both adenomyosis and leiomyomas can be identified as stasis heat with phlegm-rheum pattern, requiring administration of Ru Mo Si Wu Tang combining Wen Dan Tang adding combinations of medicinals such as Wu Ling Zhi and Pu Huang (aka Shi Xiao San), Yan Hu Suo and Mu Xiang, Gu Sui Bu and Xu Duan, Chuan Qi, Bai Zhu, Fu Ling, Ze Xie, Yu Sheng Wan, and Wan Ling Dan. Remember! It is essential that you make sure to add Bai Zhu, Fu Ling, and Ze Xie (disinhibit water by bland percolation, fortify the spleen and disinhibit dampness, and discharge heat) to promote the resolution of metabolic waste resulting from the break down and dissolution of these growths.

The break down and dissolution of these growths will be visible as an enlarged "halo" on ultrasound image. Don't worry! These "halo" perturbations will gradually shrink in size throughout the administration of this therapeutic regimen. Typically, following 3 months of administration, the growths will have shrunk by 1/3 to 1/2, in 6 months by 1/2 to 3/2, and for some patients in 8 to 9 months they may even completely disappear. It just depends on the patient, for some it may take longer than 12 months.

If necessary, the patient could consider consulting with her gynecologist for concomitant administration of a GnRH agonist (e.g., buserelin, goserelin) and oral contraception to expedite therapeutic efficacy. Remember! Even after the complete resolution of these growths, you must continue administering your TCM formula for 2 to 3 more months in order to prevent a "rebound" of these growths that may very well occur at a more rapid rate and larger extent than before.

Section 4: Pregnancy, Childbirth, and Postpartum Care

Case Study #1: Persistent Failure to Conceive – Channel Heat and Blood Heat Pattern

Q: A 38 y/o female has been married and sexually active with her spouse for many years, and despite persistent attempts she had *not* been able to get pregnant. Determined to be a mother, she decided to receive artificial insemination. This procedure resulted in an ectopic pregnancy and right-sided fallopian tube and ovarian obstruction, which required surgical resection. Two years later, she received another artificial insemination that resulted in conception and the successful birth of twin girls.

After giving birth to twins, she was able to get pregnant on 3 occasions with her husband, but unfortunately all ended in miscarriage (spontaneous abortion). To make matters worse, 3 ovarian cysts were found on her left ovary (2 of them were about 5 cm and 1 was 7.8 cm) along with a mucinous mass on her endometrium, which were all resected. This patient has never given up! Recently she received an in vitro fertilization (IVF) and embryo transfer with 3 embryos introduced into her uterus, but the embryos failed to mature, and as before, the attempt failed.

The patient's menstrual cycle comes at regular intervals every 22 to 24 days, but with scant bleeding (hypomenorrhea) and stuffiness in the chest (胸中窒 xi□ng zh□ng zhì), difficulty getting to sleep, and inability to get food down. She said that she still hopes to have another child before she gets too old. I prescribed Ru Mo Si Wu Tang adding Huang Qin, Shan Yao, Ai Ye, and Xu Duan. Do you think this is a good formula?

A: Mhh!...A parous and multigravida woman with a regular menstrual cycle of 22 to 24 days who received an IVF and embryo transfer, but the procedure did *not* bear fruit. This can be identified as latent heat in the thoroughfare and controlling vessels and thoroughfare and controlling vessel stasis obstruction with blood heat pattern.

All you need to do is focus on *extending* the menstrual cycle (start of menses) and this patient should be able to conceive and go on to give a successful birth. It's *not* necessary to take hormone injections that stimulate ovulation—excessive administration of hormone injections may lead to ovarian atrophy, endometrial hyperplasia (or atrophy), endometriosis, and even breast cancer.

As for TCM treatment, I would prescribe a blood-nourishing blood-quickening, stasis-dispelling pain-relieving, and network vessel-freeing channel (menstruation)-regulating formula such as Ru Mo Si Wu Tang adding large doses of The Three Yellows, Mu Dan Pi, and Zhi Zi. It really is*n't* necessary to add Shan Yao (boosts qi and nourishes yin, supplements the spleen, lung, and kidneys, and secures essence and checks discharge), Ai Ye (warms the channels and stanches bleeding, dissipates cold and regulates menstruation, and quiets the fetus), and Xu Duan (mildly warm in nature, supplements the liver and kidney, quickens the blood and transforms stasis, and quiets the fetus) for this patient. However, you could add Niu Xi (quickens the blood and frees the channels, supplements the liver and kidney, strengthens sinew and bone, disinhibits water and frees strangury, and conducts fire (blood) downward).

Remember! The key here is *extending* the menstrual cycle in order to allow the patient's natural hormone feedback mechanisms adequate time to promote a healthy endometrial environment for implantation. To do this, you must cool the blood and abate heat!

Case Study #2: Infertility – Psychological Factors

Q: A 25 y/o female patient visited me with a history of excessive menstrual bleeding (menorrhagia) and painful menstruation (dysmenorrhea), and a longstanding allergic reaction to greasy and oily foods manifesting as maculopapular eruptions over her entire body that occasionally even necessitates a rush to the emergency room (ER) for medical assistance. Since getting married 1 year ago, she has been trying to have a baby but *without* any luck.

I prescribed Ru Mo Si Wu Tang adding Huang Qin (8 qian), Ban Xia (3 qian), Fu Ling (3 qian) San Leng (3 qian), and E Zhu (3 qian). After only 4 weeks of administration, she successfully conceived!

This was great news in itself, but then her older sister (27 y/o and married for 3 years) visited me explaining that she had also been trying to get pregnant ever since she got married. Once again, I administered this same formula, and after a relatively short period of 6 weeks, she also got pregnant. I don't doubt the efficacy of TCM medicinals in the treatment of infertility, but these "immediate" results really did surprise me. What do you think is going on here?

A: It depends on the etiology of infertility, and whether it involves the female, male, or both. Of course, it is possible that your accurate identification of stasis heat with phlegm-rheum obstructing the uterus pattern and prescription of a corresponding formula was able to successfully regulate the constitution and resolve her condition.

However, *psychology* was most likely involved as well. Stress, pressure, and anxiety are all major contributing factors in infertility. It would appear that these patients really trusted their doctor and thus felt assured and at ease, an emotional state that promoted a physiological response. What a wonderful outcome, the joy of bringing life into this world!

Case Study #3: Low Amniotic Fluid (Oligohydramnios)

Q: I have a 29 y/o patient who is in her 8th month (3rd trimester, week 27–40) of pregnancy. Recently, during a routine prenatal examination she was diagnosed with low amniotic fluid (oligohydramnios), which is defined as an amount of amniotic fluid < 500 mL (amniotic fluid index (AFI) < 5) in the 3rd trimester. She is worried that this condition may lead to fetal abnormalities and complications during childbirth.

This is my first case of treating a pregnant woman with this specific pathocondition. Not completely sure what I should or could do for this patient, I advised her to get plenty of rest and make sure to eat lots of protein. How would you treat this patient?

A: The most common causes of oligohydramnios are leaking or rupture of membranes, placental insufficiency, birth defects, and maternal conditions (e.g., hypertension, dehydration, preeclampsia, chronic hypoxia). If low amniotic fluid occurs in the 2nd trimester, there is a much worse prognosis. Your patient is already in the 3rd trimester so the chances of birth complications are much lower. Western medicine will typically try to treat the underlying cause, and if necessary, go ahead with delivery if the fetus is close to term.

As for TCM treatment, you can consider prescribing either a blood-quickening blood-supplementing, qi-boosting spleen-fortifying, and kidney yang-supplementing formula, such as Shi Quan Da Bu Tang, or a spleen-fortifying qi-supplementing, blood-quickening, and yang-upbearing fall-raising formula, such as Bu Zhong Yi Qi Tang. These types of formulas will help increase the blood supply to the uterus and promote an optimal environment for fetal development.

Case Study #4: Placenta Previa and Placenta Accreta

Q: A 29 y/o patient is in her 9th month of pregnancy. Following a routine prenatal ultrasound examination, her obstetrician informed her that placenta previa was discovered and explained that this condition has a high risk of hemorrhage (rupture of placental vessels), both during pregnancy (antepartum) and delivery.

Right now, the patient does *not* have any symptoms. What types of medicinals would you prescribe for this patient?

A: A woman diagnosed with *placenta previa* who is in her 9th month of pregnancy will typically either go ahead with induction of labor (e.g., oxytocin infusion, early amniotomy) or possibly undergo the safer approach of cesarean section.

Placenta previa occurs when a portion of the placenta covers the neck of the uterus (cervical os), and presents as either completely covered (complete previa) or partially covered (marginal previa). Patients with this condition have a higher risk of hemorrhage (rupture of the placental vessels) and obstructed labor. However, the prognosis is typically very good, with*out* any fetal distress and a normal recovery after delivery by the mother.

You should also be aware of the possibility your patient may have abnormal placental attachment (i.e., *placenta accreta* in most cases), which makes detachment and separation of the placenta after birth difficult and can lead to serious complications (e.g., severe vaginal bleeding, infection, need for hysterectomy). This is the type of pathocondition that the master TCM physician Fu Shan (style: Fu Qing-Zhu) designed the classic formula Sheng Hua Tang (生化湯 /Engendering Transformation Decoction) for!

Previous cesarean section, previous placenta previa, a history of uterine surgery (e.g., endometrial ablation, dilation and curettage) are all risk factors for both *placenta previa* and *placenta accreta*. For *placenta accreta* in particular, I would prescribe Sheng Hua Tang (expels stasis and engenders the new, quickens the blood and dispels stasis, and warms the channels and relieves pain).

Case Study #5: Itchy Papules in Pregnancy

Q: Recently, I have had 2 separate cases involving a pregnant female patient with itchy skin.

One is a 34 y/o who complained of itchy skin over her entire body, for which I prescribed Blood Desiccation Formula adding Huang Qin and Long Yan Rou. I am still waiting to find out the results during her follow-up visit.

The other is a 32 y/o who is pregnant with her second child and complained of intense itch on the buttocks, inner thighs, armpits, and shoulders as well as small ballpoint pen-sized red papules (*no* fluid inside and *no* heat). She explained that the itch became more intense around 8 pm, causing her to vigorously scratch to the point her pores were irritated and swollen. A dermatologist prescribed antihistamines, but it did *not* relieve the itch.

I decided to prescribe Xian Fang Huo Ming Yin combining Ma Xing Yi Gan Tang and adding Di Gu Pi, but this was *not* effective either. Now, it is winter and her skin is even itchier, causing her to scratch so hard that excoriations with pus appear. I changed the formula to Blood Desiccation Formula combining Ma Gui Ge Ban Tang and adding Sheng Shi Gao and Huang Qin. Again, I am still awaiting her follow-up visit to find out if it was effective.

Please share your experiences in treating itchy skin during pregnancy. How do you treat this condition?

A: Itchy skin during pregnancy is *not* at all uncommon, especially over the abdomen and legs. The skin over the abdomen stretches, the endocrine and autonomic nervous system undergo dramatic changes, and this time in a woman's life can be a very emotional experience overall. In my clinical practice, I have treated patients with existing eczema that either returns or is further exacerbated by pregnancy.

In many other cases, I believe that the psychological and emotional challenges of pregnancy may be just as relevant as the physical changes, causing psychosomatic symptoms of itching. For instance, your patient whose itch intensifies at around 8 pm could very well be a result of dry skin from taking a hot shower at that time every evening. Try to find out what she is usually doing at 8 pm and you may have your answer.

A blood-nourishing yin-enriching and liver-emolliating dryness-moistening formula such as Blood Desiccation Formula adding Gan Cao and Long Yan Rou sounds like a good approach for these patients. Huang Qin may *not* be imperative, but come to think of it, if you wanted to add Huang Qin, then you might as well add in other fetus-quieting miscarriage-preventing medicinals such as Bai Zhu, Shan Yao, Xu Duan, and Ai Ye.

For many of my patients who present with itchy skin during pregnancy, I will prescribe Blood Desiccation Formula adding Mu Dan Pi (cools the blood), Zhi Zi (clears heat, drains fire, and cools the blood) and Di Gu Pi, Qing Hao, and Zhi Mu, (enrich yin and downbear fire, cool the blood and clear vacuity heat, and eliminate steaming bone). For patients whose etiology is obviously psychosomatic, I may even prescribe Gan Mai Da Zao Tang Combining Ban Xia Hou Po Tang along with a dose of positive encouragement and advice on resolving stress and staying healthy.

Remember! There is one *very rare* (< 1% of pregnant women) pathocondition that may also present with itchy skin called intrahepatic cholestasis of pregnancy (ICP), which is also known as obstetric cholestasis (OC). This itching usually affects the palms of the hands and soles of the feet, itching is often worse at night, there is *no* rash, and the patient may notice dark urine and pale-colored stool. It usually occurs during the third trimester of pregnancy. Patients with this pathocondition should be closely monitored by their GYN/OBN doctor because it increases the risk for pregnancy complications (e.g., preterm birth, stillbirth).

Case Study #6: Postpartum Itchy Eczema – Hypersensitivity Reaction

Q: After giving birth, this 27 y/o woman with a history of atopic dermatitis in her youth broke out in an itchy, maculopapular rash on her back, abdomen, neck, and upper and lower limbs. When it first appears, the itch is so intense that her scratching causes bleeding and leaves a lingering excoriation which takes a long time to heal. She went to see a dermatologist, who prescribed antihistamines to control the allergic (type I hypersensitivity) reaction and relieve the itch, which worked at first, but over time has become completely ineffective.

The patient suspects she has a case of "malign blood (惡血 è xuè)" in her body as a result of pregnancy. This is a commonly used colloquial saying, though technically inaccurate, that people often use here in attempts to pin down a specific cause of a malady when one is uncertain. What do you think I should prescribe for this patient?

A: Itchy skin and rashes (dermatitis/eczema) are common postpartum skin pathoconditions, especially if the patient has an atopic history. She could call it "malign blood" if she wants to, but it is simply a hypersensitivity reaction triggered by the emotional and physiological stressors of pregnancy.

As for treatment, I would prescribe an yin-enriching liver-emolliating and blood-nourishing dryness-moistening formula such as Blood Desiccation Formula adding The Three Great Yang-Supplementers, Huang Qin, Ma Huang, Yi Yi Ren, and Sheng Shi Gao. This formula should bring positive results. And for intense itchiness, you can also bleed Da Zhui (GV14) (above, on, and below), Cun Kou (Tai Yuan (LU9)), and Wei Zhong (UB40); and needle Feng Chi (GB20), Tian Zhu (UB10), He Gu (LI4), Shen Men (HT7), Zu San Li (ST36), Tai Chong (LV3), San Yin Jiao (SP6), Yin Ling Quan (SP9), and Xue Hai (SP10).

Since this patient already has an atopic predisposition and the itch is particularly intense, I doubt that this is a case of postpartum visceral agitation (depression) manifesting as psychogenic itchy skin (urticaria). However, I have had many postpartum mothers present with this *psychogenic* type of condition. For these patients, I would typically prescribe either a center-harmonizing agitation-calming and stagnation-dissipating phlegm-transforming formula, such as Gan Mai Da Zao Tang Combining Ban Xia Hou Po Tang adding Long Yan Rou; or Blood Desiccation Formula adding The Sweets (Gan Cao, Da Zao, and Long Yan Rou). These formulas will quickly resolve the itchy skin.

Case Study #7: Uterine Bleeding (Spotting) and Anemia in Pregnancy

Q: A 27 y/o primaparous woman currently in her 9th week of pregnancy with her second child explained that she had been incurring light uterine bleeding (spotting) ever since the 5th week of pregnancy. I prescribed Dang Gui San variant for 1 week with*out* any noticeable efficacy. What is the best approach for this patient going forward?

Another patient, a 29 y/o in her 6th month (2nd trimester) of pregnancy initially visited me 2 weeks ago bringing in her most recent blood test results: hemoglobin (Hb) 10 (F, 12–16 g/dL). She says she feels fatigue and malaise and believes she has anemia. After taking calcium and iron supplements, she noticed a dramatic improvement in sleep, appetite, and energy level. Do you think it is necessary for me to prescribe medicinals for this patient?

A: Light bleeding (spotting) during the first 12 weeks (1st trimester) of pregnancy is quite common and typically does *not* signal that there is a problem. The main cause of spotting in the 1st trimester is simply implantation bleeding. Heavy bleeding during the 1st trimester, on the other hand, *does* warrant concern since there may be a problem that could result in miscarriage, especially if it is accompanied by abdominal cramping, back pain, and tissue passing through the vagina with the blood.

As for treatment, I would also prescribe a blood-nourishing stasis-transforming and blood-cooling fetus-quieting formula such as Dang Gui San adding Ai Ye (1 liang) and Huang Qin (3 qian). If qi vacuity pattern is pronounced, then you could prescribe Bu Zhong Yi Qi Tang adding Huang Qin, Du Zhong, Shan Yao, Xu Duan, and Ai Ye. If this is *not* effective, then try including large doses of Huang Qi and possibly small doses of The Three Great Yang-Supplementers.

Anemia and hypovolemia commonly present during pregnancy. The TCM pharmacopoeia offers an array of effective options for the treatment of these types of prenatal and postpartum conditions. I like to prescribe You Gui Yin adding Ren Shen (powder), Xi Lu Rong (powder), and Ji Nei Jin. Also, right after giving birth and during the initial postpartum phase, you could advise the patient to suck on sliced Ren Shen decocting pieces (a minimum of 5 qian up to 1 liang per day) like a "lozenge" until it moistens, dissolves, and the remaining fibers can be swallowed. This will provide strength and energy, boost the immune system, and prevent a broad spectrum of postpartum complications, including heat (low-grade fever), malaise, and generalized pain.

Remember! Ren Shen is only for uncomplicated cases of qi, blood, and yin vacuity pattern (e.g., anemia due to excessive blood loss during delivery) that present with symptoms such as low-grade fever (~ 38 C°), malaise, and generalized pain. Obviously, if there is high fever (≥ 39 C°) along with other signs and symptoms of overt infection, then you should *not* prescribe Ren Shen in this manner. Either determine the source of the infection yourself or advise the patient to get a thorough examination and proceed from there.

Case Study #8: Idiopathic Thrombocytopenic Purpura Diagnosed During Pregnancy

Q1: A 35 y/o female patient visited me with the following history: Last year (34 y/o) she was pregnant with her first child and 2 months into pregnancy she incurred an episode of heavy uterine bleeding, prompting her to get it checked out. Test results revealed thrombocytopenia: platelets (PLT) 80,000 (normal range 150,000–400,000 μL). She was diagnosed with idiopathic thrombocytopenic purpura (ITP), was administered corticosteroids, and went on to give birth via cesarean section.

Her condition seemed to be under control up until about 3 months after giving birth, when she incurred an episode of extremely heavy menstruation (hypermenorrhagia). Her doctor recommended she receive intravenous immunoglobulin (IVIG) in hopes of getting the PLT under control again (prior to that episode of hypermenorrhagia the patient's PLT had been normal at 200,000).

That's when she decided to give TCM a try coming in for an initial consultation. Her PLT had dropped down to 44,000 by that time. I decided to prescribe Sheng Yu Tang adding The Three Great Yang-Supplementers (5 qian each), Huang Qin (3 qian), Zhu Jie Qi (1 qian), Tu Si Zi (8 qian), Ren Shen (3 qian), Lu Rong (2 qian), and Han Lian Cao (2 qian). After taking this formula for 1 month PLT dropped further down to 27,000.

Do you think adding yin-enriching fire-downbearing, blood-cooling vacuity heat-clearing, and steaming bone-eliminating medicinals such as Qing Hao, Zhi Mu, and Di Gu Pi would be effective? After I get PLT under control and stabilized at relatively normal levels, I plan on having her gradually reduce the dosage of corticosteroids by 1/3. At that time, is it necessary to add in blood-stanching medicinals such as Ai Ye and Ce Bo Ye? Thank you for your advice and guidance.

A: In TCM classical texts on pathology, ITP corresponds with descriptions of presenting symptoms that include spontaneous bleeding (衄 nu) in various parts of the body (e.g., teeth, nose, gums, ears, flesh).

Remember! These types of skin manifestations should *not* be confused with the hyperpigmentation (i.e., chloasma, linea nigra, darkened nipples) some women experience during pregnancy, which may persist months after giving birth and may eventually resolve spontaneously; or the uterine bleeding (spotting) manifestations that occur during the first 12 weeks (1st trimester) of pregnancy, which are typically just caused by implantation bleeding that will also resolve spontaneously.

Hmm!...an episode of flooding (血崩 xuè b□ng) 3 months after pregnancy, persistently low PLT, and Sheng Yu Tang (supplements and regulates blood, cools the blood and dispels stasis, and nourishes yin and supplements qi) has *not* been effective. I would try changing to either Sheng Hua Tang (expels stasis and engenders the new, quickens the blood and dispels stasis, and warms the channels and relieves pain) or Dang Gui San (nourishes blood and transforms stasis and cools the blood and quiets the fetus).

Just make sure to add The Three Great Yang-Supplementers (return and reinforce yang, "boost" the metabolism and immune system, and bolster right qi), Ren Shen (powder) (greatly supplements original qi and stems vacuity desertion, engenders liquid, promotes an increase in the transport of oxygen and nutrients in the blood, and protects cells by slowing down the rate of apoptosis), Xi Lu Rong (powder) (invigorates kidney yang, boosts essence-blood, regulates the thoroughfare and controlling vessels, and promotes hematopoiesis), Zhu Jie Qi (clears heat and resolves toxin, quickens the blood and relieves pain, disinhibits water and disperses swelling, and increases platelet count), and Huang Bo (clears heat, dries dampness, resolves toxin, and eliminates steaming. Ai Ye (warms the channels and stanches bleeding and dissipates cold and regulates menstruation) is included in Dang Gui San, and yes, you could add it into Sheng Hua Tang as well, but you definitely do *not* need to add Qing Hao, Zhi Mu, and Di Gu Pi at this time.

Q2: I am still trying to get this patient's ITP under control. Despite being administered prednisolone and IVIG, and then finally going ahead with the invasive procedure of splenectomy, she still has only been able to maintain PLT at levels of 5,000 to 20,000. I prescribed Dang Gui San adding Ai Ye, Tu Si Zi, Zhu Jie Qi, The Three Great Yang-Supplementers, Ren Shen, and Xi Lu Rong. After taking this formula for 2 weeks, her PLT went from 21,000 to 26,000, but 2 weeks later it dropped back down to 5,000.

I know that if PLT is not maintained at > 30,000 there is a considerable risk of spontaneous bleeding. What can I do to help this patient get her PLT up to safer levels and allow her to lead a healthy, symptom-free life?

A: Just as in other pathoconditions, you must accurately identify the pattern as the basis for determining treatment. In my clinical practice, the majority of ITP cases have been *liver blood vacuity* pattern (about 70% of my cases), requiring administration of a formula such as Si Wu Tang, Sheng Yu Tang, Dang Gui San, Qi Bao Mei Ran Dan, or Blood Desiccation Formula.

If the patient presents with fatigue, poor appetite, and malnutrition, then this can be identified as *spleen qi vacuity* pattern (about 10 to 15% of my cases), requiring administration of a formula such as Xiang Sha Liu Jun Zi Tang or Shen Ling Bai Zhu San.

If the renal production of thrombopoietin is insufficient, resulting in hypoplasia and fibrosis of the marrow, then this can be identified as *kidney yang vacuity* pattern (about 15 to 20% of my cases), requiring administration of a formula such as Shen Qi Wan or You Gui Yin.

For patients with splenomegaly and those who have undergone a splenectomy, this can be identified as *dual heart and spleen qi and blood vacuity* pattern, requiring administration of a formula such as Gui Pi Tang, Jia Wei Gui Pi Tang (if heat is pronounced), Ren Shen Yang Rong Tang, or Shi Quan Da Bu Tang. Just make sure to include Zhu Jie Qi, Ren Shen, Lu Rong, The Three Great Yang-Supplementers (unless, of course, heat is pronounced!), and Huang Qin (or Huang Bo).

In patients with a *poor appetite*, you can prescribe combinations of the stomach-opening medicinals such as The Digestants (Cang Zhu, Shan Zha, Gu Ya, Mai Ya, Ji Nei Jin, and Shen Qu), or spleen-fortifying dampness-percolating medicinals such as Shan Yao, Bu Zhu, and Fu Ling. This therapeutic approach will increase the patient's PLT count and maintain levels that will allow her to lead a healthy, symptom-free life.

Case Study #9: Postpartum Hair Loss – Psychological Stress

Q: A 33 y/o female patient visited me explaining that she began "losing hair" (thinning) after giving birth to her second child earlier this year during the summer. She took medication for a while, which seemed to help halt thinning and rejuvenate growth. To her dismay, when autumn rolled around the thinning recurred, shedding 100 to 150 strands of hair each day in the shower, along with reddening of both cheeks, ungratifying defecation (大便不爽 dà biàn bù shuang), bilateral rib-side pain and tenderness upon palpation, and a shortened menstrual flow (menses lasting only 3 days as opposed to her normal 5–6 days).

I prescribed Xiao Chai Hu Jia Long Gu Mu Li Tang adding Mu Dan Pi and Zhi Zi. Do you think this is a good treatment approach?

A: This sounds to me like a classic case of psychogenic hair loss (alopecia), a diagnosis further supported by her other stereotypical somatic disorder symptoms. So for this case, yes, I think your approach is right on the mark. Prescribing a Shao Yang-harmonizing and fright-settling spirit-quieting formula such as Xiao Chai Hu Tang adding Long Gu, Mu Li, Mu Dan Pi, and Zhi Zi should be effective. I would also add Yu Sheng Wan as well.

If this formula is *not* effective, then you could consider changing to a center-harmonizing agitation-calming and stagnation-dissipating phlegm-transforming formula, such as Gan Mai Da Zao Tang Combining Ban Xia Hou Po Tang, or a blood-nourishing liver-emolliating and yin-enriching dryness-moistening formula, such as Blood Desiccation Formula combining Si Ni Tang and adding Fu Ling.

After about 1 month of administration, hair loss (shedding) will resolve and in about 3–5 months hair growth will rejuvenate (sprouts of hair popping up!). For hair loss, particularly if it is concentrated in patches, but not limited to, I sometimes also apply a topical medicinal paste made of Ai Ye (Mugwort Leaf) and Dang Gui (Chinese Angelica Root) (or Bai Zhi (Dahurian Angelica Root)) on the affected area of the scalp and shine the beam of an infrared lamp over it for about 20–30 minutes. This will promote local blood circulation and enhance therapeutic efficacy.

Case Study #10: Postpartum Hair Loss Is Common – It Will Grow Back!

Q: Recently, I had another case of hair loss in a postpartum female patient. This 27 y/o received epidural anesthesia to relieve pain while giving birth last month. After a successful pregnancy, she began experiencing hair loss that her doctor diagnosed as telogen effluvium.

I identified this as yang vacuity pattern and prescribed You Gui Yin variant, but this formula has *not* been effective. Please offer your advice and suggestions.

A: Epidural anesthesia may cause transient hair loss in some people, but it is relatively rare. I tend to believe that the *psychological* stress involved in the patient "believing" that the anesthesia (a type of *physiological* stress) is the culprit, dwelling on this "overwhelmingly daunting reality" ad infinitum. She may even harbor fragmented subconscious doubts about her decision to receive this type of anesthesia, because it could have harmed her baby in some way—I have had a patient like this before!

As for treatment, yes, you could go with a kidney yang-supplementing formula, such as Shen Qi Wan or You Gui Yin, or a blood-quickening qi-supplementing formula, such as Bu Yang Huan Wu Tang.

But remember! The key here is providing the patient with emotional support and encouragement. Explain to her that postpartum hair loss is something that many women experience, and has nothing to do with the epidural anesthesia. It is the combination of physiological and psychological stressors involved with pregnancy and childbearing that cause many women to incur this temporary annoyance. Explain to her that she is still young and vibrant; her hair will grow back quickly and be even fuller and more radiant than before. Don't worry…just relax…and let your hair grow!

Case Study #11: Postpartum Joint Pain and Cold and Numbness of the Extremities

Q: Since accumulating more experience in treating prenatal and postpartum patients, I have discovered that a lot of women experience joint pain and cold and numbness of the extremities following child birth. For these types of patients, I usually prescribe Shi Quan Da Bu Tang variant, but unfortunately, I have not had much success. How do you treat these types of postpartum ailments?

A: Shi Quan Da Bu Tang (quickens and supplements the blood, boosts qi and fortifies the spleen, and supplements kidney yang) is one possibility for these types of aches, pain, coldness, and numbness. However, depending on the specific quality and location of symptoms, you could also consider prescribing other liver- and kidney-supplementing, qi- and blood-supplementing, and dampness-eliminating pain-relieving formulas such as Gui Qi Jian Zhong Tang, San Bi Tang, Du Huo Ji Sheng Tang, or You Gui Yin.

As a general rule, for joint pain and cold and numbness of the extremities, I like to prescribe either Gui Qi Jian Zhong Tang (supplements qi, blood and kidney yang) or Dang Gui Si Ni Tang (nourishes blood and dissipates cold and warms the channels and frees the vessels), making sure to include Huang Qi (large dose), Wu Zhu Yu, and Gan Jiang. And in colder climates or during the winter months, I make sure to add larger doses of The Three Great Yang-Supplementers, Wu Zhu Yu, Ma Huang, and Chuan Jiao.

If the patient presents with generalized aches and pain throughout the entire body and/or separated symphysis pubis, then I would prescribe Du Huo Ji Sheng Tang (supplements the liver and kidney, supplements qi and blood, and eliminates dampness and relieves pain). Du Huo Ji Sheng Tang is a major formula (大方 dà f□ ng) that is very bulky when decocting pieces are prescribed for decoction (as opposed to extract powder/granules) and also contains some very expensive medicinals such as Ren Shen, Shou Di Huang (traditional yellow wine and sun-dried processing method), Gui Ban, and Bie Jia.

Remember! Postpartum depression (aka "baby blues") is another consideration that you must rule out. In TCM, this condition can be classified as visceral agitation, and for these patients you should add large doses of The Sweets (Gan Cao, Da Zao, and Long Yan Rou) and Yu Sheng Wan to your formula.

Case Study #12: Postpartum Hives

Q: A 28 y/o female patient visited me explaining that 2 months after giving birth she began breaking out in hives. A dermatologist diagnosed her with urticaria (hives) and prescribed antihistamines, which resolved the condition for 1 to 2 days, but then the hives returned again. A severe episode would include difficulty swallowing (possibly angioedema involving the mucus membranes of the throat) along with erythematous, oval-shaped wheals and papules on her buttocks, abdomen, back, neck and inner aspects of her elbows. She also said that eating greasy food seemed to trigger and exacerbate the outbreaks.

I have prescribed Blood Desiccation Formula adding Ma Huang, Qing Hao, Zhi Mu, Di Gu Pi, and Lian Qiao for 1 month now, but the patient still gets the hives! How would you treat this patient?

A: Yes, this certainly sounds like a hypersensitivity reaction, possibly prompted by a combination of blood vacuity, inadequate nutritional intake, and hormonal changes from pregnancy. In TCM, this can be classified as construction-defense disharmony (營衛不調 yíng wèi bù tiáo), resulting in either exterior wind-heat pattern at the onset (or during flare-ups) that may evolve into blood desiccation pattern later on in the postacute and chronic stages.

You have identified this patient's condition as blood desiccation pattern with blood heat. During the patient's next visit, make sure to verify that this is the correct pattern and modify your formula accordingly.

Remember! For postpartum patients, you must always consider the possibility of visceral agitation (postpartum depression) as well. Thus, you could also try a center-harmonizing agitation-calming and stagnation-dissipating phlegm-transforming formula such as Gan Mai Da Zao Tang Combining Ban Xia Hou Po Tang (including large doses of Hong Zao) adding Long Yan Rou (large dose), Ma Huang, Xing Ren, Rou Gui, Lu Lu Tong, and Yu Sheng Wan. This approach should effectively address both the physiological and psychological aspects of postpartum hives.

Case Study #13: Postpartum Urinary Retention

Q: One week ago, a 29 y/o female gave birth via vaginal delivery, with subsequent postpartum urinary retention. The obstetrician in charge went ahead with the standard protocol of catheritization to induce urination. When the patient returned home 48 hours later, she still was unable to urinate normally (only voided a small volume despite ample fluid intake and felt distention in the lower abdomen).

Her husband sought my consultation to treat this condition and regulate her constitution. I prescribed (Yu Sheng) Wu Ling San (Nephritis Formula) including large doses of Fu Ling, Bai Zhu, and Ze Xie. Do you think this is the right approach?

A: Postpartum urinary retention (aka postpartum voiding dysfunction) is a relatively common complication in women who give birth via vaginal delivery, which is likely caused by trauma to the bladder and pelvic floor muscles and nerves during delivery. In classical TCM pathology, this condition corresponds with shifted bladder (轉胞 zhuan b□ o).

As for treatment, the first thing you can do to promote micturition is simply needle the acupoints San Yin Jiao (SP6), Tai Chong (LV2), and Zu San Li (ST30). In the majority of cases, this will be effective. If you still need to prescribe a formula, I would prescribe a water-disinhibiting dampness-percolating, yang-warming qi-transforming, qi-moving blood-quickening, and pain-relieving formula such as (Yu Sheng) Wu Ling San (Calculi Formula)—*not* (Nephritis Formula)!—for its capacity to disinhibit water by bland percolation and promote smooth muscle contractions in the urinary tract. This should do the trick!

Note: Shifted bladder is a TCM classical pathologic term that specifically refers to urinary stoppage in pregnancy (妊娠小便不通 rèn sh□ n xiao biàn bù t□ ng), occurring when the fetus compresses on the mother's urinary bladder and resulting in lower abdominal distention with mild pain and urinary stoppage. However, Dr. Lee applies a broader interpretation and application of the term to encompass the postpartum complications of urinary retention (stoppage) as well.

Case Study #14: Persistent Postpartum Urinary Retention

Q: Right now, I have another patient with postpartum urinary retention. A residual urine volume of as much as 1,500 ml was measured, prompting her to receive continuous catheritization for 2 weeks until she was able to urinate on her own. The problem is that she can only void 80 ml to 140 ml of urine at a time, and she still has dribbling urinary block (癃閉 lóng bì).

This situation has been going on for 8 months already. How can I help this patient regain normal urination?

A: Prolonged labor, epidural analgesia, episiotomy, instrumental delivery, nulliparity, vaginal and perineal laceration, fetal macrosomia (newborn has a birth weight of more than 4,000 grams (8 pounds, 13 ounces)), or a previous history of voiding difficulty are risk factors for postpartum voiding dysfunction. Urinary retention is a rather common complication of pregnancy (10–15% of pregnancies depending on how it is defined) with most cases resolving either spontaneously or following catheritization.

In these types of patients with urinary retention and dribbling urinary block despite receiving catheritization, you must also rule out the possibility of frequent urination resulting in a relatively small urine volume during each micturition (which adds up!). Naturally, you must take into consideration physiological absorption of water: for instance, if 3,000 ml is ingested and 1,200–2,000 ml is excreted, then this is normal; but if only 800–1,000 ml is excreted, then this would be considered pathological, requiring treatment.

If the total urine volume is normal, but each urine volume is too small, then this may be caused by neurogenic bladder (i.e., flaccid, spastic, or mixed) that results in uncoordinated bladder contraction and urinary sphincter synergy (i.e., detrusor-sphincter dyssynergia). To correct this imbalance (dyssynergia), I like to prescribe a qi-moving counterflow-downbearing, stagnation-dissipating phlegm-transforming, and liver-coursing depression-resolving formula such as Gan Mai Da Zao Tang Combining Ban Xia Hou Po Tang, Wen Dan Tang, Xiao Yao San, Si Qi Tang, or Qi Qi Tang.

Remember! You should also monitor BUN and CR levels to determine if there is any renal damage. High residual urine volume (1,500 ml is high!) could lead to hypovolemia and result in insufficient blood supply to the kidneys (renal hypoperfusion). If renal function has been compromised, then consider prescribing either a kidney yang-supplementing formula variant, such as Shen Qi Wan or You Gui Yin, or a kidney yang-warming qi transformation-promoting and bland-percolating dampness- and water-disinhibiting formula, such as Wu Ling San (Nephritis Formula).

If there is frequent urination with only small amounts excreted each time (total volume remains low), along with sagging distention in the lower abdomen, then this suggests the possibility of uterine prolapse or bladder prolapse (cystocele), which can be identified as qi vacuity pattern, requiring administration of Bu Zhong Yi Qi Tang or Gui Zhi Ren Shen Tang.

Case Study #15: Separated Symphysis Pubis

Q: A 33 y/o multiparous female patient visited me seeking consultation and treatment for a separated symphysis pubis (aka pubic symphysis diastasis) that occurred during delivery of her third child. She gave birth about 1 month ago, but she said the pain in her pelvis is so bad sometimes that she can't even stand up from a sitting position.

My wife just recently gave birth to our first child, and I can imagine how much the additional discomfort and pain of this type of condition could put a damper on a happy newborn household. I prescribed Bu Zhong Yi Qi Tang variant. Do you think this is a good approach? What about adding other medicinals?

A: Definitely! A spleen-fortifying qi-supplementing, yang-upbearing fall-raising, and blood-supplementing and -quickening formula like Bu Zhong Yi Qi Tang is the right approach for this mother with a separated symphysis pubis.

However, I would also make sure to include a large dose of Huang Qi (supplements qi and upbears yang and disinhibits water and disperses swelling) and add Du Zhong and Xu Duan (serve as lumbus (spine) and lower limb conductors, supplement the liver and kidney, and strengthen sinew and bone), Yan Hu Suo and Mu Xiang (quicken the blood, move qi, and relieve pain), The Three Great Yang-Supplementers (warm the channels and free the network vessels, supplement fire and assist yang, dissipate cold and relieve pain), and Huang Qin (counterbalances the heat). And you should also perform acupuncture on these acupoints: Tai Chong (LV3), San Yin Jiao (SP6), Cheng Jiang (CV24), and Bai Hui (GV20).

Remember! For some patients presenting with postpartum lumbar pain, you must also consider the possibility of commonly presenting postpartum conditions, such as depression ("baby blues"), which can be classified as a type of *visceral agitation* (臟躁 zàng zào), and *anemia*.

For *visceral agitation* that presents with aching pain, I would consider prescribing a spleen- and stomach-supplementing, phlegm-damp-transforming, and blood-nourishing wind-stabilizing formula such as Ban Xia Tian Ma Bai Zhu San adding Du Zhong and The Sweets.

If the postpartum lumbar pain extends through to the lower abdomen and down around the pubic symphysis and ischium, then it may be caused by excessive blood loss after delivery (postpartum hemorrhage) that results in low blood volume (hypovolemia) and *anemia*. Patients with low blood volume may present with symptoms of a high fever, headache, chills, and body aches, especially in cases of profuse lochia (vaginal discharge) after delivery. In cases of severe *anemia*, pronounced chills with pain will present, so intense that the patient will feel the need to sleep covered up with a heavy blanket even in the sweltering heat of the summer.

That's exactly what happened to my wife after giving birth to our first child. So right after she gave birth to our second child, I immediately prescribed a simple regimen of an *exceptionally* large daily dose (approximately 4 liang (150 g)) of sliced Ren Shen decocting pieces for about 4 to 5 days up until her symptoms resolved and she was discharged from the hospital. She took the sliced Ren Shen pieces throughout the day like a "lozenge"—placed in the mouth until it moistens, can be chewed on, and eventually dissolves, with the remaining fibers swallowed or spit out. Ren Shen greatly supplements original qi and stems vacuity desertion, supplements the spleen and boosts the lung, engenders liquid, and quiets the spirit. From a modern physiological perspective, it has the capacity to promote an increase in the transport of oxygen and nutrients in the blood and protect cells by slowing down the rate of apoptosis.

Plus, I had Du Huo Ji Sheng Tang (boosts the liver and kidney, supplements qi and blood, dispels wind-damp, relieves impediment pain) stewed with either turtle meat (boosts yin and supplements the blood) or lamb (boosts qi and supplements vacuity and warms the center and mildly precipitates) prepared as *medicinal food* for her to eat throughout the month-long postpartum rest and recuperation period (坐月子 zuò yuè zi). And I also prescribed You Gui Yin (warms and supplements kidney yang, quickens the blood and dissipates stasis, strengthens sinew and bone, and eliminates dampness and relieves pain) to take as a *medicinal decoction*

This second pregnancy went smoothly without any postpartum complications. This therapeutic approach was able to give her body the extra boost she needed, regulating her constitution to quickly regain strength and vitality. We applied this approach during her third pregnancy with the same successful results.

Case Study #16: Bad Breath After Pregnancy

Q: A 35 y/o primiparous mother recently came with the chief complaint as follows: Ever since giving birth 2 months ago she has had uncharacteristic bouts of bad breath every time she eats white radish (*Raphanus sativus* L. var. longipinnatus Bailey) and chili peppers and when she has an empty stomach and feels nervous. She also has hard and irregular stools (1 stool/3–5 days), nasal congestion, and an enlarged thyroid gland. The patient thinks that hormonal changes during pregnancy are the cause of her bad breath and general malaise.

These changes may be a factor, but I think some of her problems could be caused by postpartum depression ("baby blues"). I prescribed Wen Dan Tang adding Da Huang, but her symptoms remained the same. Then, I switched to Ru Mo Si Wu Tang combining Gui Zhi Fu Ling Wan (to treat blood amassment in the lower burner), but this was also *not* effective. Could this be a problem with the nose or olfactory function? What do you think?

A: After giving birth, the mother is in a state of hormonal flux as the body gradually works its way back to normal. Estrogen and progesterone levels *drop* dramatically, which for some women may result in the "baby blues" (postpartum depression), while oxytocin (the "bonding hormone") *soars*, making the mother susceptible to anxiety.

In rare instances, thyroid hormone levels also *increase* following pregnancy, resulting in hyperthyroidism at first and then evolving into hypothyroidism (*low* thyroid hormone levels) later on with the possible manifestation of goiter and other symptoms. And then there are the physical changes to the body…really a lot of things going on in the woman's life! For some women, these challenges are compounded by the emotional factors faced with family (e.g., spousal, in-laws) and/or career pressures.

These hormonal fluctuations and changes in pH levels may make some more susceptible to bad breath. A simple way to treat this is by advising the patient to drink lots of water (try adding some fresh lemon and mint!), rinse her mouth with water frequently, and brush her teeth after every meal. Depending on whether you have a decent rapport with the patient and she feels like talking about her family situation and environment, you could try to further suss out if there are any underlying pressures or stressors going on in her life, such as strained relationships with her in-laws, unfulfilled expectations involving the tradition of valuing male offspring and belittling females, etc. Maybe you can be of some emotional support and assistance, encouraging her to stay positive and work through the challenges.

If you determine that your initial assessment of postpartum depression ("baby blues") is at the heart of her ailments, then I would prescribe a center-harmonizing agitation-calming and stagnation-dissipating phlegm-transforming formula such as Gan Mai Da Zao Combining Ban Xia Hou Po Tang (for the "baby blues" and enlarged thyroid) adding Sheng Shi Gao and Huang Qin (for the stomach heat), Ma Huang, Bai Zhi, and Xin Yi (or Xi Xin) (for the nasal congestion), and Long Yan Rou and Yu Sheng Wan (for the anxiety).

Remember! You must also rule out gum disease (e.g., periodontitis) and gastrointestinal disorders (e.g., gastric, duodenal, and esophageal ulcers, gastroesophageal reflux disease (GERD)). If the patient notices bleeding gums (牙衄 yá nu) when eating or brushing her teeth, then this suggests gum disease, which can be identified as stomach heat or kidney yin vacuity pattern. Gastrointestinal disorders can similarly be identified as stomach heat and center burner heat pattern, resulting in putrid belching (噯氣腐臭 □i qì fu chòu), sour belching (噯酸 □i su□n), or belching of sour putrid qi (gas) (噯氣酸腐 □i qì su□n fu).

Naturally, you will need to accurately diagnosis the condition and conduct pattern identification as the basis for determining treatment.

If she hasn't already, it may be a good idea to advise her to make a trip to the dentist to get her gums checked out.

Case Study #17: Low Breast Milk Supply

Q: A few days ago a couple in their early 30's came to visit me explaining that the woman recently gave birth and had been breastfeeding the baby without any problems. Then, she began taking antibiotics for the treatment of periodontitis and noticed a drastic drop in breast milk supply (hypogalactia). She said there wasn't enough milk to feed her baby.

I prescribed Gui Qi Jian Zhong Tang adding Ren Shen and Niu Bang Zi and will see the patient again next week for a follow-up. How would you treat this patient?

A: I have had many mothers come in with claims of reduced milk production after taking various medications, including antibiotics, but I am *not* convinced there is a direct correlation. Most likely the patient is either not milking properly or there is some other underlying cause (e.g., insufficient glandular tissue). Milk must be removed often and well, on a supply and demand basis—meaning the more milk that is extracted from the breasts (and the more often), the more milk the breasts will produce.

However, you should remind patients that for almost any type of infection and inflammation, whether it be during the breastfeeding period or otherwise, TCM treatment can provide be administered *instead* of Western medicine antimicrobial (e.g., antibiotics) and anti-inflammatory (e.g., corticosteroids) agents. For instance, it is relatively common for breastfeeding mothers to incur mastitis, requiring administration of Xian Fang Huo Ming Yin adding Huang Qin, Pu Gong Ying, Zhi Zi, Mu Dan Pi, Fu Ling, and Ze Xie. Taking TCM medicinals will provide exceptional efficacy at resolving the infection, alleviate any concerns of adverse effects on the quality and quantity of milk, and preserve rotund breast shape (no sagging!).

Remember! Huang Lian Jie Du Tang, which includes The Three Yellows, provides exceptional broad-spectrum antimicrobial and anti-inflammatory action for the treatment of infection and inflammation throughout the entire body.

If the patient really does have a low supply of milk and you determine it is caused by insufficient glandular tissue (IGT) (aka mammary hypoplasia), then I would consider prescribing either a blood-quickening blood-supplementing, qi-boosting spleen-fortifying, and kidney yang-supplementing formula, such as Shi Quan Da Bu Tang, Gui Qi Jian Zhong Tang, or Ren Shen Yang Rong Tang; or a kidney yang-supplementing formula, such as You Gui Wan or Shen Qi Wan. Just make sure to include Gan Jiang, Fu Zi, Huang Qi, Niu Bang Zi, Dan Shen, and Dang Shen (or Ren Shen). This will effectively stimulate glandular tissue and promote the production of milk.

While we are on the topic, I think it is worth mentioning that nowadays most people have major misconceptions that breastfeeding somehow causes the breasts to become smaller afterwards. Actually, in my experience, the reality is entirely the opposite. The breasts are at their fullest and most vibrant during the postpartum stage when the mother is breastfeeding—the more the mother nurses the infant, the more the mammary glands and breast tissue will expand. I would recommend to mothers that if they wanted to have fuller and larger breasts, then by all means, breastfeed! The milk secreted by the mammary glands and fed to the infant comes from the nutrients absorbed and metabolized from the mother's diet, not from her glandular and adipose tissue, so her breasts will not get smaller! Remember! The "size" is based on the breasts prior to pregnancy and *not* the size of the engorged breasts after pregnancy and during the nursing period. Naturally, the breasts may be "smaller" relative to when breastfeeding, but *not* in comparison to original size!

Plus, some women, especially professional women with careers to get back to, opt to receive galactagogue injections (i.e., containing factors that regulate lactation such as prolactin and oxytocin) to promote lactation in order to get back to work right after the month-long postpartum rest and recuperation period (坐月子 zuò yuè zi). These types of drugs increase hormone levels (either indirectly or directly) to *dramatically* boost milk production, but also bring the risk of mammary gland atrophy and other side effects (some severe!), such as abdominal cramps, diarrhea, nausea, hives, hyperprolactinemia, hypogonadism, menstrual irregularities, ventricular arrhythmias, and infant toxicity.

Thus, unless absolutely necessary, I would discourage patients from receiving quick-fix hormone injections or taking drugs; otherwise, what started out as plump "steamed buns" may turn into shriveled "dumplings" or even flat "pasta." The best way to stimulate prolactin production in the body and promote lactation is the natural way, by eating a healthy, well-rounded diet. Some foods that are known to naturally increase breast milk production are whole grains, papaya, chives, Chinese yam, dandelion root, Brewer's yeast, asparagus, garlic, red beets, and many types of seeds (e.g., sesame, poppy, anise, coriander).

Section 5: Other Gynecological Disorders

Case Study #1: Iron Deficiency Anemia

Q: Many patients, especially women, have sought treatment for iron deficiency anemia (IDA). The most common symptoms are shortage of qi (lack of energy), heavy body, inability to get food down, glomus and oppression below the heart, stuffiness in the chest, scant menstrual flow (with many blood clots), difficult defecation (constipation), dizziness, and a predisposition to contracting interstitial cystitis (lower abdominal spasms).

In most patients, symptoms will improve when they are taking iron and vitamin supplements, but once they stop, the symptoms return again. In the past, I have usually prescribed Ban Xia Tian Ma Bai Zhu San variant to supplement the spleen and stomach, transform phlegm-damp, and nourish the blood and stabilize wind.

But recently, I have thought about how IDA can also be identified as a type of blood desiccation pattern, and thus have included a large dose of Dang Gui in the formula. What do you think about this treatment approach?

A: For patients with IDA (a type of microcytic anemia), the most effective formula I have prescribed is either You Gui Yin (warms and supplements kidney yang, quickens the blood and dissipates stasis, strengthens sinew and bone, and eliminates dampness and relieves pain) or Sheng Yu Tang (supplements blood and qi, dispels stasis, and nourishes yin). Just make sure to include The Three Great Yang-Supplementers, Huang Qin, Ren Shen/Chuan Qi Powder, and Xi Lu Rong (powder).

Though I seriously *doubt* there is any correlation between the two, if your patient does happen to have interstitial cystitis, then you could also add Long Dan Cao, Zhi Zi, and Pu Huang. And for the constipation, though Gan Di Huang and Dang Gui do contain stool-softening actions, as long as you add Da Huang the patient will most certainly be good to go!

Yes, I agree with the blood desiccation classification. You could try prescribing an yin-enriching liver-emolliating and blood-nourishing dryness-moistening formula such as Blood Desiccation Formula, Qi

Bao Mei Ran Tang, or Di Huang Yin Zi. Just make sure to include The Three Great Yang-Supplementers, Huang Qin, Ren Shen/Chuan Qi Powder, and Xi Lu Rong (powder). If this approach is *not* effective, then I would change the formula to You Gui Yin variant.

On a related topic, recently I have been treating a patient with aplastic anemia caused by bone marrow insufficiency (spinal tap revealed myelofibrosis). Despite trying the gamut of therapeutic modalities, it has been necessary for the patient to receive regular blood transfusions. If the patient goes only 2 weeks without a transfusion, the hemoglobin (Hb) drops down to 5 (F, 12–16 g/dL) and platelets (PLT) < 50,000 (150,000–400,000 μL). However, after prescribing a 2-week regimen of You Gui Yin adding The Three Great Yang-Supplementers, Huang Qin, Ren Shen/Chuan Qi Powder, and Xi Lu Rong (powder), with the same amount of blood transfusion, the patient has already been able to maintain blood Hb levels of between 6.3–6.5. This is encouraging progress that the patient and I hope to continue building on!

Case Study #2: Intensely Itchy, Milky Grayish-Colored Vaginal Discharge with a Fishy Odor

Q: A 28 y/o female patient visited me with a history of vaginal itching and discharge that she said got so bad at times that she didn't even want to leave the house. Her gynecologist prescribed a topical antibiotic cream, and after 2 months of application, the itch and discharge completely resolved. But not long after, the condition returned and was even worse than before: more intensely itchy and the discharge turned into a milky grayish color with a fishy odor so profuse it required her to change her underwear 3–4x/day.

She went back to see her gynecologist and this time she was administered both oral and topical medication, which reduced the amount of vaginal discharge, but the itch and odor remained. Examination of her vaginal fluid revealed insufficient levels of commensal bacteria, likely killed off by the antibiotics, resulting in an altered vaginal microbiota that is making it difficult for her body to fight infection. Seems like she may be caught up in a vicious ("viscous") cycle!

To break that "viscous" cycle, I decided on a dual treatment approach, consisting of Bu Zhong Yi Qi Tang combining Long Dan Xie Gan Tang adding Ku Shen. Fortifying the spleen and supplementing qi can help boost the immune system and promote the growth of commensal bacteria, while draining liver-gallbladder repletion fire and clearing damp-heat in the lower burner can fight any residual microbial infection.

After taking this formula for 1 week, the patient came back for follow-up and said that her symptoms had improved. Do you have any suggestions or advice on modifying this formula going forward? What would you prescribe for this type of patient?

A: Intensely itchy, milky grayish-colored vaginal discharge (vulvovaginitis) with a fishy odor can be identified as liver channel damp-heat pouring downward pattern. In our modern industrialized world with access to excellent nutrition and healthcare, it would be an exceptionally rare case for a patient to present with spleen qi vacuity pattern. Plus, sexual promiscuity is much more socially accepted nowadays than in times of antiquity when the TCM classics were scribed, so we must also take that into consideration when evaluating etiology and pathomechanisms.

Thus, for this type of patient, Long Dan Xie Gan Tang variant is the optimal selection. If itch is pronounced, then add She Chuang Zi, Ci Zi Li, and Zao Jiao Ci. If the itch has resolved, but there is still profuse and viscous white vaginal discharge (leukorrhea), then you can consider adding Jin Ying Zi, Sheng Long Gu, and Sheng Mu Li (or simply combining Jin Suo Gu Jing Wan to your formula instead). If this condition persistently recurs, then the patient's sexual partner(s) should also be examined and treated if necessary. Otherwise, this problem will just keep going back and forth like ping pong!

Remember! For quicker results, you can also consider prescribing (Yu Sheng) Vaginal Suppository (clears heat and resolves toxin, kills worms and relieves itch, and dispels wind and eliminates dampness), an effective way to help fight the infection and resolve the itch. This multifaceted approach will provide the best possible treatment.

I would only consider prescribing a spleen-fortifying qi-supplementing formula such as Bu Zhong Yi Qi Tang if the patient presents with *extremely* profuse, thin, watery discharge that soaks through repeated pad changes. In this type of case, the excessive loss of fluid could lead to qi vacuity fall (氣虛下陷 qì x□ xià xiàn), uterine prolapse, or even hypovolemic shock.

Case Study #3: Bowenoid Papulosis

Q: A couple brought their 10 y/o girl in for a visit, explaining that she had multiple white papules on her labia and following a thorough medical examination (including biopsy) she was diagnosed with bowenoid papulosis (BP). Her doctor told the parents there was a chance for these lesions to become cancerous and thus advised that the child be administered drug therapy and consider laser ablation. The parents were devastated by this news.

The parents wanted to try other methods of treatment first so I prescribed Long Dan Xie Gan Tang variant and am awaiting their return for follow-up in 1 week. What do think about this case? How did the girl contract these lesions in the first place? Is it necessary to undergo laser ablation? What formula would you prescribe?

A: Just as many other pathologies, including genital warts, this pathocondition is likely caused by a virus (e.g., human papillomavirus (HPV)), which is often transmitted by sexual contact, but can also be transmitted vertically from the mother to baby and possibly even fomites (e.g., objects such as towels). The vast majority of cases are benign (about 97%) and many cases spontaneously resolve, though recurrence is possible. Thus, I would definitely take a wait-and-see approach. You can try to reassure the parents that malignant transformation is exceedingly rare, and if possible, to not worry too much about it.

As for TCM medicinals, yes, my first choice would be a liver and gallbladder repletion fire-draining and lower burner damp-heat-clearing formula such as Long Dan Xie Gan Tang variant. However, if the taste is too bitter for the girl to stomach, then you could also prescribe a heat-clearing toxin-resolving, swelling-dispersing hardness-breaking, and blood-quickening pain-relieving formula such as Xian Fang Huo Ming Yin. Just make sure to add She Chuang Zi, Ci Ji Li, and Yi Yi Ren into your formula.

I would also add Wan Ling Dan (resolves toxin and disperses welling-abscesses and lowers the viral load in the blood), which includes a small dose of Xiong Huang (potent antimicrobial and anticancer actions) in its composition. Start out at a dosage of 1 pill/1x/day and gradually increase to 3 pills/3x/day. You can also consider adding Xiao Ji and Da Ji (dissipate stasis, resolve toxin, and disperse welling-abscesses). And if there is scarring left behind from the healing process, then you can add Ma Huang, Xing Ren, and Yi Yi Ren.

Remember! Typically, an adult dosage is prescribed for a patient who weighs ≥ 40 kg, and that includes children and adolescents as well. However, for infants and children who weigh < 40 kg, you must adjust the dosage accordingly! For example, if your 10 y/o patient with a viral infection weighs 20 kg, then I would prescribe half the normal adult dosage of all the medicinals included in your formula. That means for Wan Ling Dan, instead of starting out at 1 pill/3x/day, I would start out at .33 pill/3x/day and gradually increase to a maximum of 1 pill/3x/day.

Case Study #4: Prepubescent Girl with White Vaginal Discharge

Q: A mother brought in her 9 y/o girl who has white, malodorous vaginal discharge (usually thin fluid, but occasionally foamy in consistency). She had been treated by several other TCM doctors previously with*out* effectiveness, and now she wants to see if I can help.

I prescribed a week's prescription of Long Dan Xie Gan Tang adding Qian Shi, She Chuang Zi, Ku Lian Zi, Mu Li, and Xiong Huang, and will find out if there has been any improvement in symptoms during her next visit. Do you think this is a good formula?

A: Vaginal discharge is very common in young girls—lack of estrogen, neutral pH, hygiene issues, and fecal contamination are all factors that make prepubescent girls more susceptible to infection and inflammation. Malodorous, foamy, white vaginal discharge certainly indicates infection, which is most likely bacterial (e.g., streptococcus, *E. coli*, *Gardnerella vaginalis*, *Haemophilus influenzae*), but could also be a yeast infection (i.e., *Candida albicans*).

Regardless of the type of evil qi (邪氣 xié qì) (aka pathogenic factor), genitourinary tract infections such as vulvovaginitis can be identified as liver channel damp-heat pouring downward pattern. So, yes, Long Dan Xie Gan Tang will definitely provide effective treatment. However, if you wanted to modify the formula, then I would consider including a large dose of Long Dan Cao (drains repletion heat in the liver and gallbladder and clears and eliminates lower burner damp-heat) and adding combinations of heat-clearing blood-cooling medicinals (e.g., Mu Dan Pi, Zhi Zi, Pu Gong Ying) and dampness-disinhibiting medicinals (e.g., Fu Ling, Lian Xu, Fu Ping)

You do *not* need to add She Chuang Zi (unless itch is pronounced) or Qian Shi, Ku Lian Zi, Long Gu, and Mu Li (unless there is profuse and viscous white vaginal discharge (leukorrhea)), and Xiong Huang is definitely *not* advisable for oral administration, especially for a young patient with a mild pathocondition such as this. If necessary, you could prescribe Antimicrobial Wash (clears heat and resolves toxin, kills worms and relieves itch, dispels wind and eliminates dampness, and closes sores and engenders flesh), an immersion and wash therapy that includes the potent toxin-resolving worm-killing (antimicrobial) medicinals Xiong Huang and Liu Huang, but is safe, because it is only for topical application.

Case Study #5: Genital Warts – Depressed Heat Toxin Brewing in the Liver Channel

Q: A 31 y/o female patient tested positive for human papillomavirus (HPV) during a routine gynecological examination when she was 25 y/o. Four years later, at the age of 29, she developed genital warts (condylomata acuminata). At that time, she was administered a topical medication that eventually resolved the cauliflower-like lesions. But a year later, at the age of 30, the lesions returned, and this time the topical medication was *not* effective. Thus, she decided to have a laser ablation procedure performed.

Recently, the genital warts grew back again, and that is why she came to see me for help. Based on her history, how would you treat this patient?

A: Typically, infection with HPV that manifests in genital lesions can be identified as depressed heat brewing in the liver channel pattern. The first-line formula for this type of pathocondition is a liver and gallbladder repletion fire-draining and lower burner damp-heat-clearing formula such as Long Dan Xie Gan Tang or Dang Gui Long Hui Wan. If itch is pronounced, then you should add Ci Ji Li, Zao Jiao Ci, and She Chuang Zi.

For cases of recalcitrant anogential warts and when symptoms are particularly problematic, I would also recommend adding Wan Ling Dan (resolves toxin and disperses welling-abscesses, soothes the sinews and quickens the blood, dispels wind and relieves pain, and effectively lowers the viral load in the blood). And once the brunt of the lesions have resolved, you can also consider adding Ma Huang, Xing Ren, and Yi Yi Ren to promote suppleness of the tissue and prevent scarring.

Additionally, you could prescribe (Yu Sheng) Antimicrobial Wash (clears heat and resolves toxin, kills worms and relieves itch, dispels wind and eliminates dampness, and closes sores and engenders flesh), an immersion and wash therapy that includes potent toxin-resolving worm-killing (antimicrobial) medicinals, to fight the virus both inside and out.

In certain cases, I have also prescribed Xian Fang Huo Ming Yin adding Long Dan Cao (large dose), Ru Mo Si Wu Tang adding Huang Qin and Long Dan Cao (large doses of each), and Xiao Chai Hu Tang adding Long Dan Cao (large dose). These approaches have also provided effective treatment. Just make sure to include Long Dan Cao, an essential liver and gallbladder repletion heat-draining and lower burner damp-heat-clearing and -eliminating medicinal.

Case Study #6: Menopausal Transition – Loss of Libido

Q: This 46 y/o female patient had been experiencing vaginal dryness, inability to become sexually aroused, and a complete lack of sexual desire for at least the past 6 months. Worried that this might have a negative impact on her marriage, she went in for a gynecological examination. Her gynecologist diagnosed her with ovarian insufficiency, likely resulting from menopausal transition, and recommended hormone replacement therapy (HRT) (estrogen and progestin).

However, she was concerned about the potential side effects of HRT and decided to see if TCM could help. What is the best approach for treating this patient?

A: These types of symptoms involving loss of libido—vaginal dryness, painful intercourse (dyspareunia), inability to become sexually aroused, and lack of sexual desire—are very common in women as they approach the mid-century mark when menopausal transition usually begins to take place. For patients who do *not* want to risk the potential side effects of long-term HRT administration (e.g., increased risk of uterine cancer, breast cancer, stroke, heart attacks, blood clots, and stress urinary incontinence), I like to prescribe the yin and yang neutrally-supplementing, subduing and settling, and securing and astringing formula Gui Zhi Jia Long Gu Mu Li Tang adding Zi He Che and Yu Sheng Wan. And during cold weather months, I will add Gan Jiang, Fu Zi, and Huang Qin.

You could also consider prescribing (Yu Sheng) Vaginal Suppository (or Antimicrobial Wash), which includes She Chuang Zi (warms the kidney and invigorates yang) and Liu Huang (supplements fire and reinforces yang). If this approach does not provide effective results, then try changing to an yin-enriching liver-emolliating and blood-nourishing dryness-moistening formula such as Blood Desiccation Formula adding She Chuang Zi and Yin Yang Huo. And if the condition is recalcitrant, then consider adding Liu Huang (powder).

In times of antiquity, a much more common cause of loss of libido in women was sacroiliac tuberculosis. Nowadays, with the widespread availability of healthcare services and the use of antibiotics, this is very rare in advanced industrialized societies. Nowadays, a problem I see arising more frequently is the excessive use of antibiotics that kill off the "healthy" vaginal flora (microbiota) and alter the capacity of the mucous membranes to secrete adequate amounts of vaginal lubricating fluid. This results in painful intercourse and potentially the loss of interest in sexual activity.

For patients who have a history of excessive use of antibiotics, I will typically prescribe a liver-coursing qi-rectifying and Shao Yang depressed heat-clearing formula, such as Xiao Chai Hu Tang, or a blood-nourishing yin-enriching and heat-clearing blood-cooling formula, such as Di Gu Pi Yin. Just make sure to include medicinals that nourish yin, engender liquid, and moisten dryness (e.g., Tian Men Dong and Mai Men Dong) and that enrich yin and downbear fire, cool the blood and clear vacuity heat, and eliminate steaming bone (e.g., Qing Hao, Zhi Mu, and Di Gu Pi).

Case Study #7: Can TCM Medicinals Increase Breast Size?

Q: When I was in high school and college, I remember going on dates with one young woman in particular who it seemed did not have any mammary glands or adipose tissue on her chest whatsoever, just nipples. We got along fairly well, but our relationship never really developed very far for various reasons, *not* the breasts! After studying traditional Korean (Chinese) medicine and Western medicine, and going on to become a doctor, this was never really a topic on my mind, either personally or professionally.

Well, that was until recently, when to my surprise, I have had a number of adolescent and young women (high school and college) come to visit me asking whether or not TCM can help increase the size of their underdeveloped breasts (micromastia). I really don't have experience at treating this condition and am not sure that TCM can help. What is your perspective on this?

A: Naturally, you must first assess the body type (tall, thin, stocky, or rotund). Sometimes we just have to play with the genetic cards that have been dealt and accept the fact we "can't make mountains out of molehills." A patient in late adolescence or young adulthood, who is physically healthy and strong with relative moderate body fat in other parts of her body, has a good chance of successfully increasing breast size through a combination of lifestyle and dietary modifications, and if the patient chooses, the administration of TCM medicinals.

You should advise these types of patients to get 8 to 10 hours of sleep a night, massage their chest area and breasts while showering, and eat a well-rounded diet that includes plenty of eggs, liver, brain, seafood, all types of nuts, brown rice, soybeans, and of course Si Shen Tang.

As for TCM treatment, you can prescribe medicinals that supplement the spleen, stomach, and kidney, boost qi, engender essence, and promote digestion. The medicinals I have found most effective are Shan Yao, Niu Bang Zi, Zi Su Zi, and Zi He Che. Another option is to have the patient drink a small daily amount (30–50 ml) of Lu Rong Medicinal Wine* for at least 6 months to 1 year, or possibly even longer. If the patient doesn't like to drink alcohol, then you could consider simply prescribing a regimen of Xi Lu Rong (powder) (5 fen/3x/day) and Ren Shen/Chuan Qi Powder (3 g/3x/day) and advise the patient to eat plenty of fresh burdock root

(Niu Bang), kudzu root (Ge Gen), Chinese yams (Shan Yao), and oysters (Mu Li), along with a well-balanced diet as mentioned above. Over time, these approaches should provide effective results.

*Note: Lu Rong Medicinal Wine (鹿茸藥酒/Deer Antler Medicinal Wine)—steep fresh Xi Lu Rong and Shi Quan Da Bu Tang in white liquor or rice wine for at least 1 year.

Case Study #8: Mastitis – Xian Fang Huo Ming Yin Variant

Q: About 2 months ago, Mrs. Jiang, a 43 y/o female patient, had a contraceptive implant placed in her left upper arm. Two weeks later, she suddenly began feeling an aversion to cold and redness and swelling around her left areola. She was super stressed out and nervous about it, and rushed over to see me for a clinical visit.

I diagnosed her with mastitis and prescribed Xian Fang Huo Ming Yin variant. Do you think this is a good approach? Also, do you think it may be possible that the contraceptive implant could have caused this infection in her breast?

A: Contraceptive implants have been in use for a long time now and from my clinical experience and what I have read in news reports, journals, and papers, I have never heard of these little devices causing mastitis. It seems unlikely, but possible, that the patient could have been infected with bacteria (e.g., *Staphylococcus aureus*, *E. coli*, Streptococcus) upon implantation, but *not* directly caused by the implant itself.

Regardless of how the patient became infected, you are definitely on the right track by prescribing this heat-clearing toxin-resolving, swelling-dispersing hardness-breaking, and blood-quickening pain-relieving formula. Just make sure to add large doses of Pu Gong Ying, Jin Yin Hua, Huang Qin, Huang Bo, Lian Qiao, and Niu Bang Zi.

This therapeutic approach will quickly resolve the inflammation and swelling and get the infection under control, so it does *not* exacerbate into pain and generalized symptoms.

Case Study #9: Urinary Incontinence in Young Girl

Q: A couple brought in their 6 y/o girl explaining that 1 week ago they discovered that their daughter had discharged a large amount of viscous secretion from her vagina, and after that episode she began having trouble with urinary incontinence. At that time, I started administering Bu Zhong Yi Qi Tang including Huang Qi (2 liang) and adding Shan Yao, The Three Great Yang-Supplementers, Dang Shen, and Ren Shen.

After taking this formula for 2 months, the urinary incontinence has almost completely resolved; but now, sometimes after urinating and while sitting cross-legged, she still has dribbling and a bit of urine excretion. How would you go forward from here?

A: My first impression is that the "large amount of secretion from her vagina" is in fact coming from the urinary bladder. Obviously, prior to treating this patient, you must rule out urinary tract infection (UTI) (e.g., urinary bladder infection (cystitis)), which may present with symptoms such as pain upon urination (dysuria), frequency, urgency, and hematuria. However, it appears that the spleen-fortifying qi-supplementing, yang-upbearing fall-raising, blood-supplementing and -quickening formula Bu Zhong Zi Qi Tang variant has been working, so it must *not* be an infection!

What I would do going forward is add some securing and astringing medicinals (e.g., Bai Guo, Jin Ying Zi, Sheng Mu Li) and qi-moving bind-dissipating and genitourinary system conductor medicinals (e.g., Long Yan He, Ju He, Li Zhi He). This should provide the right formula you need to get the girl's "pee pee" working properly!

Just for reference, if the girl did happen to have a UTI that presented with urinary incontinence or urinary calculi (very rare) that resulted in infection, then this can be identified as damp-heat pouring downward pattern. And for children and adolescents in particular, you must also rule out the possibility of Tourette syndrome, which may manifest as a type of "urinary tract tic." For cases involving patterns such as qi vacuity, qi vacuity downward fall (prolapse), and kidney yang vacuity, you could also add Xi Lu Rong (powder). However, downward fall (prolapse) and kidney yang vacuity pattern would be much more likely to present in middle-aged and older women who have pelvic organ prolapse or neurogenic bladder.

Case Study #10: Interstitial Cystitis

Q: Mrs. Li has suffered from chronic, noninfectious cystitis (interstitial cystitis) for many years, with symptoms of urinary frequency, urgency, and lower abdominal discomfort. Recently, recurrent episodes have been occurring every time she feels nervous or overworked. Her urologist recommends behavioral modifications (e.g., avoiding triggers) and also said she could try oral medications (e.g., tricyclic antidepressants), or even more invasive procedures if necessary. She is trying to avoid triggers, but she does not want to take those kinds of drugs or undergo invasive procedures.

That's why she came to visit me. Can TCM provide effective treatment for this pathocondition?

A: The actual cause of interstitial cystitis is unknown, but there are many hypotheses proposed such as autoimmune processes, vascular occlusions, hormonal irregularities, and psychogenic factors. In my clinical practice, I simply classify this pathocondition as a *psychogenic disorder* caused by anxiety, which correlates with *visceral agitation* in classical TCM pathology.

For the majority of my patients, I will prescribe Gan Mai Da Zao Tang Combining Ban Xia Hou Po Tang (harmonizes the center and calms agitation and dissipates stagnation and transforms phlegm), Wen Dan Tang (harmonizes the gallbladder and stomach and dispels phlegm turbidity harassing the inner body), or Si Shen Tang (fortifies the spleen, secures essence, nourishes the heart and quiets the spirit, and boosts the immune system). Just make sure to include Da Zao, Long Yang Rou, and Yu Sheng Wan.

For patients presenting with signs and symptoms that can be identified as effulgent yin vacuity pattern, I would prescribe Zhi Bo Di Huang Tang; for Shao Yang vacuity heat with hyperactivity of liver yang pattern, I would prescribe Xiao Chai Hu Jia Long Gu Mu Li Tang; for vacuity taxation with dual vacuity of yin and yang pattern, I would prescribe Gui Zhi Jia Long Gu Mu Li Tang; and for foot Tai Yin channel disease with phlegm-damp obstruction pattern, I would prescribe Ban Xia Tian Ma Bai Zhu San adding Gan Cao and Long Yan Rou. Just as above, you should make sure to include Da Zao,

Long Yang Rou, and Yu Sheng Wan in your formula.

Remember! Unless it has already been administered as a prescription, I would advise the patient to include the medicinals (ingredients) in Si Shen Tang (Four Spirits Decoction)—Fu Ling, Shan Yao, Qian Shi, Lian Zi, and Yi Yi Ren—along with Da Zao, Long Yan Rou, and Gou Qi Zi in dishes as a regular part of her daily diet. Also, advise the patient to avoid potential triggers (e.g., tobacco, alcohol, foods with high potassium content, spicy foods), get regular exercise and plenty of sleep, and try Kegel exercises to strengthen the pelvic floor.

Case Study #11: Frequent Urination – May Lead To Uterine and Bladder Prolapse

Q: Mrs. Wang, a 60 y/o female, has been having problems with frequent urination, which has been gradually worsening over the past couple of years. It doesn't matter if it is the daytime or nighttime, she has to urinate every 30 minutes or so. After urinating, she feels heaviness and pain in the lower abdomen (*no* burning sensation) and like there is residual urine still in her bladder. Plus, she has glomus below the heart, constipation (1 stool/3–4 days), dry mouth, no thought of food and drink (不思飲食 bù s□ yin shí), cold fingers, a fear of cold (畏寒 wèi hán), and every morning she feels like her face and fingers are slightly swollen. Do you think these symptoms could be psychosomatic?

A: As people age, our genitourinary system goes through changes, and in women these changes may include increased urinary frequency and urgency, increased risk of urinary tract infections (UTIs), vaginal atrophy, and pelvic organ prolapse (i.e., protrusion of bladder, rectum, intestines, uterus, cervix, or vaginal apex into the vaginal vault). The genitourinary system symptoms that your patient presents with suggest the possibility of uterine or bladder prolapse, which is compressing the ureters and causing frequent urination, heaviness and pain in the lower abdomen, residual urine in the bladder, and maybe constipation. As for the other symptoms, it is possible that these are psychosomatic; however, we can prescribe a formula that will effectively remedy *all* of her symptoms.

In TCM, prolapse can be identified as qi vacuity downward fall (氣虛下陷 qì x□ xià xiàn). As for treatment, you can administer a spleen-fortifying qi-supplementing and yang-upbearing formula such as Bu Zhong Yi Qi Tang (including a large dose of Huang Qi) adding The Three Great Yang-Supplementers, Huang Qin, Fu Ling, Ze Xie, a small dose of Da Huang (add incremental doses of 5 fen up until the patient maintains 1–3 stools/day), and Ji Nei Jin and Shan Zha.

Huang Qi and The Three Great Yang-Supplementers will remedy the swollen feeling in her face and fingers and fear of cold; Chen Pi, Sheng Ma, and Chai Hu will remedy the glomus below the heart, Da Huang will remedy the constipation, and Ji Nei Jin and Shan Zha will remedy the no thought of food and drink. Plus, once she starts drinking and eating again, the dry mouth will resolve spontaneously as well.

Case Study #12: "All Sorts of Ailments" After Giving Birth

Q: Mrs. Xie, a 33 y/o female, explained that ever since giving birth 5 years ago she has been having "all sorts of ailments": sloppy stool, abdominal pain, flushing and profuse facial sweating, and excessive tearing.

I prescribed a 2-week prescription of Bu Zhong Yi Qi Tang adding Ren Shen, Bai Zhu, and Fu Ling, and will see the patient again on her next follow-up visit. Do you think this formula will be effective?

A: As for the excessive tearing, you must distinguish whether the "tearing" is viscous yellow eye matter or thin and watery as in tearing on exposure to wind. Does it involve nasolacrimal duct obstruction (dacryostenosis) in which tears well up, spill out, and result in excessive tearing (epiphora)?

If viscous yellow eye matter presents with redness of the conjunctiva, then this can be identified as externally contracted wind-heat pattern and classified as *wind-fire red eye* (風火赤眼 f□ng huo chì yan) (aka *conjunctivitis*). If so, then you would want to first treat the infection with an exterior-effusing, heat-abating, and wind-extinguishing formula such as a Yang Dan Tang, Ge Gen Tang, or Ma Huang Tang. Just make sure to include heat-clearing toxin-resolving medicinals such as The Three Yellows, Jin Yin Hua, Pu Gong Ying, and Lian Qiao. Plus, you should bleed Zan Zhu (UB2), Si

Zhu Kong (SJ23), Cun Kou (Tai Yuan) (LU9), and Da Zhui (GV14) (above, on, and below); and needle Feng Chi (GB20), Tian Zhu (UB10), Wan Gu (GB12), and He Gu (LI4).

If the thin, watery tears of tearing on exposure to wind present, then this can be identified as spleen yang vacuity (or kidney yang vacuity) with exterior pattern and classified as *tearing on exposure to wind.* Thus, you could administer either a qi-boosting spleen-fortifying, qi-moving phlegm-transforming, exterior-resolving nasal orifice-freeing, and wind-dispelling cold-dissipating formula, such as Tearing on Exposure to Wind Formula adding Gan Jiang and Fu Zi; or a kidney yang-warming and -supplementing, blood-quickening stasis-dissipating, sinew- and bone-strengthening, and dampness-eliminating pain-relieving formula, such as You Gui Yin adding Bai Guo and Wu Wei Zi (constrain the lung and sweat, check discharge and diarrhea, engender liquid and astringe essence, and quiet the heart and calm the spirit), and Ma Huang, Bai Zhi, Xi Xin, and Xin Yi (diffuse the lung and resolve the exterior, free the (nasal) orifices, dispel wind and dissipate cold, and serve as respiratory tract conductors).

If the case involves *nasolacrimal duct obstruction* resulting in excessive tearing, then this can be identified as stomach heat, requiring administration of a formula such as Qing Wei San, Liang Ge San, or Qing Shang Fang Feng Tang.

The same goes for the symptoms of *sweating* and *flushing*. You must first distinguish whether the sweating is spontaneous sweating or night sweating, and whether the flushing is tidal reddening, pink colored, or dark (purplish) red colored. Tidal reddening of the cheeks indicates Shao Yang channel heat pattern or steaming bone vacuity heat pattern; pink colored indicates a wide range of possibilities, including emotional distress, high blood pressure, and drug side effects (e.g., corticosteroids, antituberculosis medication); and dark (purplish) red indicates static blood pattern and blood heat pattern.

The Bu Zhong Yi Qi Tang (fortifies the spleen, supplements qi, and upbears yang) variant you prescribed will provide effective treatment for pathoconditions that can be identified as qi vacuity pattern. However, you must also take into consideration the *profuse* sweating by including a large dose of Huang Qi (supplements qi and upbears yang and boosts defense and secures the exterior) and adding Long Gu and Mu Li (calm the liver and subdue yang, quiet the spirit, and astringe and secure), Ma Huang Gen (astringes and checks sweating), and Qing Hao and Zhi Mu (enrich yin and clear vacuity fire). This therapeutic approach will effectively supplement qi, while also nourishing yin, subduing yang, securing the essence, and preventing damage to fluids.

Case Study #13: "Chronic PID"? *No*, It's Running Piglet!

Q: This 30 y/o unmarried female recently visited her family doctor who referred her to a gastroenterologist and a gynecologist to find out why she has been experiencing episodes of pain below the umbilicus and in the lower abdomen. The pelvic and transvaginal ultrasound, computed tomography (CT) scan, and lab tests all turned out to be normal, and she was eventually diagnosed with chronic pelvic inflammatory disease (PID). I am not sure if this was a diagnosis by default or there was some basis for making this determination, such as adnexal or cervical motion tenderness upon manual vaginal examination.

Since then, she has received both Western medicine (i.e., antibiotics) and TCM (i.e., medicinals, acupuncture, and moxibustion) treatment, which have *not* provided effective results. Now, the condition has intensified with 2 or 3 painful episodes every week that usually occur in the late afternoon around 4 to 5 p.m. She said that sometimes she feels a cramping (gripping) pain in the lower abdomen at first, which then extends throughout the lower cinnabar field (下丹田 xià d□ n tián) as an aching pain that is particularly sensitive to any type of pressure. The only sure-fire way she has found to reduce the pain of these episodes is by taking a hot bath or shower. What do you think is wrong with this patient?

A: Cases of acute PID, for which a definitive bacterial infection is identified by culture and increased WBC and ESR levels, can be identified as damp-heat pouring downward pattern, requiring administration of a liver and gallbladder repletion fire-draining and lower burner damp-heat-clearing formula such as Long Dan Xie Gan Tang variant. However, in cases of "chronic PID" such as this, with *no* abnormal lab test results (i.e., WBC and ESR levels) or imaging study findings (e.g., abscess in the fallopian tubes, hydrosalpinx, adhesions), and antibiotics have *failed* to relieve symptoms, I would definitely have to question the validity of this diagnosis.

"Chronic PID" has become an easy *fallback* diagnosis that gynecologists resort to when they are uncertain about the etiology of a clinical presentation. Patients want to know what is wrong with them, so "chronic PID" is a way to provide them with an answer.

In TCM, this pathocondition can be classified as running piglet (奔豚 b□ n tún) or insensitivity below the umbilicus (臍下不仁 qí xià bù rén), and does *not* have anything to do with inflammation or infection.

You can prescribe Ling Gui Zao Gan Tang*—Fu Ling (1.5 liang), Gui Zhi (8 qian), Da Zao (20–30 pieces sliced open), and Gan Cao (8 qian)—adding Long Yan Rou (a large dose of at least 1 liang). Or, you could consider prescribing Dang Gui Shao Yao San (nourishes the blood and regulates the liver and fortifies the spleen and disinhibits dampness for the treatment of all types of lesser abdominal pain), Gui Zhi Fu Ling Wan (quickens the blood and transforms stasis and disperses accumulations and concretions), or Shen Qi Wan (supplements the kidney and assists yang for the treatment of hypertonicity of the lesser abdomen (少腹拘急 shao fù j□ jí)).

Regardless of the formula, you should also add Yu Sheng Wan (2–3 pills/day) to promote cerebral collateral circulation, recalibrate autoregulation in the brain, and quiet the spirit and calm the nerves.

*Note: Ling Gui Zao Gan Tang is a *Treatise on Cold Damage and Miscellaneous Diseases* formula specifically designed for the treatment of running piglet.

Case Study #14: Reversal Cold of the Extremities – Pattern Types

Q: We most certainly have cold weather here in South Korea during the winter, but it seems that a lot of female patients in particular present with a feeling of cold extremities all year round, especially at night while sleeping. Most of these patients only feel cold at the very distal extremities (toes and fingers).

What do you think the reason is for this phenomenon? Can it be cured?

A: In TCM pathology, a feeling of cold extremities can be classified as reversal cold of the extremities (手足厥冷 shou zú jué l□ng) and identified as a type of reversal pattern (厥證 jué zhèng). Reversal pattern manifests in the symptoms of cold extremities, warm (hot) extremities, and sudden loss of consciousness. For this case, we will only focus on the symptoms of the extremities—*heat reversal* (熱厥 rè jué) and *reversal cold* (厥冷 jué l□ng).

Reversal pattern encompasses a wide array of pathoconditions that involve compromised microvasculature (capillaries, arterioles, and venules) and macrovasculature (arteries and veins) that inhibit circulation, including atherosclerosis (e.g., peripheral artery disease (PAD)), thrombosis (e.g., deep vein thrombosis (DVT)), autoimmune disorders (e.g., Raynaud's, vasculitis, dermatomyositis), metabolic disorders (e.g., diabetes), and trauma.

In the great majority of cases, especially in female patients such as yours, this phenomenon can be attributed to a mild case of inhibited qi dynamic (mechanism) (氣機 qì j□), or to put it in layman's terms—a lack of physical activity and cardiovascular/aerobic exercise! Most of these types of patients can be identified as simply qi vacuity pattern or possibly as qi vacuity with mild yang vacuity and mild cold stasis pattern.

As for treatment, you can start out by prescribing mild versions of the reversal cold formulas presented below and perform acupuncture on corresponding acupoints of the affected extremities (warm needle during the winter for common cases and all year round for chronic, recalcitrant cases). Most importantly, advise these patients to get into a basic cardiovascular/aerobic exercise routine, whether it's the gym, on a treadmill at home, swimming, bicycling, jogging, or just going for long walks.

Obviously, you must closely evaluate the clinical presentation of each patient: Is there ulceration? What color is the skin on the affected extremities? Purplish-red coloration indicates *heat* and blackish- purple indicates *cold*. Do they look like iced jujubes (Da Zao)? Do the vessels appear sapphire in color and the flesh present with a cold, lusterless complexion like slabs of boiled pork belly?

If *heat* presents, then this can be classified as *heat reversal* (熱厥 rè jué) and identified as *exterior-interior heat* pattern. For this pattern, you can prescribe a formula that resolves both the exterior and interior, such as Ge Gen Qin Lian Tang, Huang Lian Jie Du Tang, Ma Huang Tang, Ge Gen Tang, Gui Zhi Tang, Bai Hu Tang, or even Xian Fang Huo Ming Yin. Just make sure to include combinations of the following medicinals: The Three Yellows (clear heat and resolve toxin); Sheng Shi Gao (drains fire); Ma Huang, Fang Feng, and Bai Zhi (resolve the exterior); and Ge Gen (resolves the flesh). If swelling and pain present, then this can be identified as *stasis heat* pattern, requiring administration of a blood-nourishing and -quickening, stasis-dispelling pain-relieving, network vessel-freeing channel-regulating, and swelling-dispersing formula such as Ru Mo Si Wu Tang adding Huang Qin, Huang Lian, Jin Yin Hua, and Pu Gong Ying (clear heat and resolve toxin, course wind and dissipate heat, and disinhibit dampness).

If *cold* presents, then this can be classified as *reversal cold* (aka *cold reversal* (寒厥 hán jué)), and identified as *qi and yang vacuity with cold stasis* pattern. For this pattern, you can prescribe a qi-, blood-, and kidney yang-supplementing formula such as Gui Qi Jian Zhong Tang, Shi Quan Da Bu Tang, Bu Yang Huan Wu Tang, and Dang Gui Si Ni Tang. Just make sure to include Fu Zi (returns yang and stems counterflow, assists yang and supplements fire, and frees the channels and network vessels), Gan Jiang (warms the channels and the center and frees the channels and network vessels), Wu Zhu Yu (dissipates cold, relieves pain, and warms the center), Xi Xin (dissipates cold and frees the orifices), and Huang Qin (counterbalances the great heat nature of the other medicinals). By the way, during the blistering cold weather months in places like South Korea, you likely do *not* need to add Huang Qin!

In rare cases, you may come across a patient presenting with a *blood desiccation* pattern type. For this pattern, you can prescribe an yin-enriching liver-emolliating and blood-nourishing dryness-moistening formula such as Blood Desiccation Formula, Qi Bao Mei Ran Dan, or Di Huang Yin Zi. Or, you could also prescribe a blood-nourishing stasis-dispelling and blood-quickening qi-supplementing formula such as Sheng Yu Tang, Bu Yang Huan Wu Tang, or Ru Mo Si Wu Tang. Just make sure to include The Three Great Yang-Supplementers, Xi Xin, Mu Tong, Wu Zhu Yu, and Huang Qin in your formula.

IX. PEDIATRICS

In many ways pediatrics is the most rewarding specialization of all. The toughest part often revolves around trying to deal with the emotions—anxiety, fear, and expectations—of parents who bring in their children for a visit. Fortunately, the great majority of the maladies and disorders that children present with are just a part of the developmental process: they can be effectively treated and will improve over time with an excellent prognosis. As Dr. Lee likes to say: "When treating children, a doctor simply needs to hold the child's hand and help them get through the tough time."

Section 1: Common Pediatric Disorders

Case Study #1: Profuse Sweating – During Sleep and Upon Awakening

Q: Recently a 6 y/o girl visited with a chief complaint of profuse sweating (hyperhidrosis) over the entire body. Her parents explained that it *only* occurs about 30 minutes after awakening from sleep and is most intense on her hands, feet, and neck, while the rest of the time she is perfectly normal.

I prescribed Wen Dan Tang combining Huang Lian Jie Du Tang, but was considering Jian Ling Tang combining Huang Lian Jie Du Tang. Which approach do you think is the best?

On a related note, while treating this pediatric patient with hyperhidrosis, I began to think about my son who is now 6 months old. Recently, when he wakes up from sleep his head is soaked with sweat. This further irritates his existing atopy (skin hypersensitivity) issues by causing him to scratch even more, which leaves behind a trail of large erythematous patches. What can I do to resolve this condition?

A: Children commonly present with spontaneous sweating. The 6 y/o girl you are treating most likely is going through a period in which the thermoregulatory (perspiration) center in the hypothalamus that controls sweating is not fully developed yet, thus resulting in the autonomic neuronal dysfunction of excessive sweating (hyperhidrosis).

As for treatment, I would try prescribing a liver-settling wind-extinguishing and yin-enriching yang-subduing formula such as Jian Ling Tang (including Gan Cao) adding Long Yan Rou, Qing Hao, Zhi Mu, Di Gu Pi, Huang Bo, Ma Huang Gen, Shan Zha, and Ji Nei Jin. These medicinals will help to subdue the overactivity of the regulatory control centers in the brain and regulate the constitution, giving the body the support and impetus it needs to fully develop its self-regulation capacities. The excessive sweating will gradually resolve, so don't sweat it!

For your son's case of waking up with a head full of sweat that intensifies the existing itchy skin problems, I think this may be a simple case of "wearing too many clothes to bed." You should try reducing the amount of clothing and see if the situation improves. As parents, we worry about protecting our children from the elements so they won't catch a cold, but sometimes we can overdo it. Too much heavy clothing that does not "breathe" prevents air from circulating and creates a veritable "steam room" inside the layers of insulation, which naturally results in excessive sweating with the heat rising to the top, effusing in the form of sweat on the head and permeating to the surface as damp, itchy skin.

So the key is to just wear enough to keep warm, especially nowadays when most people have heating in their homes: it's often unnecessary to wear so much clothing. If the itchy skin is really intense, then you could prescribe an exterior-resolving dampness-eliminating and lung qi-diffusing and -disinhibiting formula such as Ma Xing Yi Gan Tang, which will quickly resolve the itchiness.

Case Study #2: Why Does Four-Year-Old Still Drool?

Q: A 4 y/o boy still frequently drools, prompting his mother to bring him in for evaluation and treatment. I identified this condition as spleen vacuity copious drool with kidney yang vacuity pattern and prescribed Wu Ling San (Nephritis Formula). He has taken this formula for 1 month now, but there really hasn't been any improvement. Please offer your advice and guidance.

A: Indeed, children usually stop drooling by the time they are about 18 months old. However, a small percentage of kids may continue to drool up until they are anywhere from 4 to 6 years old, so it's *not* necessarily abnormal. Kids will usually *grow out* of it sometime along the path of development.

This sounds like a simple case of drool (涎 xián) and spittle (唾 tuò), also referred to as drool-spittle. Based on TCM theory, drool is the humor of the spleen and spittle is the humor of the kidney. Drool has a thin consistency, with the main function of moistening the mouth, and spittle has a thicker consistency, with the main function of aiding in the digestion of food.

As for treatment, I would consider prescribing a qi-boosting spleen-fortifying formula such as Xiang Sha Liu Jun Zi Tang (moves qi and transforms phlegm), Shen Ling Bai Zhu San (harmonizes the stomach and percolates dampness), or Li Zhong Tang (warms the center and dispels cold). Naturally, if possible, it would be best to stir-fry (炒 chao) process these medicinals prior to decoction to further enhance the formula's spleen-fortifying action.

For reference, before prescribing a formula, I would always first conduct a detailed observation of the color and consistency of the fluid, along with any other distinguishing signs and symptoms. In TCM, the terms saliva (口水 kou shui), drool (涎 xián), spittle (唾 tuò), phlegm-drool (痰涎 tán xián), and phlegm-rheum (痰飲 tán yin) can be used to describe fluid that flows from the mouth. For starters, you should answer these questions: Is the fluid watery or viscous with stringy strands? Is it malodorous? Does spittle (frothy, milky color) form? Is the fluid so viscous that it forms the consistency of phlegm-rheum? In general, viscous, malodorous, and dark-colored fluid indicates *heat* and can be identified as *stomach heat* pattern; while clear, thin, odorless fluid indicates *cold* and can be identified as *qi vacuity* or *yang vacuity water flood* (水泛 shui fàn) pattern.

If spittle (frothy, milky color) presents, then this can typically be identified as *kidney yang vacuity water flood* or *spleen and stomach vacuity cold* pattern.

- For *kidney yang vacuity water flood* pattern, you can prescribe a formula that warms kidney yang and promotes qi transformation and disinhibits dampness and water by bland percolation, such as Wu Ling San (Nephritis Formula).
- For *spleen and stomach vacuity cold* pattern, you can prescribe a formula that boosts qi and fortifies the spleen and harmonizes the stomach and percolates dampness, such as Xiang Sha Liu Jun Zi Tang, Li Zhong Tang, Bu Zhong Yi Qi Tang, or Shen Ling Bai Zhu San.
- If the spittle is malodorous, then this indicates *heat*, so you should consider adding medicinals that clear heat and resolve toxin, such as Pu Huang, Lian Qiao, Huang Qin, and Huang Lian.

Most of the patients I treat present with the *spleen and stomach vacuity cold* pattern type!

Case Study #3: Sudden Decrease of Vision

Q: A mother brought her 9 y/o son in with the chief complaint of sudden decrease in vision. One year ago, his vision score was 1.0 and during a recent check up his vision had dropped down to 0.3. What do you think is going on here?

A: Obviously, you should ask to see the results of a comprehensive ophthalmological examination: this could result from a wide range of abnormalities from astigmatism and myopia to cataract, glaucoma or retinopathy. That does sound like a rather dramatic decrease in visual acuity in just 1 year for sure, and is on the lower extreme of mild vision loss (< 0.8 to ≥ 0.3).

Based on the limited information you have provided, my initial impression is this could simply be the result of an exterior with phlegm-heat pattern. Thus, I would first consider prescribing a heat-clearing phlegm-transforming formula such as Wen Dan Tang adding Ma Huang, Di Long, Chuan Qi, and Lai Fu Zi.

If this approach is *not* effective, then I would prescribe a blood-nourishing yin-enriching and heat-clearing blood-cooling formula, such as Di Gu Pi Yin, or a blood-nourishing stasis-dispelling and network vessel-freeing channel-regulating formula, such as Ru Mo Si Wu Tang. Just make sure to include The Eye Brighteners (Qian Li Guang, Mi Meng Hua, She Tui, and Chan Tui), Tian Ma, Fu Ling, and Gou Qi Zi.

If this approach is *still* not effective, then you can approach this as a case of optic nerve atrophy or macular degeneration, requiring administration of a blood-quickening qi-supplementing formula such as Bu Yang Huan Wu Tang adding The Eye Brighteners, Fu Ling, and Chuan Qi (powder).

Case Study #4: Fetal Hydronephrosis and Fetal Pelviectasis

Q: This 11 y/o boy was diagnosed with right-sided *fetal hydronephrosis* (swelling of the kidney) when he was a 7-month-old fetus in his mother's womb. After birth, it was necessary to receive urethral catheterization for continuous drainage of urine, but the kidney was severely damaged and it had to be resected.

The child does *not* have any discomfort or functional impairment, but the mother still worries and wonders if TCM supplementing medicinals would ensure a better outlook for the future. Do you think it is necessary to treat this patient even if there are *no* presenting signs or symptoms?

On a related note, my son is now 9 months old. He was diagnosed with an enlarged renal pelvis before birth (*fetal pelviectasis*) on the left side, which is a much milder version of the extreme enlargement characterized by *fetal hydronephrosis*. At that time, I took your advice and began administering my wife the kidney-supplementing yang-assisting formula Shen Qi Wan in attempts to regulate the fetal constitution via the placental circulation route.

Previous ultrasound of my son showed normal renal pelvis size on both sides: left 0.9 cm and right 0.8 cm. Last week we got the results back on the most recent ultrasound, which revealed enlarged renal pelvis on the left side and what appears to be narrowing of the ureter (*ureteral stricture*), but the overall size of the kidneys are symmetrical and within the normal range.

Right now there does *not* seem to be any pain or discomfort and the urine volume is normal. Do you think it is necessary to treat this condition?

A: The 11 y/o patient with *fetal hydronephrosis* can be classified as insufficiency of earlier heaven (先天不足 xi□ n ti□ n bù zú). The vast majority of people with only a single kidney lead perfectly normal lives with no long-term complications or shortening of life expectancy. It's really *not* necessary for this type of patient to be treated with TCM medicinals unless he consumes nephrotoxic medication and foods or incurs traumatic injury to the remaining kidney that causes renal damage or failure. This is the same situation for a kidney donor, who gives up one for the sake of another and goes on living a normal life. Just remember to advise the patient to eat a healthy well-balanced diet, drink lots of water, and don't overdo it on the salty and processed foods.

As for your son's enlarged renal pelvis (*pelviectasis*) and possible left-sided narrowing of the ureter (*ureteral stricture*), it does *not* sound like something you need to worry about. On the other hand, if this were a case of *hydronephrosis*, which may cause infection, renal damage, and renal failure, it obviously would warrant concern, aggressive treatment, and follow-up. *Hydronephrosis* occurs when blockage of the ureter (ureteropelvic junction obstruction (UPJO)) is severe enough to cause obstruction of the free flow of urine out of the kidney, which will result in enlargement of the pelvis and the entire kidney ballooning from the pressure, along with possible retrograde flow of urine from the bladder into the ureter (vesicoureteral reflux).

If his condition still worries you, then you could classify it as insufficiency of earlier heaven, just as you did before, but have your son take the decoction instead. Since the kidney is the root of earlier heaven (the congenital constitution), I would administer small dosages of either Shen Qi Wan (supplements the kidney and assists yang) or Shi Quan Da Bu Tang (quickens and supplements the blood, boosts qi and fortifies the spleen, and supplements kidney yang). These formulas will regulate the constitution and promote organ development.

Additionally, you could periodically have lab tests conducted to follow up on BUN, CR, Hb, and T-Pro. If there are *no* abnormalities in these results, then it really is *not* imperative to aggressively treat this condition.

Case Study #5: Pulmonary Artery Aneurysm in an Infant

Q: Today a couple brought in their cute little 1-year-old daughter. They explained that it wasn't until she was 6 months old that her ductus arteriosus finally closed. This resulted in irregular transmission of blood between the aorta and pulmonary artery, creating pressure and causing the formation of an 8 mm pulmonary artery aneurysm (PAA) to develop.

The patient does *not* present with any signs or symptoms of pathology. Is there anything I can or should do for this patient?

A: You do *not* need to worry about treatment unless the child presents with signs or symptoms (e.g., high blood pressure, chest pain). Usually, as the child grows older this type of condition will resolve on its own and never cause any problems. This goes for most congenital defects and complications, over time they will usually resolve.

If the parents really want to treat this condition, then you could consider prescribing a formula such as Shi Quan Da Bu Tang (quickens and supplements the blood, boosts qi and fortifies the spleen, and supplements kidney yang), Bu Yang Huan Wu Tang (quickens the blood and transforms stasis, cools the blood, and supplements qi), or Sheng Yu Tang (supplements the blood and qi, cools the blood and dispels stasis, and nourishes yin). These formulas will regulate the constitution and promote resolution of the aneurysm.

Case Study #6: Moyamoya Disease – Requires Monitoring and Treatment

Q: Eight months ago, this 6 y/o patient was diagnosed with moyamoya disease based on the findings of x-ray imaging, and also presented with peritoneal effusion (ascites) at that time. I have been providing her with medicinal treatment over the past six months, during which time her condition had been showing considerable improvement. However, recently her condition has taken a turn for the worse again. Can this patient be cured? How should I proceed from here?

A: Moyamoya disease is rare type of cerebrovascular occlusive disorder characterized by progressive stenosis or occlusion of the internal carotid arteries. To make up for the reduced blood flow, tiny new vessels called *collaterals* grow in attempts to compensate. These *collaterals* may temporarily help increase blood supply, but they may eventually stop working, putting the patient at risk of cognitive and developmental delays or disabilities, transient ischemic attacks (TIAs), aneurysms, stroke, and hemorrhage.

Moyamoya literally means "puff of smoke" in Japanese, describing the hazy, smoke-like appearance of these new *collaterals* drifting in the brain. This is a progressive disease that can occur at any age, but usually presents between 5 and 10 years old and 30 and 50 years old. Once diagnosed, the patient will likely be administered medication long-term to reduce the risk of stroke and/or to control seizures, and possibly be advised to undergo revascularization surgery, which is very risky, but does offer a positive long-term outlook if successful.

As for TCM treatment, in the acute stage, you would have to prescribe a blood-quickening stasis-transforming, blood-cooling, and qi-supplementing formula such as Bu Yang Huan Wu Tang (including large doses of Dan Shen and a small dose of Huang Qi) adding Mu Dan Pi (cools the blood and clears heat and quickens the blood and disperses stasis) and small doses of The Three Great Yang-Supplementers (warm the channels and free the network vessels, supplement fire and assist yang, and boost the metabolism and bolster right qi).

Continue prescribing this formula anywhere from 3–6 months, as you gradually increase the doses of Huang Qi and The Three Great Yang-Supplementers, and then go ahead and make the switch over to Bu Yang Huan Wu Tang combining You Gui Yin (warms and supplements kidney yang and quickens the blood and dissipates stasis). If BUN and Cr levels are elevated and/or ascites presents, then add Da Huang. And if an excessive amount of fluid accumulates in the abdominal (ascites) or thoracic (pulmonary edema) cavity, then change the formula to Wu Ling San (Nephritis Formula) (warms kidney yang and promotes qi transformation and disinhibits dampness and water by bland percolation) adding Huang Qi, Ting Li Zi, Ren Dong Teng, Da Huang, and Ren Shen/Chuan Qi Powder.

If the parents decide to go ahead with revascularization surgery, following surgery I would prescribe Bu Yang Huan Wu Tang adding The Three Great Yang-Supplementers and Ren Shen/Chuan Qi Powder to promote cerebral circulation and reduce the risk of ischemic complications. If increased intracranial pressure presents as a complication, then change the formula to Ban Xia Tian Ma Bai Zhu San (supplements the spleen and stomach, transforms phlegm-damp, and nourishes the blood and stabilizes wind) adding Wu Zhu Yu, Ren Shen/Chuan Qi Powder, and Yu Sheng Wan.

Remember! This disease tends to run an unpredictable course and the mortality rate is *extremely* high. In addition to intracerebral hemorrhage, associated renal artery complications may arise that lead to fluid accumulation, systemic edema, and renal failure. Stay vigilant and take extra care and precaution!

Case Study #7: "My Kid Is Too Short!" – TCM Medicinals

Q: Recently, I have had numerous parents visit me claiming that their child has developmental delays, with the usual chief complaint going something like this: "My kid is too short! Is there anything we can do to make him/her grow taller?" Many of these parents have even considered growth hormone (GN) therapy for their kids, but are concerned about the possibility of side effects from these injections. They want to try TCM instead. What is your opinion about these types of cases?

A: A general guideline for average annual growth of a child is at least 4 cm per year. If the child does *not* grow at least 4 cm per year, then the parents should have the child tested to determine whether or not growth hormone levels are normal. However, even if the child does have low growth hormone levels early on in life does *not* mean that the body won't eventually recalibrate (catch up) and incur a spurt of growth hormone secretion to reach great heights (or at least average!). Certain aspects of some people just develop slower than others and there really is no "one size fits all" basis for determination.

Administering GN therapy in children poses the risk of many unpleasant and potentially severe side effects (e.g., rash, transient fever, gynecomastia, arthralgia, insulin resistance, progression of scoliosis). Thus, in the great majority of cases, I would recommend administration of TCM medicinals over GN therapy. In TCM, just as for other types of developmental delays, the inability to meet height standards can be classified as insufficiency of earlier heaven (congenital constitution).

As for treatment, in cases where growth hormone levels are *normal*, I would simply prescribe either Xiang Sha Liu Jun Zi Tang (boosts qi and fortifies the spleen and moves qi and transforms phlegm) or Shen Ling Bai Zhu San (boosts qi and fortifies the spleen and harmonizes the stomach and percolates dampness). If necessary, you could also consider adding Shan Zha and Ji Nei Jin (disperse food and promote digestion and fortify the spleen and open the stomach) and/or Xu Duan and Gu Sui Bu (quicken the blood and transform stasis and supplement the liver and kidney). Plus, you should advise the patient to eat foods that include the medicinals (ingredients) in Si Shen Tang—Shan Yao, Qian Shi, Yi Yi Ren, Bai Guo, Lian Zi, and Fu Ling—as part of the daily diet. Prescribe this regimen for a minimum of 3–6 months. In most cases, you will observe noticeable growth and increased vitality.

In cases where growth hormone levels have been confirmed to be *low* via testing, this can be identified as yang vacuity pattern, requiring a prescription combining qi-, blood-, and yang-supplementing medicinals such as Shi Quan Da Bu Tang, Shen Qi Wan, You Gui Yin, or Gui Qi Jian Zhong Tang. Just make sure to include Ren Shen/Chuan Qi Powder, The Three Great Yang-Supplementers, and Huang Qin (counterbalances the heat). Over time, this should promote growth and development.

Remember! In times of antiquity (and in poor, underdeveloped countries of today), disharmony of later heaven (acquired constitution) (後天失調 hòu ti□n sh□ tiáo) was (is) also a major factor in causing developmental delays due to poor nutrition, lack of clean water, and hygiene problems. Even in modern, industrialized societies nutritional intake is *not* always adequate, so you must always advise the patient and parents to maintain a healthy diet, get 8–10 hours of sleep a night, and exercise regularly. But at the end of the day, some people will naturally be shorter than others, and the parents will just have to accept this reality—"it's all in your genes!"

Case Study #8: Congenital Hydrocele – Make Sure to Add Di Long!

Q: A 2 y/o patient of mine was born with left-sided hydrocele, which did not spontaneously resolve after 1 year. Following standard Western medicine protocol, his doctor recommended surgery. However, the parents are wary of surgery and want to try TCM instead.

My initial impulse was to prescribe Wu Ling San (Nephritis Formula) or Bu Zhong Yi Qi Tang variant, but then I thought that this approach may be effective in the short term, but once he stops taking it, the swelling will resume. This would be treating the "tip", but the "root" remains, and thus the condition will *not* be resolved.

This family happens to be some friends of my relatives, so I told them that I would look into this case more closely and have them come back in a few days. I remember you mentioning about using Di Long for pathoconditions of the genitalia. Is your reasoning due to its channel-freeing and network vessel-quickening actions or some other reason?

A: This reasoning is elucidated in *The Essential Herbal Foundation* (本草備要 *Ben Cao Bei Yao*) profile of Di Long (actually listed under the alternative name Bai Jing Qiu Yin (白頸蚯蚓/White-Necked Earthworm)) as follows: "…descending thus disinhibits urine…frees the channels and network vessels…. Indicated for…urinary stoppage in adults and children…."

For the treatment of hydrocele, you can definitely prescribe Wu

Ling San (Nephritis Formula) (warms kidney yang and promotes qi transformation and disinhibits dampness and water by bland percolation), but just make sure to add Di Long. Di Long enters the urinary bladder Tai Yang channel, frees the channels and quickens the network vessels, clears heat and extinguishes wind, disinhibits urine, and promotes the repair of the tunica vaginalis serous membrane pouch that covers the testes, thus expediting the resolution of edema.

Don't worry! Just continue prescribing this formula and you will see positive results. Remember! The answers can always be found in the classics! Besides, in the vast majority of cases, the child will *grow out* of these types of developmental glitches over time anyways.

Case Study #9: Infant Sleep Apnea...Cerebral Palsy?...It's Lowe Syndrome!

Q1: Recently, I received a call from a very worried and concerned father who has a 1 y/o boy with the following history: The boy was born with congenital cataracts in both eyes that severely affected vision and prompted corrective surgery when he was 9 months old. A week after being released from the hospital, his father discovered him in bed initially semiconscious with spasm over the entire body. While still in bed, he then went completely limp and eventually was *not* breathing at all, with purplish-colored distal extremities and lips. The father immediately performed mouth-to-mouth resuscitation, which stimulated respiration and brought the child back to consciousness.

Since then, the boy has been in the hospital for over 2 months now, receiving antispasmodics that have *not* proven effective, and now his Western medicine doctors really do*n't* know what to do next. That's why the father has now contacted me, asking me to visit the child in the hospital and prescribe medicinal therapy. What do you think might be the cause of this patient's erratic condition? Please offer your advice and guidance.

A: This sounds like it may be a case of infant sleep apnea with prolonged loss of oxygen to the brain (hypoxia) and excessive buildup of carbon dioxide (hypercapnia) that led to brain damage and trauma-induced spastic cerebral palsy. The anesthesia used during cataract surgery may have either caused the sleep apnea to develop or precipitated exacerbation of preexisting sleep apnea. It is also possible that the infant had cerebral palsy prior to surgery, but it just went undiagnosed, and the anesthesia from surgery exacerbated the already compromised brain structures and caused respiratory paralysis.

Regardless of etiology, cerebral palsy can be classified as five infantile limpnesses (小兒五軟 xiao ér wu ruan). As for treatment, I would prescribe a blood-, qi-, and kidney yang-supplementing formula such as Shi Quan Da Bu Tang, Gui Qi Jian Zhong Tang, or Bu Yang Huan Wu Tang. Just make sure to include The Three Great Yang-Supplementers, Huang Qin, The Three Insects (extinguish wind and settle tetany, attack toxin and dissipate binds, and free the network vessels and relieve pain), Tian Ma (extinguishes wind and checks tetany, represses the liver, dispels wind and frees the network vessels), Shan Zha, Ren Shen/Chuan Qi Powder, and Ma Huang and Di Long (nervous system conductor medicinals).

This formula will quickly resolve symptoms and stabilize the condition so that the child can leave the hospital and begin the process of overcoming any residual motor, sensory, or cognitive impairment. This is a non-progressive condition, so after the damage has occurred the patient still has ample opportunity to reach *relatively* normal functional capacity. It's just that reaching certain developmental milestones may take a bit longer, while some may never be fully actualized.

Remember! Cerebral palsy patients commonly present with ophthalmological disorders (e.g., strabismus, nystagmus, amblyopia, refractive errors, strabismus, nystagmus, amblyopia, cortical visual impairment).

Q2: I have more detailed information from the father about the history of this 1 y/o boy now. It turns out that this is a very special pediatric patient indeed. In the hospital, the boy incurred frequent episodes of fright reversal (convulsion) (驚厥 j□ng jué), fright epilepsy (驚癇 j□ng xián), stiff upper and lower extremities, toe tremor upon flexion and extension, flexion contracture of the foot, neck tremor, hypercapnia, and compulsive eating.

Following enzymatic and genetic testing, his doctors diagnosed him with a very rare genetic disorder called Lowe syndrome (aka oculocerebrorenal syndrome), which is characterized by bilateral cataracts, developmental and intellectual disability, seizures, and impaired renal function among other problems. He is currently being administered antispasmodic drugs (phenobarbital, carbamazepine, and depakine) along with antibiotics to fight a respiratory infection.

Taking into consideration your previous suggestions and the patients presenting signs and symptoms, I prescribed Bu Yang Huan Wu Tang adding Fu Ling, Ze Xie, Bai Zhu, The Three Insects, Ren Shen/Chuan Qi Powder, The Three Great Yang-Supplementers, Huang Qin, Pu Gong Ying, Ma Huang, Hou Po, and Xing Ren.

Do you think this is a good approach for this patient's condition?

A: Hmm…now that is a rare one! Yes, from my understanding, this disease involves a mutation in the OCRL1 gene. Seizures may occur, which are initially myotonic (jerks and spasms), but later become atonic (limp and still), and eventually generalized hypotonia (decreased muscle tone and strength) sets in. In many patients, it is renal disease (e.g., hyperaminoaciduria, uremia, nephritis, renal failure) that eventually brings life to an end.

This is definitely a tough case. For now, I would try the Bu Yang Huan Wu Tang variant, see how things evolve, and then go from there.

Case Study #10: Compulsive Overeating and Mild Case of Cerebral Palsy in Toddler

Q: I have another interesting case of a 1 y/o boy with compulsive overeating (his mother said "he eats as much as an adult"), hypertonicity of the toes on both feet, and a habit of toe walking. His mother has a history of depression prior to pregnancy and after giving birth the condition has worsened. Right now, she is a patient in the psychiatric ward (the third time being admitted since giving birth) and has been diagnosed with bipolar postpartum depression.

The toddler does *not* present with any other common symptoms of cerebral palsy (e.g., strabismus, joint contractures, spasticity, abnormal posture). How would you treat this toddler?

A: Children and adolescents require lots of food to support growth spurts and the rapid pace of development, so it is tough to determine if this really is a compulsive eating disorder or just appears to be one because "he eats as much as an adult." Irregular eating habits and consuming excessive amounts of food in infants and toddlers can be the result of underdeveloped brain structures that are unable to control urges and shift attention span (in this case on the act of eating). After all, eating is the most primitive and instinctual need that humans must satisfy. The hypertonicity of the toes on both feet and a habit of toe walking indicate spasm of the calf muscles and foot muscles, which suggests the possibility of mild cerebral palsy.

As for treatment, I would focus on promoting development of the earlier heaven (congenital constitution) through regulation of the constitution by prescribing a blood-, qi-, and kidney yang-supplementing formula such as Shi Quan Da Bu Tang, Gui Qi Jian Zhong Tang, or Bu Yang Huan Wu Tang.

Just make sure to include The Three Great Yang-Supplementers (return and reinforce yang, "boost" the metabolism and immune system, and bolster right qi), Huang Qin, Ren Shen/Chuan Qi Powder (supplements original qi, engenders liquid, stems vacuity desertion, quickens the blood and transforms stasis, and stanches bleeding), Di Long (clears heat and checks tetany, calms the liver and subdues yang, frees the channels and quickens the network vessels, and calms panting and disinhits urine), Lai Fu Zi (disperses food and eliminates distention and downbears qi and transforms phlegm), and Hai Piao Xiao (powder) (controls acid and regulates hunger feedback controls).

In the majority of cases, kids simply *grow out* of these types of conditions; once their bodies have fully developed, the dysregulation and dysfunction naturally works its way into homeostasis.

If the compulsive overeating does *not* resolve as the toddler gets older and develops, then you must consider the possibility of postinfectious (external contraction) sequela that has caused metabolic waste buildup along the neurological pathways (neuromuscular junctions), resulting in dysregulation and dysfunction. For this type of scenario, you must consider prescribing a gallbladder- and stomach-harmonizing and phlegm turbidity harassing the inner body-dispelling formula, such as Wen Dan Tang, or a Shao Yang-harmonizing and fright-settling spirit-quieting formula, such as Chai Hu Jia Long Gu Mu Li Tang. Just make sure to add Hai Piao Xiao (powder) and Lai Fu Zi, and possibly Si Ni Tang or The Three Great Yang-Supplementers.

In the case of the mother, postpartum depression can be classified as visceral agitation in classical TCM pathology. For this condition, you can prescribe a center-harmonizing tension-releasing and spirit-quieting agitation-calming formula such as Gan Mai Da Zao Tang Combining Ban Xia Hou Po Tang (including a large dose of Da Zao sliced open) adding a large dose of Long Yan Rou (8 qian–1 liang). Boil down to a thick decoction and have the patient drink as a beverage throughout the day. This approach should lead to marked improvement and allow the mother to return home and fully embrace the joy of motherhood!

Case Study #11: Torticollis – Insufficiency of Earlier Heaven

Q: This 6-month-old boy was born with torticollis (neck twists to the right side). His father is a family doctor and explained that the infant was positioned abnormally in the womb (breech position), making it a difficult labor and delivery process. He has tried prescribing anticholinergics, but this has *not* been effective.

Now, he wants to know if I can do anything to help his son regain normal neck function. How would you treat this patient?

A: Torticollis can be acquired or congenital and results from tightness, thickening, and shortening of the sternocleidomastoid muscle. This is a case of infant torticollis, which can be classified as insufficiency of earlier heaven (congenital constitution), requiring administration of a combined qi-, blood-, and yang-supplementing formula such as Shi Quan Da Bu Tang, Gui Qi Jian Zhong Tang, or You Gui Yin. Just make sure to include Huang Qi, Tian Ma, Xi Lu Rong (powder), and Ren Shen (powder) treatment.

These medicinals, in combination with passive and active stretching performed by the parents or under the guidance of a physiotherapist, will promote a faster and more complete recovery. Plus, in the majority of cases, children will simply *grow out* of this condition by the time they turn 1 year old.

Case Study #12: Guillain-Barre Syndrome

Q: This 5 y/o girl has recently been diagnosed with Guillain-Barre syndrome (GBS). Two weeks ago, she came down with a high fever, nausea and vomiting, dizziness, sore back, urinary and fecal incontinence, and speech impairment. After being admitted into the hospital for 10 days now, the fever and flu-like symptoms have subsided. Do you think TCM can treat this pathocondition?

A: GBS is an acute postinfectious, inflammatory polyneuropathy characterized by symmetric and ascending flaccid paralysis, which most commonly manifests as acute inflammatory demyelinating polyradiculoneuropathy (AIDP). It is caused by external contraction (e.g., *Campylobacter jejuni*, cytomegalovirus, Epstein-Barr virus) and the resulting affects of autoantibodies attacking the invading antigens.

Western medicine treatment involves supportive management and administration of analgesics, antibiotics, antispasmodics, corticosteroids, autohemotherapy (autologous blood therapy), intravenous immunoglobulin (IVIg), plasmapharesis, nerve growth factor (NGF), and cyclophosphamide (chemotherapeutic agent). These therapeutic approaches are often able to quickly resolve the acute manifestations, but do *not* provide effective treatment for the neurologic deficits that are left behind.

As for TCM treatment, in the acute stage when there is *still* a high fever, you should prescribe the blood-quickening stasis-dispelling, blood-supplementing blood-breaking, and channel-freeing formula Di Long San adding large doses of The Three Yellows (clear heat and resolve toxin). However, since the fever has *subsided* now, I would prescribe the blood-quickening stasis-dispelling, blood-supplementing blood-breaking, channel- and network vessel-freeing, and kidney yang-supplementing formula Paralysis Formula #1 (Di Long San Variant) adding Ren Shen/Chuan Qi Powder (supplements original qi, engenders liquid, stems vacuity desertion, quickens the blood and transforms stasis, and stanches bleeding).

Remember! If corticosteroids *are* administered, then this can be identified as qi, blood, and kidney yang vacuity pattern, so you must change the formula to either Paralysis Formula #2 (Shi Quan Da Bu Tang Variant) or Paralysis Formula #3 (You Gui Yin Variant).

Case Study #13: Ingrown Eyelashes

Q: This 6 y/o boy with ingrown eyelashes (trichiasis) has already had 2 therapeutic procedures performed (not sure if it was epilation (lash removal), electrolysis, or cryoablation), but the condition continues to recur. How would you treat this recalcitrant condition?

A: Ingrown eyelashes (*trichiasis*) are common and typically result from infection, aging, or trauma. The rubbing irritation of the misdirected eyelash can lead to itchy irritation, pain, and in severe cases corneal damage (i.e., abrasions, ulcers).

The focus of treatment should be on resolving the orbicularis oculi muscle spasms caused by the continuous irritation of the eyelash rubbing on the cornea, which results in a vicious cycle of inflammation and infection (just as in spastic entropion!). By relieving the spasm, this will resolve the irritation, and in turn, the inflammation and infection, which in most cases will effectively remedy this condition.

Thus, I would prescribe a blood-quickening stasis-transforming and accumulation- and concretion-dispersing formula such as Gui Zhi Fu Ling Wan. If infection and purulent eye matter present, then I would add Huang Qin, Jin Yin Hua, and Lian Qiao (clear heat and resolve toxin and course wind and dissipate heat). Plus, I would also bleed Zan Zhu (UB2), Si Zhu Kong (SJ23), and Da Zhui (GV14) (above, on, and below); and needle acupoints such as Feng Chi (GB20), Tian Zhu (UB10), Wan Gu (GB12), He Gu (LI4), Nei Ting (ST44), Ting Gong (SI19), and Er Men (TB21).

Another similar, but less common, pathocondition is inverted eyelashes (*epiblepharon*), which results from extra horizontal folds of the skin on the upper or lower eyelids. *Epiblepharon* is a congenital condition that manifests in Asian children much more frequently than other ethnic groups. Most of the time kids with this pathocondition simply *grow out* of it, with the symptoms resolving spontaneously. However, some may need treatment to resolve the symptoms of irritation and intense itch that results in rubbing and/or scratching, which may cause corneal damage.

Case Study #14: Kawasaki Disease – Exterior Wind-Heat Pattern

Q: A couple brought their 7 y/o daughter in explaining that she was diagnosed with Kawasaki disease (KD) at 4 months of age. She immediately received IV immunoglobulin (IVIG) therapy and began administration of aspirin in efforts to prevent coronary artery complications. However, on a follow-up examination 1 year later, imaging studies revealed the presence of a coronary artery aneurysm.

Since then, imaging studies have continued showing the presence of coronary thrombosis, but the patient does *not* have any noticeable symptoms—appetite, weight, stool, sleep, and energy level are all *normal*. Does this patient need to be treated? If she does, how would you treat this patient?

A: KD is defined as an acute, necrotizing vasculitis, likely caused by viral infection in combination with a genetic predisposition (higher prevalence in Asians). The acute stage is marked by clinical features such as high fever, flu-like symptoms (e.g., diarrhea, fatigue, abdominal pain), erythema and edema of the extremities, generalized rash, lymphadenopathy, and inflammation of the mucous membranes (e.g., "strawberry" tongue).

In TCM, this condition can typically be identified as Yang Ming exterior wind-heat pattern, requiring administration of a sweat-effusing exterior-resolving formula such as Ge Gen Tang adding Huang Qin, Huang Lian, Pu Gong Ying, Jin Yin Hua, and Lian Qiao (clear heat and resolve toxin and course wind and dissipate heat), Ban Xia, Bai Zhu, Fu Ling, and Ze Xie.

In the post-acute and chronic stages, coronary artery complications may manifest such as coronary artery aneurysms and stenosis, which may lead to life-threatening myocardial infarction and arrhythmias. In TCM, this can be identified as qi stagnation and blood stasis pattern, requiring administration of either a blood-nourishing blood-quickening, stasis-dispelling pain-relieving, and network vessel-freeing channel-regulating formula, such as Ru Mo Si Wu Tang, or a blood-quickening stasis-transforming, blood-cooling, and qi-supplementing formula, such as Bu Yang Huan Wu Tang adding Mu Dan Pi and Zhi Zi (cool the blood and clear heat and quicken the blood and disperse stasis).

You should continue administering medicinal treatment up until the functional magnetic resonance imaging (fMRI) shows normal coronary artery patency.

Case Study #15: Bed-Wetting in Adolescence

Q: Most people think that bed-wetting is only a problem for infants in diapers and in some toddlers up to about 5 years old, but in my clinical practice I have had a few female patients in junior high school who still have problems with bed-wetting (nocturnal enuresis). A common physical feature is that they are all tall, thin, and picky eaters with spleen vacuity constitutions, who often feel tired and fatigued.

Usually, I will prescribe either Gui Zhi Jia Long Gu Mu Li Tang, Chai Hu Jia Long Gu Mu Li Tang, Shi Quan Da Bu Tang, or Shen Qi Wan. For younger children, these formulas have proven effective in improving the symptoms, and in some cases, completely resolving the condition. But these formulas have not been as effective for these junior high school girls. Do you have experience treating bed-wetting in this age group? Please offer your advice and guidance.

A: In younger children, the most common anatomical cause of bed-wetting (nocturnal enuresis) and daytime wetting (diurnal enuresis) is delayed or incomplete development of the sphincter in the bladder and urethra, which makes it impossible to hold in urine during sleep when the urge feedback sensors are literally at rest.

Naturally, you must also first rule out psychological (e.g., stress), hormonal (e.g., antidiuretic hormone (ADH) deficiency), or pathological (e.g., diabetes, urinary tract infection (UTI)) factors. However, in my clinical experience, most cases are either of psychological or anatomical etiology.

If those subduing and settling and qi-, blood- and kidney yang-supplementing formulas you typically prescribe are *not* effective, then you could consider the following approaches:

For toddlers, you can advise them to eat fresh ginkgo seeds (Bai Guo) (constrains the lung and stabilizes panting, checks discharge, and reduces urine) steamed with rice or mixed in with other dishes *before* every meal 3x/day and/or prescribe Si Ni Tang adding Xi Lu Rong (invigorates kidney yang, boosts essence-blood, strengthens sinew and bone, and regulates the thoroughfare and controlling vessels).

For adolescents in their teens, I would consider prescribing a spleen-fortifying qi-supplementing, yang-upbearing fall-raising, blood-supplementing and -quickening formula such as Bu Zhong Yi Qi Tang adding large doses of Huang Qi, Bai Guo, and Long Yan He (or Li Zhi He) along with The Three Great Yang-Supplementers and Huang Bo.

Remember! Regardless of the formula you choose, make sure to instruct the patient to take these medicinals *before* every meal (3x/day), with the last meal no later than 6 p.m.

Case Study #16: "Can't Sit Still or Pay Attention to Anything"

Q: A mother brought in her 13 y/o daughter for a visit explaining that the girl "can't sit still or pay attention to anything," has atopic dermatitis (generalized eczema, pruritis, and lichenification), and epilepsy (incurs an average of 2 seizures per week). Prior to a seizure the patient will awake from sleep and laugh out loud, and during a seizure the jaw and limbs are stiff with twitching (myoclonic and generalized tonic-clonic seizures).

This really seems like a tough case. How would you treat this patient?

A: Oh!...This does sound like a tough case! First, here is a general overview of my clinical experiences treating pediatric patients who may present with similar clinical presentations:

For the treatment of *Tourette Syndrome (TS)*—dopamine *excess*—the most effective formulas that I have tried are Wen Dan Tang, Chai Hu Jia Long Gu Mu Li Tang, Jian Ling Tang, Huang Lian Jie Du Tang, or possibly even Jian Ling Tang combining Huang Lian Jie Du Tang. But the problem with these types of cold, bitter, and acrid formulas is that you must get children to actually drink the decoction!

Thus, in light of these "unpalatable" circumstances, I may also prescribe a center-harmonizing agitation-calming, qi-moving counterflow-downbearing, and stagnation-dissipating phlegm-transforming formula such as Gan Mai Da Zao Tang Combining Ban Xia Hou Po Tang adding Huang Qin (Huang Lian or Huang Bo), Long Yan Rou, and Yu Sheng Wan*. Long Yan Rou contains bioactive constituents that promote the production and release of serotonin, which *inhibits* dopamine production and creates a balanced interplay of these pivotal hormones (neurotransmitters) that affect mood and behavior.

For the treatment of hyperactivity, impulsivity, and inattention that may present in *attention deficit hyperactivity disorder (ADHD)*, cerebral palsy, and other types of developmental delay patients—dopamine *deficiency*—you must apply a supplementing approach. I would prescribe formulas such as Shi Quan Da Bu Tang, Bu Yang Huan Wu Tang, You Gui Yin, or Shen Qi Wan, making sure to include Ren Shen/Chuan Qi Powder, The Three Great Yang-Supplementers, Huang Qin, and Xi Lu Rong (powder). And remember! For pediatric patients in particular, it is especially important to include combinations of The Digestants (Cang Zhu, Shan Zha, Gu Ya, Mai Ya, Ji Nei Jin, and Shen Qu) to disperse food, arouse and fortify the spleen, open and harmonize the stomach, and promote digestion. This will ensure that the nutrients in the diet and bioactive constituents in the medicinals are adequately absorbed and utilized.

Since your patient also has *epileptic seizures* (juvenile myoclonic epilepsy), this adds another level of complexity to the case. I would add combinations of medicinals such as Zhu Ru, Lai Fu Zi, The Three Insects, and Qi Cao to your main formula. Recently, I have been treating a 30 y/o patient by prescribing a large dose of Zhu Ru (10 pieces/day) to be decocted and drank as a beverage throughout the day along with Wen Dan Tang variant, acupuncture, and auricular acupuncture (leaving the tack in for 3–5 days at a time). This approach has produced excellent results, allowing the patient to go from nearly 100 seizures per week to about 10 now.

*Note: Yu Sheng Wan dosage based on the following body weight criteria: ≥ 40 kg = 1 pill/day, 20–40 kg = 1/3 pill/day, and < 20 kg = 1/4 pill/day.

Section 2: Tourette Syndrome

Case Study #1: Tourette Syndrome and ADHD – Bed-Wetting

Q: During the initial clinical visit, this 10 y/o boy was extremely active—to the point that he would not remain seated or stay in one place long enough to even talk with him. His parents explained that this hyperactivity makes it difficult for their son to focus on one thing long enough to complete basic tasks. They also said that the boy has never grown out of the bed-wetting (nocturnal enuresis) habit, with a frequency of 2–3 times on average and as many as 10 times a night. This has really been a tough situation for their family to deal with and they wonder if there is anything they can do.

I prescribed Jian Ling Tang adding Huang Qin (8 qian) and Long Yan Rou (1 liang), which seemed to be effective, as he now only wets the bed 1 time every 2 days. He has already taken this formula for 1 month now and neither the bed-wetting nor the hyperactivity has resolved. I am beginning to wonder if I am on the right track or not? What do you think?

A: Mhm...hyperactivity and inability to pay attention, plus bed-wetting...It sounds to me like either attention deficit hyperactivity disorder (ADHD), Tourette syndrome (TS), or TS with concomitant ADHD, both of which are neurodevelopmental disorders that present in childhood.

ADHD presents with symptoms of hyperactivity, impulsivity, and inattention, which may impair learning and impact cognitive development and social integration. In TCM, ADHD can be classified as insufficiency of earlier heaven (a type of developmental delay) and identified as qi, blood, and kidney yang vacuity pattern.

TS is characterized by motor and vocal tics and may concomitantly present with ADHD. Sleep problems such as sleepwalking, night terrors, and bed-wetting are also common. Multiple neurotransmitters (i.e., histamine, dopamine, serotonin, GABA, and glutamate) are thought to be involved in causing this pathocondition, particularly dopamine *excess* or supersensitivity of the postsynaptic dopamine receptors, which disrupts normal nerve conductance and impairs motor function. In TCM, *TS* can be identified as a type of heat pattern that includes yang hyperactivity, yang straying outward, phlegm-rheum heat, and liver and kidney yin vacuity pattern.

As for treatment, I would consider prescribing a formula such as Wen Dan Tang (harmonizes the gallbladder and stomach and dispels phlegm turbidity harassing the inner body), Chai Hu Jia Long Gu Mu Li Tang (harmonizes Shao Yang and settles fright and quiets the spirit), Jian Ling Tang (settles the liver and extinguishes wind and enriches yin and subdues yang), or even Zhi Bo Di Huang Tang (enriches yin, downbears fire, and eliminates steaming) adding Long Gu and Mu Li. Just make sure to include Gan Cao, Da Zao, Long Yan Rou, and The Three Yellows in your formula.

In some cases where the pediatric patient really can't stand the taste of the above formulas and refuses to take the medicine, I may instead resort to prescribing Gan Mai Da Zao Tang Combining Ban Xia Hou Po Tang (harmonizes the center and calms agitation and dissipates stagnation and transforms phlegm) adding The Three Yellows and Shan Zha.

If Jian Ling Tang variant has proven effective in improving the bed-wetting, then this suggests you are indeed on the right track. I would stick with it. Just make sure to add male genitourinary conductors (e.g., Long Yan He, Li Zhi He, Ju He, Shan Zha He) and astringing (e.g., Qian Shi, Lian Xu, Jin Ying Zi) medicinals to enhance effectiveness. Also, advise the parents to encourage the child to get lots of exercise and/or participate in physical activities to work up a sweat and exert some of that energy!

Case Study #2: Autism Spectrum Disorder

Q: This patient is a 6 y/o boy whose mother has a history of depression, which made her emotionally and psychologically unstable and unable to take care of her son for about 2 years after birth. Later, I found out that the child also presented with the following features: reduced intelligence compared to other children of the same age, an aversion to looking people directly in the face (no eye contact), only speaks in words and phrases (not complete sentences), an intense fascination and even fixation with water, itchiness over his entire body, and urinary and fecal incontinence. He is currently being administered methylphenidate (Ritalin) and undergoing early behavioral and educational management.

I am curious, in TCM, would this pathocondition be classified as five slowness (五遲 wu chí) and identified as spleen and kidney yang vacuity pattern, or identified as a type of yang hyperactivity of the liver with heart-kidney yin vacuity and blood vacuity pattern? I am thinking this is a case of yang hyperactivity pattern and thus considering administration of either Jian Ling Tang combining Huang Lian Jie Du Tang or Wen Dan Tang adding heavy-settling (minerals), yin-supplementing, and blood-supplementing medicinals.

A: I do*n't* see any symptoms that would indicate yang hyperactivity pattern at all! Based on the presenting symptoms, I would say this is a case of autism spectrum disorder (ASD). ASD is a neurodevelopmental disorder that can be classified as either insufficiency of earlier heaven or five slowness and identified as either dual qi and blood vacuity with yang vacuity pattern or kidney yang vacuity pattern. Thus, I would prescribe a formula such as Shi Quan Da Bu Tang, You Gui Yin, or Gui Qi Jiang Zhong Tang, making sure to include The Three Great Yang-Supplementers and Ren Shen/Chuan Qi Powder.

As for the itchiness over the entire body, you must consider the possibility of side effects from the methylphenidate (Ritalin), which include skin rash, sweating, nervousness, agitation, anxiety, palpitations, and sleep problems.

If the itchiness is accompanied by an erythematous rash, then this suggests exterior heat pattern, for which you may want to reduce the amount of yang-supplementing medicinals and add Ma Huang and The Three Yellows. If there is *no* erythema, then this suggests blood desiccation, for which you can reduce the amount of yang-supplementing medicinals and add in larger doses of blood-nourishing yin-enriching medicinals. And if the itchiness and rash continues to be a problem, you should advise the parents to talk with the patient's doctor about either adjusting the dosage or changing the prescription altogether.

Case Study #3: Tourette Syndrome vs. ADHD

Q: What are the key features that distinguish Tourette syndrome (TS) and attention deficit hyperactivity disorder (ADHD)? How do you make a differential diagnosis? How do you treat a Tourette syndrome patient who also presents with ADHD? Please offer your invaluable advice and suggestions.

A: Children with *TS* present with the characteristic features of involuntary, repeated, and intermittent movements and/or vocalizations (motor and/or vocal tics). These motor and vocal tics are sudden, rapid, involuntary, intermittent, and nonrhythmic movements and/or vocalizations without any recognizable purpose. Tics may manifest in a myriad of idiosyncrasies. Typical motor tics include eye blinking, facial grimacing, shoulder rotation, head jerking, jumping, and twisting the body among others. Typical vocal tics include throat clearing, grunting, lip smacking, coprolalia, and echolalia among others.

Technically, *TS* does *not* have a negative impact on attention span and learning capacity. It's just that the manifestation of these tics, especially if severe, may be disruptive for other students and teachers in an educational environment, and the inability to "control" these sporadic urges may take a toll on the emotional and psychological well-being of some patients. Hyperactivity, inattention, and impulsivity are not diagnostic features of this pathocondition, but it is *not* uncommon for TS patients to present with ADHD at the same time.

The key diagnostic feature of *ADHD* is the presentation of hyperactivity, inattention, and impulsivity, which does have a detrimental impact on the patient's social skills and learning capacity. It is *not* that these patients lack intelligence, it's just that they lack the ability to focus their attention long enough to engage, interact, reciprocate, and comprehend. So naturally, over time, this will take a toll on their capacity to retain information and acquire knowledge. Specialists in the field of psychology and psychiatry explain these learning difficulties as problems of *executive function*—attention, self-control, memory, and organization.

TS can be identified as a type of heat pattern that includes yang hyperactivity, yang straying outward, phlegm-rheum heat, and liver and kidney yin vacuity pattern. *ADHD* can be classified as insufficiency of earlier heaven (a type of developmental delay), which can be identified as qi, blood, and kidney yang vacuity pattern.

It is quite common for a *TS* patient to present with varying degrees of anxiety and agitation, whether it be formally diagnosed as *ADHD*, *obsessive-compulsive disorder* (*OCD*), or other related conditions. The key here is to determine the predominant behavioral abnormality based on the presenting signs and symptoms. For example, which are the most obvious and disruptive: the tics; impulsivity, hyperactivity and inattention; or obsessiveness and compulsiveness?

In my clinical practice, I most often treat *TS* patients whose predominant symptoms are tics, with relatively lesser degrees of hyperactivity and inattention (i.e., *ADHD*). Thus, for these patients, I would identify *TS* as the root and make this the focus of my treatment. Typically, if the root can be effectively treated, then the peripheral symptoms (tip) will also subside.

Case Study #4: Tourette Syndrome – Etiologies, Patterns, and Therapies

Q: Most children diagnosed with Tourette syndrome (TS) will be administered drug treatment and undergo behavioral therapy. However, usually these antipsychotics and psychostimulants only have a marginal effect on mitigating the severity of symptoms.

In the past, I have treated TS patients and those with concomitant attention deficit hyperactivity disorder (ADHD) by prescribing Jian Ling Tang variant. For some patients, this approach has proven effective at mitigating the severity of symptoms and getting the condition under control, but *not* all.

Recently, I have been treating an ADHD patient with Gui Zhi Jia Long Gu Mu Li Tang, which seems to be working well at quieting the spirit (calms anxiety), relieving impulsivity, and improving the patient's ability to pay attention. Can you share your experiences treating these types of neurodevelopmental disorders?

A: *TS* is a neurodevelopmental disorder that likely arises from a combination of environmental, social, psychological, and genetic factors. In TCM, this pathocondition can be identified as a type of heat pattern that includes yang hyperactivity, yang straying outward, phlegm-rheum heat, and liver and kidney yin vacuity pattern. For patients diagnosed with *TS* (or *TS* with concomitant *ADHD*) in the absence of other precipitating etiological factors, I would prescribe a formula such as Jian Ling Tang, Wen Dan Tang, Chai Hu Jia Long Gu Mu Li Tang, or Zhi Bo Di Huang Tang, making sure to include The Three Yellows.

TS may also present in some patients with conditions that can be classified as insufficiency of earlier heaven (e.g., *cerebral palsy*, *autism spectrum disorder* (*ASD*)) and identified as qi, blood, and kidney yang vacuity pattern. For these patients, I would prescribe a formula such as Shi Quan Da Bu Tang, Gui Qi Jiang Zhong Tang, or You Gui Yin, making sure to include The Three Great Yang-Supplementers and Ren Shen/Chuan Qi Powder.

In rare cases, *TS* may present in postinfectious (external contraction) sequelae, in which the evil has either *not* been completely eliminated (邪熱未盡 xié rè wèi jìn); or the evil has been completely eliminated, but *persists* as residual heat (餘熱未盡 yú rè wèi jìn) in the sense that it has disrupted the functional capacity of the autonomic nervous system. In the acute stage, this can be identified as exterior heat pattern, requiring administration of a formula, such as Gui Zhi Ma Huang Ge Ban Tang adding Sheng Shi Gao and Huang Qin; Bai Hu Tang; or Da Qing Long Tang. Once the initial microbial infection symptoms (e.g., fever, rash, nasal congestion, cough, malaise) have resolved, it can be identified as Shao Yang heat with phlegm-rheum pattern, requiring administration of a formula such as Wen Dan Tang, Xiao Chai Hu Tang, or Er Chen Tang.

Rarely, *TS* may present in post-traumatic sequela. For post-traumatic sequela, in the presence of elevated intracranial pressure (ICP), this can be identified as stasis heat pattern, requiring administration of a formula such as Ru Mo Si Wu Tang, Sheng Yu Tang, or Bu Yang Huan Wu Tang. Just make sure to include Huang Qin and Chuan Qi. Once the ICP has normalized, this can be identified as cold stasis pattern, requiring you to include large doses of The Three Great Yang-Supplementers.

Another rare case is for *TS* to present in complications of cerebrovascular disease, which can be differentiated into acute, post-acute, and chronic stages, and typically identified as static blood obstruction pattern with varying degrees of heat and water amassment (swelling) and stagnation with qi and yang vacuity, depending on the specific manifestations of each respective stage. Based on the staging and pattern identification, you could consider prescribing formula variants such Da Chai Hu Tang adding Chuan Qi, and Mu Li and

Long Gu (or Dai Zhe Shi and Shi Gao); Wen Dan Tang adding Tian Ma and The Three Insects; Ban Xia Tian Ma Bai Zhu San adding Dan Shen and Chuan Xiong; or Bu Yang Huan Wu Tang adding The Three Great Yang-Supplementers.

Each pattern type requires administration of a corresponding therapeutic regimen that addresses the underlying etiology and pathomechanisms.

Case Study #5: Sudden Discontinuation of Medication Results in "Rebound" Effect

Q: This 7 y/o girl who was diagnosed with Tourette syndrome (TS) has been taking fexofenadine (antihistamine) and imipramine (tricyclic antidepressant) and receiving behavioral therapy for several years now. Since the patient had been incurring some side effects (e.g., upset stomach, sweating, stomach cramps) and it did*n't* seem like she was making too much progress, her parents decided to discontinue her medication.

They came to see me after that and I began administering Wen Dan Tang variant. Well, about 1 week after discontinuing the medication and taking TCM medicinals, the girl began having some strange behavior—urinary incontinence, stealing things, and wandering off into restricted areas of her school grounds. What do you attribute these abrupt changes in behavior to?

A: TS patients who abruptly discontinue their medication most certainly risk the possibility of severe "rebound" effects that result from the sudden withdrawal of acetylcholine suppression and cause a surge of euphoric impulses. The child seems to be simply acting out these impulses in a frenzy.

Remember! You must always advise patients who are being administered Western medicine drugs to gradually reduce the dosage up until complete discontinuation. This will minimize the potential for "rebound" effects that may lead to more severe motor and vocal tics and potentially volatile and dangerous behavior.

During the process of weaning away from reliance on the drugs, it would be best for patients to concomitantly take TCM medicinals. This will ensure that therapeutic progress can continue to make headway by providing the body with the means to naturally suppress, mitigate and control the symptoms, while also regulating the constitution and putting the patient on the path towards complete resolution.

TS can be identified as a type of heat pattern that includes yang hyperactivity, yang straying outward, phlegm-rheum heat, and liver and kidney yin vacuity pattern.

For children with TS, if they are incurring *delayed* development (i.e., in reaching social, language, cognitive and physical developmental milestones), then I like to prescribe a center-harmonizing agitation-calming and stagnation-dissipating phlegm-transforming formula such as Gan Mai Da Zao Tang Combining Ban Xia Hou Po Tang adding The Three Yellows, Long Yan Rou, and Shan Zha.

For children with *normal* development, I would typically consider either a liver-settling wind-extinguishing and yin-enriching yang-subduing formula, such as Jian Ling Tang adding The Three Yellows, Shan Zha, Gan Cao, Da Zao, and Long Yan Rou; or a Shao Yang depressed heat-clearing and phlegm turbidity harassing the inner body-dispelling formula, such as Wen Dan Tang including large doses of Huang Qin (assumes sovereign medicinal role!), Gan Cao, and Da Zao.

Case Study #6: Tearing On Exposure to Wind, Sniffling, and Nose Twitching

Q: Since I began my clinical career in medicine, I have had more than 30 patients diagnosed with Tourette's syndrome (TS) visit me. And almost all of them have presented with combinations of concurrent symptoms consisting of tearing on exposure to wind, chronic rhinitis, sniffling, and nose twitching (motor tic).

Right now, I have been trying to treat this 8 y/o boy whose parents decided to discontinue administration of their son's Western medicine medication, which resulted in a severe "rebound" effect with exacerbation of symptoms. How would you treat this type of patient?

A: There are several classes of Western medicine drugs prescribed for the treatment of TS, some of which may mitigate the severity or resolve certain symptoms, but may also exacerbate other symptoms and cause troubling side effects. For instance, *antipsychotics* (e.g., haloperidol, risperidone) may help control tics, but cause side effects of involuntary repetitive movements, and discontinuing the medication may result in a disturbing "rebound" effect; and *stimulants* (e.g., Ritalin, Adderall) may help increase attention and concentration for some patients, but oftentimes these drugs exacerbate tics.

That's why the best approach is to gradually reduce the dosage of these drugs up until they are discontinued altogether. During the process of weaning away from the drugs, TCM medicinals can be concomitantly prescribed to facilitate the transition and begin making headway towards complete resolution of the condition.

In TCM, this pathocondition can be identified as a type of heat pattern that includes yang hyperactivity, yang straying outward, phlegm-rheum heat, and liver and kidney yin vacuity pattern. Depending on the presenting signs and symptoms, I would consider prescribing a formula such as Wen Dan Tang, Xie Xin Tang, Huang Lian Jie Du Tang, Jian Ling Tang, Chai Hu Jia Long Gu Mu Li Tang, Zhi Bo Di Huang Tang, Ru Mo Si Wu Tang, or Gan Mai Da Zao Tang Combining Ban Xia Hou Po Tang. Just make sure to include The Three Yellows, and for some patients with particularly severe tics, you could also consider adding The Three Insects (enter the liver channel, extinguish wind, check tetany, and free the network vessels).

As a general rule, if the nasal and vocal (throat) noises are *mild* and virtually inaudible, I tend to classify this as blockage of the nose and throat (喉中梗阻 hóu zh□ng g□ng zu), which is a type of psychosomatic disorder, and if the nasal or vocal (throat) noises are *loud* and noticeably audible, I would be inclined to classify this as the vocal tics of TS. These two phenomena must be accurately differentiated in order to conduct pattern identification as the basis of treatment.

Time and again, in my clinical practice I have come across this dichotomy: Is it mind over matter or matter over mind?

Case Study #7: Symptoms Worsen After Taking Medication

Q: This 10 y/o boy was diagnosed with Tourette syndrome (TS) at the age of 6, originally presenting with symptoms of noticeably audible snorting and visible nose twitching. After being administered Western medicine drugs, his symptoms worsened. Now, on top of the loud snorting and nose twitching, he also makes a strange grunting noise, jerks his head from side to side, shrugs his shoulders, nods his head, kicks his legs, and curses uncontrollably (coprolalia). Despite the fact that the patient's symptoms have gotten *worse* since taking the medication, his parents have decided to keep him on the same pharmaceutical regimen.

Based on my experience in treating other TS patients, I prescribed Jian Ling Tang adding The Three Yellows and Bai Jiang Can. But after taking this formula for 1 month, there were *no* noticeable improvements. This is definitely the most complex TS case I have ever attempted to treat. Do you have any advice or suggestions on treating this patient?

A: Oh!...multiple complex motor and vocal tics plus coprolalia...This certainly sounds like a challenging case. Western medicine drugs may be able to "suppress" some or all of the symptoms while they are being administered (though apparently *not* in this case!); however, they also cause troubling side effects and may result in a "rebound" effect once they are discontinued. Administration of TCM medicinals will provide the capacity not only to suppress, mitigate, and control the symptoms, but also to regulate the constitution and put the patient on the path towards complete resolution.

TS can be identified as a type of heat pattern that includes yang hyperactivity, yang straying outward, phlegm-rheum heat, and liver and kidney yin vacuity pattern. Thus, besides Jian Ling Tang, you could also consider prescribing Wen Dan Tang, Zhi Bo Di Huang Tang, or Gan Mai Da Zao Tang Combining Ban Xia Hou Po Tang. Just make sure to include The Three Yellows. For patients who present with severe tics (such as this patient!) and/or epilepsy, you should also add The Three Insects* (enter the liver channel, extinguish wind, check tetany, and free the network vessels) into your formula.

Remember! After administering this formula for 1–2 weeks, it would be optimal to begin the gradual process of discontinuing the Western medicine drugs. If the parents are *not* willing to comply, that's ok too, just continue prescribing your formula and the severity of the symptoms will eventually mitigate. One thing is for sure, treating TS patients requires *a lot* of patience from everyone. It is tough on the patient and family, and it is a challenge for doctors, but over time this condition can be brought under control and will usually completely resolve.

*Note: Wu Gong (Centipede) is a very expensive medicinal. Thus, recently I have tried substituting the much more economical Qi Cao (White Grub) in its place as one of the medicinals in The Three Insects. The results have been very good! With the exception of certain types of tumors (e.g., sarcomas) and phantom pain, for most other neuropathies that present with spasms, tremors, hypertonicity, tics, twitches, seizures, and pain, I would recommend using Qi Cao instead. Qi Cao offers more bang for the buck!

Case Study #8: Tourette Syndrome with Concomitant ADHD – Treat the Root

Q: This 13 y/o boy has a history of developmental delay since early childhood and presents with the following symptoms: a sensation of heat on his head, nasal congestion, snorting, agitation, indiscriminate cursing (coprolalia), compulsive masturbation, repeats incoherent phrases over and over (palilalia), difficulty focusing attention, does not listen to his teacher, and will not sit still (always fidgeting arms and legs).

His parents put the child through the gamut of tests and examinations and were at a loss about what to do. Eventually, a neurologist diagnosed the child with attention deficit hyperactivity disorder (ADHD) and prescribed methyphenidate (Ritalin).

Originally, I thought this was a case of insufficiency of earlier heaven or autism, and thus prescribed You Gui Yin combining Bu Yang Huan Wu Tang adding Ren Shen. After taking this formula for a period of time, in addition to the original symptoms, the patient began using insulting and abusive language towards his mother. So I tried changing the formula to simply You Gui Yin adding Huang Qi, but this only resulted in even more vulgar cursing and abusive behavior towards his mother. I am not sure what do next. How would you treat this patient?

A: It sounds to me like the more accurate diagnosis would be Tourette syndrome (TS) with concomitant ADHD. In this type of complex case, I would consider TS as the *root* and place the focus of treatment on this pathocondition.

TS can be identified as a type of heat pattern that includes yang hyperactivity (or yang straying outward), phlegm-rheum heat, and liver and kidney yin vacuity pattern. Thus, I would consider prescribing either Jian Ling Tang including Gan Cao (settles the liver and extinguishes wind and enriches yin and subdues yang), or Gan Mai Da Zao Tang Combining Ban Xia Hou Po Tang (moves qi and downbears counterflow and dissipates stagnation and transforms phlegm). Just make sure to add large doses of The Three Yellows—Huang Qin and Huang Bo (8 qian each), and Huang Lian (5 qian).

The key to determining which approach to take is based on whether the patient presents with normal development (i.e., reaching social, language, cognitive and physical developmental milestones).

For patients with *normal* development, I like to prescribe Jian Ling Tang variant, which directly suppresses the secretion and/or uptake of dopamine, controls symptoms, and regulates the constitution to resolve the condition.

For patients with *abnormal* development, I like to prescribe Gan Mai Da Zao Tang Combining Ban Xia Hou Po Tang variant, which increases serotonin levels (thus functions to reduce dopamine levels), controls symptoms, supplements the center and promotes development, and regulates the constitution to resolve the condition.

Obviously, if you keep stimulating this patient with qi- and kidney yang-supplementing medicinals, the agitation, cursing, and masturbating will continue intensifying!

TS patients with concomitant ADHD may face major obstacles for learning and social integration due to severely disruptive tics, impulsivity, hyperactivity and inattention. Over time, this will likely lead to developmental delays and the inability to stay on pace with their peers. These patients may be unable to contain the "uncontrollable" urge to make strange noises and erratic movements, utter obscene language (coprolalia), or say things over and over again (palilalia). These patients may even inadvertently break things and injure others or themselves. Their "strange," socially unacceptable behavior may cause their peers to reject them, resulting in the inability to foster relationships with others and for some may lead to self-injurious behavior.

Remember! You must differentiate between TS, autism, and developmental delay.

TS—unless it occurs concomitantly with another pathocondition such as ADHD, obsessive-compulsive behavior (OCD), or conduct disorder (CD)—presents with normal mood and behavior, but with "uncontrollable" motor and vocal tics.

Autism patients tend to be difficult to communicate with (except possibly for the few people closest to them), do not like to "make eye contact" with others, make repetitive movements (e.g., stereotyped hand movements), have fixation for certain objects, and are prone to sensory meltdowns (patient is completely unaware of their actions) that may manifest as screaming, breaking things, attacking others, and self-injury.

Developmental delay (e.g., cerebral palsy) results from insufficiency of earlier heaven and manifests as physical and/or cognitive abnormalities.

Case Study #9: Head and Neck Tics

Q: This 6 y/o girl has a history of head and neck tics (involuntary, intermittent, and jerky movements), prompting her parents to have her undergo a thorough physical and psychiatric examination. Eventually, she was diagnosed with Tourette syndrome (TS) and administered haloperidol for an extended period, which did *not* remedy the tics at all.

Recently, another motor tic has popped up: rapid torso twisting movements that occur frequently (2 to 3 times per minute!). These tics even occur in her sleep sometimes, which makes it difficult to get a good night's rest.

Do you think it's possible that this child was misdiagnosed? Could this be some type of cerebral palsy?

A: No, this sounds like a case of TS to me. If it were cerebral palsy (five limpnesses), then the symptoms would have presented either at birth or when she was a toddler ($\leq$ 3 years of age).

TS can be identified as a type of heat pattern that includes yin vacuity due to hyperactivity of yang with phlegm-heat and yang straying outward. Thus, I would prescribe formulas such as Zhi Bo Di Huang Tang, Wen Dan Tang, Jian Ling Tang, Gan Mai Da Zao Tang

Combining Ban Xia Hou Po Tang, or Ling Gui Zao Gan Tang. Depending on the specific pattern presentation, you may also need to include Sheng Long Gu and Sheng Mu Li (secure the essence and subdue yang) and The Three Yellows (clear heat and resolve toxin). Typically, tics only occur at the onset of sleep and disappear completely during the deeper stages of sleep, but if symptoms do manifest during sleep then you can add The Three Insects (enter the liver channel, extinguish wind, check tetany, and free the network vessels).

Remember! You should also advise the patient to eat lots of sweet foods (natural sweets without granulated sugar and preservatives are best!) such as dates, sugar cane, jujubes, longan fruit, raisins, and dried fruits. Naturally, sweet foods will supplement and boost the heart and spleen and nourish the blood and quiet the spirit. Also, advise the patient to get in as much physical activity and exercise as possible in order to exert the body and mind of excess energy. This holistic therapeutic approach will help the patient make a quicker and smoother transition towards a tic-free life.

Case Study #10: Autism Spectrum Disorder

Q: This 14 y/o patient was diagnosed with autism spectrum disorder (ASD) as a child. Growing up he has participated in special educational and behavioral management programs. However, he still has repetitive movements, and language, communication and intellectual abilities that lag behind others in his age group.

During his initial clinical visit, he presented with the following symptoms: difficulty focusing and paying attention, repeats words and phrases over and over again (palilalia), impulsive behavior that sometimes results in violent episodes, a fixation with masturbation, and nasal congestion. Based on my understanding, this condition can be classified as insufficiency of earlier heaven and identified as dual qi and blood vacuity with kidney yang vacuity pattern. Thus, I prescribed You Gui Yin combining Bu Yang Huan Wu Tang. Do you think this is the right approach?

A: ASD is a neurodevelopmental disorder characterized by impaired social interaction and communication, and repetitive stereotyped behavior, interests, and activities. It can be subdivided into autistic disorder (aka childhood autism or Kanner syndrome), which presents with marked language, social interaction, and intellectual impairment, and Asperger syndrome, which presents with normal language skills and intellectual capacity, and often exhibiting exceptional talents in specific areas.

In TCM, ASD can be identified as spleen and kidney yang vacuity and dual qi and blood vacuity pattern. It is difficult for autism patients to participate in the educational and learning process. This may cause problems later in life with employment and social integration. Yes, I agree with your approach, but you must make sure everyone understands that treating this condition will require patience and a lot of time (likely 2 to 3 years before noticeable results will become evident).

A general outline of some other pathoconditions that commonly affect behavior, physical, emotional, and/or intellectual development in pediatric patients are as follows: Tourette syndrome can be identified as a repletion heat with yang hyperactivity pattern; the five limpnesses (五軟 wu ruan) (aka cerebral palsy) can be identified as qi, blood, and yang vacuity pattern; epilepsy can be identified as stasis heat pattern; autoimmune brain diseases (e.g., encephalitis, central nervous system vasculitis) can be identified as heat with blood stasis pattern that over time will evolve into qi vacuity pattern; uremic encephalopathy can be identified as cold damp with static blood and phlegm-rheum pattern; and bacterial encephalitis can be identified as heat or yin vacuity fire effulgence (陰虛火旺 y□n x□ huo wàng) pattern.

X. PSYCHOLOGY & PSYCHIATRY

Anxiety and stress are of epidemic proportions in our modern industrialized society. Psychological or psychiatric imbalances may lead to the manifestation of physical maladies with*out* any identifiable physiological etiology (e.g., plum-pit qi (梅核氣 méi hé qì)), which are commonly referred to as *psychogenic disorders* (aka *somatic symptom disorder* or *somatoform disorder*). Similarly, psychological or psychiatric imbalances can exacerbate an existing physical illness *with* an identifiable physiological etiology (e.g., gastritis, asthma), or a physical illness may lead to the manifestation of psychiatric symptoms (e.g., depression in chronic illness), which are commonly referred to as *psychosomatic disorders*. For simplicity, unless a particular case warrants otherwise, throughout this chapter the umbrella term *psychosomatic disorder* (or *symptom*) will be used to denote maladies that may be caused by or exacerbated by the mind.

Section 1: Psychosomatic Disorders

Case Study #1: Mind Over Matter or Matter Over Mind?

Q: A woman in her 40s came to see me saying, "Recently, I just haven't felt right all over." It started out with abnormal uterine bleeding, then gastrointestinal reflux disease (GERD), and now aching pain in the right shoulder and back and aching pain upon palpation in the rib-side and upper abdominal region. This aching pain upon palpation is even more intense after exercising, so she doesn't exercise as much anymore. She said that the uterine bleeding was *not* a problem anymore and the acid reflux has improved except for indigestion (dyspepsia) sometimes after eating.

Honestly, I am not certain if she ever underwent an examination and received a diagnosis of GERD or not. She sounds pretty distraught and stressed out about everything. I decided to prescribe Ban Xia Tian Ma Bai Zhu San adding Huang Qin, Dan Shen, Chai Hu, Gan Cao, and Da Zao. After taking this formula for 1 month now, she has *not* noticed any improvements in her symptoms.

A: Yes, it does sound as if the rib-side and abdominal aching pain upon palpation, and possibly the other symptoms, may be of psychosomatic etiology. Typically, only these types of patients would be compelled to pat (or even briskly slap!) their body for no apparent reason (though some people may do this as a type of "massage," claiming it promotes local circulation) other than anxiety.

I frequently have patients with similar complaints whom come in patting or even slapping their bodies. Obviously you must try to rule out other possible causes, but most of the time it is simply anxiety. What I do is tell these patients: "Of course it hurts if you incessantly pat (or slap) your skin, sinews, and organs!" in a jovial tone to try to get them to relax and understand that I am *not* being hypercritical or reprimanding them. I have actually seen some patients slap their bodies so hard that they could cause muscle aches and soreness, bruising, and hematomas, or even damage organs.

Psychosomatic disorders are tough. You can't really say it *is* a disease, nor can you say it is*n't* a disease. Is it mind over matter or matter over mind? It is difficult to discern—a dichotomy, the mind and body indivisible and mutually interactive. Should the mind and body be treated separately with counseling, behavioral therapy, and medication, respectively? Or, should a multimodal therapeutic approach be administered all at the same time? If medication is prescribed, what types of drugs or medicinals can treat both the mind and body? These are tough questions that the medical community and society as a whole must confront and answer.

Chinese medicine has a long history, likely rooted as far back as the Neolithic Period (at least 5,000 BCE), accumulating thousands upon thousands of years of clinical experience. By applying pattern identification as the basis for determining treatment, innumerable formula variants can be composed and administered to effectively treat psychosomatic disorders.

For this patient, I would continue prescribing a spleen- and stomach-supplementing, phlegm-damp-transforming, and blood-nourishing wind-stabilizing formula such as Ban Xia Tian Ma Bai Zhu San adding Gan Cao, Long Yan Rou, Yan Hu Suo, Mu Xiang, Du Zhong, and Yu Sheng Wan. This approach will provide effective relief of symptoms and regulate the constitution to resolve the condition.

Case Study #2: Stress and Anxiety – Gastrointestinal Symptoms

Q: This 35 y/o male patient has a very nervous personality. About 5 years ago, he began having gastrointestinal problems which varies in severity throughout the year, sometimes *not* bothering him at all and sometimes causing considerable discomfort. The most common symptoms are inability to get food down, poor appetite, repetitive belching, flatulence (though when he has a stomachache he can*not* pass gas), glomus below the heart, and pain in the middle of the chest and umbilical region. Plus, a few times a year he gets bouts of diarrhea that he says tend to occur when he is stressed out, and usually once the diarrhea (*no* blood present) subsides a stomachache will set in.

I prescribed Xiang Sha Liu Jun Zi Tang combining Huang Lian Jie Du Tang. The patient has taken this formula for 1 month so far without any improvement. How would you treat this patient?

A: Naturally, you must first rule out the possibility of pathoconditions such as irritable bowel syndrome (IBS) and inflammatory bowel disease (IBD) (includes Crohn's disease (CD) and ulcerative colitis (UC)). IBS is defined as a functional gastrointestinal disorder, with more of a subjective diagnosis that is either induced by or exacerbated by anxiety and stress. IBD can be physically diagnosed via laboratory tests and imaging studies.

However, this sounds to me like it could be a stereotypical psychosomatic disorder. Typically, in these patients, the pain around the umbilical region derives from intestinal spasm (colicky pain, cramps) caused by autonomic hyperactivity amping up the speed of peristalsis (smooth muscle contractions) until the smooth muscles completely tighten up.

If the patient is particularly nervous with a lot of anxiety, then I would consider prescribing a liver-calming depression-resolving formula such as Xiao Chai Hu Jia Long Gu Mu Li Tang, Xiao Yao San, Si Ni San, or Yi Gan San. Just make sure to include Sheng Mu Li, Sheng Long Gu, and Yu Sheng Wan. If diarrhea is mild (3–4x/day), then simply add a small dose of Cang Zhu and Fu Ling to your formula, but if diarrhea is severe (6–7x/day), then add Fu Ling and Cang Zhu to your main formula, or consider changing your formula to Yue Qu Wan or Tian Tai Wu Yao San.

You could also advise the patient to eat Gan Cao Fen (Licorice Powder) as a snack or boil Da Zao (Jujubes) and Long Yan Rou (Longan) together to drink as a beverage. And naturally, the patient needs to lead a healthy lifestyle—eating a well-balanced diet, exercising regularly, and getting at least 8 hours of sleep a night. Over time, this holistic approach will relieve his anxiety and stress and effectively resolve the psychosomatic symptoms.

Case Study #3: Cystic Growths in the Kidney and Lung – Generalized Soreness, Aches, and Malaise

Q: Over the preceding 10 years, cystic growths were discovered in the kidney and spleen of this 61 y/o female patient, which required her to undergo left radical nephrectomy (kidney and adrenal gland) and splenectomy. Recently, a positron emission tomography (PET scan) was performed that revealed cystic growths on the right upper lobe of the lung and right kidney.

She presented with the following symptoms: left-sided hemilateral impediment pain, generalized soreness and aches, malaise, a feeling of heaviness, dry mouth, shortage of qi (lacks energy), and poor quality sleep (awakens easily). Many of these sound like stereotypical psychosomatic symptoms to me. What do you think? How would you treat this patient?

A: Uhm…cystic growths that required resection of the entire left kidney and spleen, and recently cystic growths of the lung have been discovered…This sounds like some type of diffuse polycystic disorder. Indeed, if the cysts have already been resected, then those symptoms do sound like they may be of psychosomatic nature, but it would be best to find out if the patient has been diagnosed with an underlying disorder (e.g., autosomal dominant polycystic kidney disease (ADPKD)).

Psychosomatic symptoms do *not* mean that the symptoms are imaginary. They may manifest as clear as a bright sunny day, it's just that the cause is rooted in the mind-body complex.

The best therapeutic approach would be to focus on eliminating the cysts by prescribing either Chai Ling Tang (clears heat and transforms phlegm-damp, disinhibits water, moves qi and quickens the blood, and relieves pain) or Ban Xia Tian Ma Bai Zhu San (supplements the spleen and stomach, transforms phlegm-damp, and nourishes the blood and stabilizes wind). Just make sure to include Niu Xi, Xu Duan, Gu Sui Bu, Qian Cao, and Chuan Qi (break blood, free the channels, relieve pain, and supplement the liver and kidney) and Yu Sheng Wan (quiets the spirit, calms the nerves, promotes cerebral collateral circulation, and recalibrates autoregulation in the brain).

Remember! Polycystic lesions of the kidney can lead to renal injury and kidney failure, and lung cysts can lead to emphysema, pulmonary edema, and pleural edema. Advise the patient to periodically have renal function tests (e.g., BUN, CR) and imaging studies performed and her blood pressure checked. The psychosomatic symptoms will resolve with effective treatment of the underlying condition. Stay vigilant!

Case Study #4: Lymphadenectomy – Postsurgical "Complications"

Q: Following the surgical removal (lymphadenectomy) of a lingering swollen lymph node on the left side of her neck (cervical lymphadenitis), this 43 y/o female patient explained that she began feeling tongue pain, right-sided hemilateral headache, nausea, the feeling of something stuck in the throat (globus pharyngis) with*out* difficulty swallowing (dysphagia), and insomnia.

I prescribed Xiao Chai Hu Tang adding Qing Hao, Zhi Mu, Di Gu Pi, Sheng Pu Huang, and Yu Sheng Wan. After taking this formula for 2 weeks, the patient returned saying that now she has "dizziness" in addition to her other symptoms. I am not sure what to do for this patient. Please offer your advice and guidance.

A: Cervical lymphadenopathy is likely caused by some type of microbial infection (bacteria or virus). Complications (e.g., damage to the cranial, accessory, vagus, and phrenic nerves) arising from surgical removal of a node in the lateral aspect of the neck are possible, but exceedingly rare.

In TCM, this condition can be identified as liver qi depression and Shao Yang heat with residual heat pattern, which may further be exacerbated by anxiety from worrying too much about her condition. Under these circumstances, she would be prone to bouts of psychosomatic "dizziness" and other "complications."

I like your formula! Just continue prescribing your original formula adding Tian Ma (calms the liver, extinguishes wind, and frees the network vessels), and Da Zao and Long Yan Rou (supplement the spleen and heart, nourish blood, and calm the spirit). Additionally, you should advise the patient to eat sweet foods (preferably natural sweets!) and exercise regularly. This therapeutic approach will ensure that the patient gets on the path towards a healthy mind and body.

Case Study #5: Anxiety Induces Left-Sided Hemilateral Impediment Pain

Q: This 41 y/o female explained that ever since her husband's company went bankrupt 10 years ago, whenever she gets nervous the left side of her body aches, with the pain so bad that sometimes she even cries.

Over the past 3 months, I have tried prescribing Gan Mai Da Zao Tang Combining Ban Xia Hou Pou Tang, Bu Yang Huan Wu Tang, and Gui Qi Jian Zhong Tang, making sure to add Yu Sheng Wan. However, these formulas have only provided slight improvement in her symptoms. This is a strange case. I am not sure where to go from here. What would you do?

A: It sounds to me like the impediment pain (痹痛 bì tong) may be at least partially, or possibly entirely, caused by a psychological "impediment"—anxiety and depression! Thus, I would approach this as either Shao Yang depressed heat (少陽鬱熱 shao yáng yù rè) pattern, prescribing Wen Dan Tang (clears heat and transforms phlegm and harmonizes the gallbladder and stomach and dispels phlegm turbidity harassing the inner body), or liver depression and qi stagnation (肝鬱氣滯 g□n yù qì zhì) pattern, prescribing Ban Xia Tian Ma Bai Zhu San (supplements the spleen and stomach, transforms phlegm-damp, and nourishes the blood and stabilizes wind). Just make sure to add Gan Cao, Long Yan Rou, Yu Sheng Wan, and possibly Sheng Long Gu and Sheng Mu Li, to your formula.

Naturally, you need to advise the patient to regularly exercise (e.g., taking walks, aerobics, yoga), eat healthy, and get an adequate amount of sleep every night. If these approaches still fail to make headway, then you may need to refer the patient to a neurologist and/or psychiatrist for psychotherapy or pharmacotherapy.

Case Study #6: Aching Neck, Nape, and Shoulder – Structural or Psychological?

Q: This 25 y/o male patient first began having a stiff neck, which later spread down to the upper back (nape) and left shoulder upon neck extension (bends neck backwards). Thorough examination and imaging studies have *not* revealed any structural abnormalities.

Recently, I have seen quite a few patients presenting with a similar type of clinical picture. What do you think the cause of this aching pain could be?

A: Naturally, you will first need to rule out the possibility of muscle strains from trauma or postural fatigue and structural anomalies that may compress the spinal cord (cervical myelopathy) or spinal nerves (cervical radiculopathy), such as degenerative disc disease (disc protrusion, herniation, and sequestration). The latter can usually be clearly diagnosed via imaging studies.

However, hypertonicity and pain of the nape and neck upon neck extension are also a common psychosomatic manifestation. In the majority of cases, psychological factors do indeed play a causal role in the development of these symptoms. These patients are typically under a lot of stress, do not get enough sleep or exercise, and have unhealthy diets. The most important part of the therapeutic regimen is to make sure the patient gets 8–10 hours of sleep a night (best to get to bed early!) and keep the body warm.

As for treatment, I would prescribe Ban Xia Tian Ma Bai Zhu San adding Gan Cao, Long Yan Rou, Yu Sheng Wan, and large doses of Ge Gen (and/or Tian Ma). Perform acupuncture on acupoints such as Feng Chi (GB20), Tian Zong (SI11), Fei Shu (UB13), Jian Jing (GB21), Ju Gu (LI16), Jian Zhen (SI9), Wai Guan (SJ5), and Hou Xi (SI3). And, if you have the time, perform message therapy (tui na) (推拿 tu□ ná) on the head, neck, and upper back regions.

Case Study #7: Cervical Lymph Node Biopsy Complications – Phantom Pain

Q: Three months ago, a 48 y/o female patient noticed an enlarged lymph node (lymphadenopathy) on the right side of her neck. The lymph node swelling was painless and had *not* resolved after 1 month. She went in for a follow-up examination and her doctor recommended performing a biopsy to rule out the possibility of malignancy. The good news is that the test results came back clean (no malignancy!), but ever since then she has been experiencing the following symptoms:

- Aching pain on the right side that extends from the mouth up to the temple (Tai Yang (EX-HN5)) and around to the back of the head (Feng Chi (GB20)) down her neck and nape
- Plum-pit qi, which manifests as a feeling of the throat being burnt by scalding hot tea
- And most recently, tongue pain, which began after eating hot, spicy soup, and has continued to get worse since then

Over the past 6 weeks, I have tried prescribing Wen Dan Tang adding Qing Hao, Zhi Mu, and Di Gu Pi; Gan Mai Da Zao Tang Combining Ban Xia Hou Po Tang; and Bu Yang Huan Wu Tang adding Qing Hao, Zhi Mu, and Di Gu Pi. But these formulas have *not* been effective at all in resolving, or even reducing the severity, of her symptoms.

A: Iatrogenic accessory nerve damage is a *possible* complication of lymph node biopsy, but this would typically affect the sternocleidomastoid and trapezius muscles, causing muscle weakness and impaired range of motion of the shoulder. Iatrogenic damage to the cranial, vagus, and phrenic nerves is also *possible*, but exceedingly rare.

Based on the history and symptoms, I would diagnose this as phantom pain (or phantom heat), which in this case can be identified as Shao Yang depressed heat with vacuity heat pattern. To treat this condition I would prescribe Xiao Chai Hu Tang adding Qing Hao, Zhi Mu, and Di Gu Pi (enrich yin and downbear fire, cool the blood and clear vacuity heat, and eliminate steaming bone), and Mu Dan Pi, Zhi Zi, and Sheng Pu Huang (cool the blood and stanch bleeding and quicken the blood and disperse stasis). You could also consider instructing the patient to decoct Sheng Pu Huang (1 liang) (cools the blood and stanches bleeding and quickens the blood and disperses stasis) separately and drink it throughout the day just like a beverage, holding onto each mouthful (as long as possible) like a mouthwash and then swallowing it.

Remember! If the pain "persists" even at rest, with*out* any stimulating factors, then you can also consider adding The Three Insects (extinguish wind and settle tetany, attack toxin and dissipate binds, and free the network vessels and relieve pain) and Yu Sheng Wan (quiets the spirit and calms the nerves, promotes cerebral collateral circulation, and recalibrates autoregulation in the brain). If the pain only presents *with* stimulating factors (e.g., eating, moving the mouth, brushing teeth), then you do *not* need to add these.

Case Study #8: Ants Crawling Under the Skin Sensation and Hand Tremors – Mental Delusions or Physical Disorder?

Q: During her initial clinic visit, this 40 y/o female was visibly nervous and "antsy" and reeled off a litany of what appeared to be the run-of-the-mill psychosomatic symptoms. In addition to plum-pit qi, running piglet, and paranoid insecurities about her mother-in-law, she also feels the sensation of ants crawling under the skin of her left arm (at times, saying it almost felt as if water was flowing up and down her left arm when she moves it), tremor in both hands, and distention in the chest.

To me, it really seems like all of these symptoms may really be in her head, so I administered a 2-week prescription of Gan Mai Da Zao Tang Combining Ban Xia Hou Po Tang adding Tian Ma. I will see if this formula has had any positive effects when she comes back for a follow-up visit. What is your impression of this case?

A: Well, yes, many of these can be interpreted as stereotypical psychosomatic symptoms, and some may be. However, for the sensations of ants crawling under the skin (formication), hand tremor, and hallucinatory thoughts, you must rule out the possibility of a lesion (or tumor) in the cerebrum, brainstem, or cervical spine, and also postinfectious polyneuropathy involving inflammation and demyelination (e.g., Guillain Barre syndrome (GBS) and its subtypes).

Once you have ruled out the possibility of neurological deficits, then you could continue prescribing Gan Mai Da Zao Tang Combining Ban Xia Hou Po Tang (harmonizes the center and releases tension, quiets the spirit and calms agitation, moves qi and downbears counterflow, and dissipates stagnation and transforms phlegm).

Depending on the specific presentation of symptoms and pattern identification, you could consider adding combinations of the following medicinals to your formula: Huang Qi (supplements qi and upbears yang, boosts defense and secures the exterior, disinhibits water and disperses swelling) and The Three Insects (extinguish wind and settle tetany, attack toxin and dissipate binds, and free the network vessels and relieve pain); Long Gu and Mu Li (secure the essence and subdue yang) and Di Long (frees the channels and network vessels); or Qing Hao, Zhi Mu, and Di Gu Pi (enrich yin and downbear fire, cool the blood and clear vacuity heat, and eliminate steaming bone).

Or you could even consider changing the formula to Gui Zhi Ren Shen Tang (warms the center, resolves the exterior and alleviates dampness, and boosts qi and disperses glomus) adding a large dose of

Fu Ling (up to 1.5 liang) (disinhibits water and percolates dampness and fortifies the spleen and quiets the spirit).

Case Study #9: Array of Ailments – Cover a Lot of Ground with One Formula

Q: A 26 y/o female patient visited me with an array of ailments: insomnia, profuse dreaming, intermittent bouts of diarrhea and constipation, aching fingers (second, third and fourth) on both hands, pronounced aversion to cold, tearing on exposure to wind, headache (aching pain around the head and sometimes over the entire scalp), poor appetite (sometimes better than other times), heart palpitations (commonly occur), dry eyes, dry lips, and her menstrual cycle only comes 1 time per year.

Oh! With all of these symptoms, where do I begin?

A: Hmm! A 26 y/o woman with aversion to cold, headache, tearing on exposure to wind.... It sounds to me like a combination of reversal cold, foot Tai Yin phlegm reversal headache, and insufficient fluid intake leading to yin vacuity. As I have mentioned before, whenever such a broad spectrum of symptoms and patterns present all at once, there is a good chance that the *root* of the problems may be in the mind (i.e., psychosomatic disorder or somatoform symptom disorder).

Based on the combination of these presenting symptoms, I would likely prescribe Dang Gui Si Ni Jia Wu Zhu Yu Sheng Jiang Tang (nourishes the blood and frees the network vessels and dissipates cold and downbears counterflow) adding Pu Huang, Tian Men Dong, Mai Men Dong, Tian Hua, Huang Qin (large dose), Long Yan Rou, and Yu Sheng Wan. The addition of these yin-nourishing liquid-engendering, heat-clearing toxin-resolving, spleen- and heart-supplementing, and blood-nourishing spirit-calming medicinals will further help to resolve her insomnia, dry eyes, dry mouth, and palpitations.

As for her menstrual cycle only coming 1 time per year, just because she is *not* menstruating does *not* mean that she can*not* ovulate (i.e., infertility). There are many factors that could cause menstrual irregularities; some may be more simple to deal with (e.g., stress, diet, medication, excessive exercise, hormonal imbalance), while others (e.g., ovarian cysts, polycystic ovarian syndrome (PCOS)) may require more effort. Regardless of whether she wants to get pregnant or not, if she hasn't done so, you should advise her to go in for a thorough gynecological examination to find out what exactly is going on.

Remember! The composition of Dang Gui Si Ni Jia Wu Zhu Yu Sheng Jiang Tang variant I recommended above is very similar to Wen Jing Tang (quickens the blood and dispels stasis, warms the channels and dissipates cold, and boosts qi and nourishes blood), a formula that treats female infertility. So don't get too overwhelmed by all of the symptoms—you can cover a lot of ground with one formula!

Case Study #10: Low Body Mass Index – Anxiety and Melancholic Tendencies

Q: Recently, I have treated a number of thin, slight-statured 40 to 60 y/o male patients (some clearly underweight with body mass index (BMI) well below the normal range). The odd thing is that they all shared similar symptoms—distended abdomen with minimal if any fat issue, normal appetite, no belching or gastric reflux, normal stools (1x/day), a feeling of distention in the lower abdomen, and sometimes abdominal urgency and rectal heaviness (tenesmus)—and despite showing noticeable improvements, they all stopped taking their formula regimens before the condition had completely resolved.

I tried administering several formulas for these patients—Ban Xia Tian Ma Bai Zhu San, Xiao Chai Hu Tang, Da Chai Hu Tang, and Xiang Sha Liu Jun Zi Tang—but the one that worked the best was Xiao Chai Hu Tang.

What is your impression of these thin, slight-statured middle- to older-aged males with mild, but lingering, gastrointestinal symptoms?

A: There definitely does seem to be a tendency for people with thin, slight-statured body types (low BMI) to feel anxiety and melancholy. This correlation was well established long ago in reference to the seven affects (七情 q□ qíng) (joy, anger, anxiety, thought, sorrow, fear, and fright) and five minds (五志 wu zhì) (joy, anger, anxiety, thought, and fear) discussed in *The Yellow Emperor's Inner Canon.*

The fact that Xiao Chai Hu Tang variant turned out to be the most effective formula aligns with these underlying theoretical principles. The *root* of the condition can be identified as liver depression and qi stagnation pattern, thus prescribing a formula such as Xiao Chai Hu Tang, Chai Hu Long Gu Mu Li Tang, Si Ni San, Xiao Yao San, Jia Wei Xiao Yao San, Yi Gan San, or Wen Dan Tang should be effective. Just make sure to include Chai Hu! For people with nervous or high-strung personalities, who may even be a bit on the "neurotic" side, it is particularly important to focus on balancing the mind, body, and spirit, and also boosting morale and breaking through the mental barriers.

Remember! For males in this age group, don't forget to rule out the possibility of an enlarged prostate causing the distention in the lower abdomen. If the patient does have an enlarged prostate, then you can add combinations of the following medicinals to your formula: Fu Ling, Zi Xie, Zhu Ling, and Bai Zhu (disinhibit water by bland percolation, fortify the spleen and disinhibit dampness, and discharge heat); Bai Guo, Shan Yao, Wu Wei Zi, Shan Zhu Yu, and Sheng Mu Li (astringe and promote contraction); Long Yan He, Li Zhi He, Ju He, and Chuan Lian Zi (secure essence); Huang Qi, Dang Shen, and Yu Zhu (supplement qi and tauten the "slack" or "lax" glandular tissue); Chuan Qi, Niu Xi, Du Zhong, Gou Ji, and Di Long (quicken the blood, resolve stasis, and disperse the depressed blood (鬱血 yù xuè) in the pelvic cavity); Tu Si Zi, She Chuang Zi, Sha Wan Zi, Huang Jing, Suo Yang, and Lu Rong (supplement the kidney, boost essence, increase the production of prostate gland secretions, and promote blood flow); and Pu Huang, Zhi Zi, Lian Xu, Qian Shi, and Long Dan Cao (eliminate damp-heat).

Case Study #11: High-Strung People – Prone to Blood Pressure Fluctuations

Q: In my clinical practice, I have noticed that people who suffer from anxiety and stress are much more likely to present with psychosomatic symptoms. For instance, every time this 42 y/o male patient of mine is under a lot of pressure, he feels stuffiness in the chest (胸中窒 xi□ ng zh□ ng zhì), distention in the rib-side, stiffness in the nape and neck, and vice-like pressure in the temples (Tai Yang (EX-HN 5)), along with difficulty sleeping (awakens easily) and dry eyes.

I have tried prescribing Ban Xia Tian Ma Bai Zhu San, Xiao Chai Hu Tang, Chai Ling Tang, and Gan Mai Da Zao Tang Combining Ban

Xia Hou Po Tang for various durations. The only formula that has been effective at relieving symptoms has been Xiao Chai Hu Tang. Plus, in subsequent visits, he has also mentioned that sometimes his blood pressure is too high. Do you think I should prescribe medicinals specifically focused at regulating his blood pressure?

In another case, when this 32 y/o male is under a lot of pressure, his throat will suddenly feel swollen and distended as if it locked up, making it difficult for him to breathe and necessary to be rushed to the emergency room. He continues to be administered H1 antihistamines for its antiallergic and sedative actions. What do you think is the best approach for treating this patient?

A: High-strung people with nervous personalities are prone to fluctuations in blood pressure, sometimes a bit too high and sometimes a bit too low. Unless the hypertension or hypotension is persistent and pronounced, then I would *not* worry about it. Prescribing Xiao Chai Hu Tang variant is a good choice, but I would make sure to add Sheng Mu Li and Sheng Long Gu (calm the liver and subdue yang, quiet the spirit, and astringe and secure) as well.

As for the 32 y/o patient, it sounds to me like he should be on anxiolytics (e.g., benzodiazepines, antidepressants) *not* antihistamines. I would prescribe a spleen- and stomach-supplementing, phlegm-damp-transforming, and blood-nourishing wind-stabilizing formula such as Ban Xia Tian Ma Bai Zhu San adding Gan Cao, Da Zao, Ma Huang, Xing Ren, and Yu Sheng Wan.

These therapeutic approaches will be able to effectively improve the symptoms, but to ultimately cure the condition, in the long run these patients will have to confront the underlying problem—overcoming and resolving their anxiety.

Case Study #12: Panic Attacks and Anxiety Disorder

Q: The majority of patients who visit me for treatment of panic attacks and anxiety disorders are female. The following are two stereotypical cases that come to mind.

One is a 35 y/o female with the chief complaint of excessive sweating (hyperhidrosis), which occurs every time she feels nervous, exercises, or gets into enclosed and crowded spaces, and the sensation of pronounced generalized heat at night when she goes to bed.

I prescribed Jian Ling Tang adding Qing Hao, Zhi Mu, Di Gu Pi, Huang Qin, and Huang Lian, but this was *not* effective in remedying the symptoms at all. Do you have any advice on treating this patient?

Another case is of a 46 y/o female, who feels an overwhelming oppression in the chest and has panic attacks every time she gets in enclosed spaces. But the strange thing is that it only happens during the summertime. Is this also a type of visceral agitation? She is currently being administered the benzodiazepine Alprazolam (Xanax). How would you treat this patient?

A: The 35 y/o woman with excessive sweating and the sensation of heat can be classified as a type of secondary hyperhidrosis caused by panic attacks or anxiety disorder. Thus, the focus of treatment should be on resolving the underlying distress and anxiety.

For this type of patient, I would prescribe a Shao Yang depressed heat-clearing phlegm turbidity harassing the inner body-dispelling formula, such as Wen Dan Tang; a Shao Yang-harmonizing and -resolving formula, such as Xiao Chai Hu Tang; or a center-harmonizing agitation-calming and stagnation-dissipating phlegm-transforming formula, such as Gan Mai Da Zao Tang Combining Ban Xia Hou Po Tang. Just make sure to include Qing Hao, Zhi Mu, Di Gu Pi, Mu Dan Pi, and Huang Bo in your formula.

Remember! For this type of patient in a hyperfunctional state, you should *not* prescribe Yu Sheng Wan, because of its anticholinergic actions that may exacerbate the existing heat (hyperpyrexia)!

As for the 46 y/o woman with panic attacks (panic disorder), I typically identify this condition as one of the following three general pattern types:

- Visceral agitation pattern—serotonin deficiency: In Taiwan, this type can be found mostly in people who go on fasting diets, Buddhists who strictly uphold The Eight Precepts by not taking food after noon, those suffering from illnesses who lose their appetite or are on restricted diets, anorexics, and as a side effect in those taking neuroleptic drugs (e.g., antidepressants, tranquilizers).

  For this type, I like to prescribe the center-harmonizing agitation-calming and stagnation-dissipating phlegm-transforming formula Gan Mai Da Zao Tang

Combining Ban Xia Hou Po Tang (including a large dose of Da Zao (20–30 pieces) or Long Yan Rou (1–2 liang), and in severe cases you may need to add The Three Great Yang-Supplementers and Ren Shen. In my clinical practice, I am seeing more and more of these types of patients.

- Kidney yang vacuity pattern—dopamine deficiency: For this type, I like to prescribe either a kidney yang-supplementing formula, such as You Gui Yin or Shen Qi Qan; a blood-quickening and -supplementing, qi-boosting spleen-fortifying, and kidney yang-supplementing formula, such as Shi Quan Da Bu Tang; or a qi-boosting construction-nourishing and heart-supplementing spirit-quieting formula, such as Ren Shen Yang Rong Tang.
  These formulas function to promote the secretion of adrenocorticotropic hormone (ACTH), serotonin (5-HT), and dopamine, as well as increase the patency of neurotransmitter release from synaptic vesicles across the synaptic cleft and the reception on the membrane of the postsynaptic neuron.
- Phlegm-rheum obstruction pattern—obstruction of the synaptic cleft that inhibits the release and reuptake of acetylcholine (ACh): For this type, I like to prescribe the spleen- and stomach-supplementing, phlegm-damp-transforming, and blood-nourishing wind-stabilizing formula Ban Xia Tian Ma Bai Zhu San.

Regardless of the pattern type, you can add The Sweets (boost qi and supplement the spleen and heart and nourish the blood and calm the spirit), and if necessary, You Gui Wan (powder). Remember! Be aware that *insufficiency* is the root of panic attacks (disorder) and *excess* is the root of agitated mania.

Patients who take anxiolytic drugs (e.g., benzodiazapines, antidepressants), such as alprazolam (Xanax), in excessive doses and/or over long durations are prone to the adverse effects of extreme mood fluctuations that ranges from bouts of mania (agitation, fright, and fear) and depression to hallucinations (mental, visual, and auditory), phantom pain, ataxia, residual urine, dysuria, frequent urination, constipation, diplopia, and abdominal urgency and rectal heaviness (tenesmus).

That's why I always tell patients it is safer and more effective to take Chinese medicine for the treatment of these conditions.

Case Study #13: Protect Yourself Against Malingerers and Mentally Disturbed Patients

Q: A 46 y/o divorced female patient visited me with some rather ambiguous descriptions of a sore back and lumbus. While she was in the waiting room before I called her in, my staff informed me that this patient was fiddling with objects in the room and for no apparent reason pronounced: "The doctors in this clinic are great, but the nurses are terrible!" Not only did she ridicule the staff, she also pilfered coffee bags, a couple of books, and a few items from the nurses desk. She then told me directly and indignantly that she was going to go on line and tell everyone how bad our clinic is. I couldn't bear it any longer, so I told her in a commanding tone to go find a more capable doctor and don't come back here again.

Our clinic on average has one or two female patients every month who come in without any discernible health problems and linger about the clinic long after their consultation, sometimes even refusing to leave altogether. Their presence disturbs other patients, who are seeking assistance for tangible illnesses that require urgent attention, and consumes the time and resources of our entire staff. I am not sure about the best way to handle this. Do you have any advice or suggestions?

A: Beware of malingerers and mentally disturbed patients, and since you are a male doctor, especially females. Diligently record everything that has been said and transpired during the visit, so you can use this as evidence in the horrible circumstance a patient tries to sue you for sexual harassment or some other type of malpractice.

Remember! Be very focused and conscious of your tone of voice and mannerisms at all times. Your intentions of showing concern for the patient may be intentionally or unintentionally misconstrued as "heartfelt" feelings of procuring love, but when that "love" never actualizes, the patient may try to accuse you of sexual harassment. Yes, this could happen. Don't be overly paranoid about it, just be professional and vigilant at all times!

Case Study #14: People on Strict or Fasting Diets – Add The Sweets

Q: Recently, several female patients aged between 20 to 30 years old have visited me, all presenting with a similar constellation of symptoms that include nausea, vomiting, aching pain around the navel and abdominal region, shortness of breath, shortage of qi (lacks energy), heaviness of the body, anxiety, insomnia, and poor appetite.

Have you noticed a trend for these types of patients in your clinic? How would you treat these types of patients?

A: Yes, I have noticed a trend for these types of patients in my clinic. The first things I would do is find out if they have any menstrual irregularities, check for anemia, and rule out the possibility of other underlying pathoconditions (e.g., gynecological, gastrointestinal, food allergies, drug side effects).

However, I have had many young women come in who are on strict calorie restriction or fasting diets. In the pursuit of a "perfect" slender figure, they virtually starve themselves in efforts to realize that "ideal." The extreme dieting goes on for too long and "very real" physical (body) and mental (mind) imbalances can develop, as the body becomes sluggish, the mind distorted, and the spirit deflated.

At the onset, I would prescribe a spleen- and stomach-supplementing, phlegm-damp transforming, and blood-nourishing wind-stabilizing formula, such as Ban Xia Tian Ma Bai Zhu San adding Gan Cao, Da Zao, and Ren Shen (powder). Once the brunt of the symptoms have resolved and the patient feels a lot better, I would then change to a kidney yang-warming and -supplementing, blood-quickening stasis-dissipating, sinew- and bone-strengthening, and dampness-eliminating pain-relieving formula, such as You Gui Yin or Shen Qi Wan, in order to promote the secretion of hormones and neurotransmitters.

Remember! Regardless of the formula you choose, make sure to include The Sweets (Gan Cao, Da Zao, and Long Yong Rou) to boost qi and supplement the spleen and heart and nourish the blood and calm the spirit.

Case Study #15: Hot Flashes – Sign of Male Menopause?

Q: This 63 y/o male patient explained that starting about 3 months ago he began feeling weak and fatigued, so he went to see a TCM doctor who told him that he had an intermittent (regularly interrupted) pulse. The doctor said that based on his experience this type of pulse indicates "sluggish" blood perfusion, and in addition to weakness and fatigue, patients with this pulse commonly present with dizziness.

Recently, he has had hot flashes, facial flushing, cold extremities, a tingling sensation in his lips, numbness on the tip of his tongue, stuffiness in the chest, and sometimes dizziness.

I am not sure about this patient. I am wondering if these symptoms may be caused by male menopause, cardiovascular disease, or if they are simply psychosomatic.

A: Although men also go through a type of menopause, it is exceedingly *rare* for men to present with hot flashes and facial flushing, whereas it is common in women. Male menopause is a gradual process of testosterone decline (about 1% each year after the age of 50), as opposed to the abrupt drop off in estrogen levels in females (typically between the age of 45 to 55). The most common symptoms of male menopause are lack of energy, decreased motivation, depression, reduced self-confidence, difficulty concentrating, and difficulty sleeping.

It is also *unlikely* that the isolated tingling sensation in the lips, numbness of the tip of the tongue, and occasional dizziness are signs of an impending cerebrovascular accident (CVA). The warning signs of stroke would develop rapidly, and may also be associated with loss of balance, headache, blurred vision, speech difficulties, unilateral drooping face, and weakness of the arm or leg on the affected side.

Most *likely* this is a case of anxiety-induced psychosomatic disorder, drug side effects, or a combination of the two. Thus, make sure to ask if the patient is taking any other medication and determine if these "symptoms" are in fact drug side effects. I see so many of these types of patients in my clinical practice nowadays. That is why I always keep an updated drug reference manual on hand, so I can go through the potential side effects of drugs with my patients. Patients have a tendency to believe the official manual more than the TCM doctor, and they can see clearly for themselves the reality of what may indeed be the root of their problems.

This is particularly prevalent with the wide-ranging applications and "overprescription" of drugs, such as *benzodiazepines* (e.g., Xanax, Valium), which are prescribed for all sorts of conditions from anxiety disorders and sleep disorders to Meniere's disease, and *antidepressants* like selective serotonin uptake inhibitors (SSRIs) (e.g., Prozac), which are prescribed for the treatment of depression and anxiety. These drugs have a cascade affect on the regulation and balance of a myriad of hormones and neurotransmitters in the brain, especially serotonin, dopamine, gamma-aminobutyric acid (GABA), acetylcholine (ACh), and adrenocorticotrophic hormone (ACTH). Patients who take these drugs may present with a host of side effects including confusion, impaired motor coordination, forgetfulness, lack of concentration, drowsiness, gastrointestinal problems, and respiratory depression.

As for treatment, I would consider prescribing Ban Xia Tian Ma Bai Zhu San (supplements the spleen and stomach, transforms phlegm-damp, and nourishes blood and stabilizes wind), Zhi Bo Di Huang Tang (enriches yin, downbears fire, and eliminates steaming), or Wen Dan Tang (clears Shao Yang depressed heat and dispels phlegm turbidity harassing the inner body). Just make sure to include Qing Hao, Zhi Mu, and Di Gu Pi (enrich yin and downbear fire, cool the blood and clear vacuity heat, and eliminate steaming), Tian Ma (calms and represses liver yang and dispels wind and frees the network vessels), The Sweets (boost qi and supplement the spleen and heart and nourish the blood and calm the spirit), and possibly Long Gu and Mu Li (calm the liver and subdue yang and quiet the spirit).

Naturally, you could also consider prescribing comparable formulas, such as Jia Wei Xiao Yao San, Jia Wei Xiao Chai Hu Tang, and Chai Hu Jia Long Gu Mu Li Tang, as long as the composition corresponds with the identified pattern.

Case Study #16: A Litany of Minor Ailments and Symptoms

Q: A 59 y/o female visited me with a chief complaint of generalized puffy swelling, which she said was more noticeable in the mornings and went down a bit by afternoon. Aside from this, she went on to mention other ailments as follows: headache with a sensation of heat on the vertex, aching pain in both shoulders, dry eyes, eye floaters, lumbar pain, knee pain, stool like sheep's droppings, colon polyps (have already been removed), and slight swelling and pain in the finger joints of both hands. She explained that when the puffy edema is severe, even taking diuretics does not reduce the swelling.

What are your impressions of this case? How would you treat this patient?

A: Naturally, you would have to try your best to rule out the possibility of an underlying etiology for the presentation of these symptoms. However, based on my clinical experience, whenever a patient comes in with a litany of minor ailments and symptoms that seem to compound into an overall clinical picture of general discomfort, stress, and anxiety, I would consider the strong possibility of psychogenic or psychosomatic origins.

Oftentimes, these patients will have been or are still being administered various anxiolytics (e.g., antidepressants, benzodiazepines) that regulate neurotransmitters. Antidepressants, such as selective serotonin reuptake inhibitors (SSRIs) (e.g., Zoloft), increase serotonin, dopamine, and norepinephrine levels; benzodiazepines (BDZs) (e.g., Xanax, Valium) increase GABA levels; and tricyclic antidepressants (TCAs) (e.g., imipramine, amitriptyline, clomipramine) increase serotonin and norepinephrine levels and decrease acetylcholine levels.

These drugs may be effective for *some* patients, but *not* all, and they all come with the risk of side effects, dependency, and withdrawal symptoms. Typically, these patients can be identified as the following patterns (or combinations/variations of these): liver depression and qi stagnation, liver depression and blood vacuity, yin vacuity with yang hyperactivity, Shao Yang depressed heat and phlegm turbidity harassing the inner body, spleen-stomach disharmony, and ascendant hyperactivity of liver yang (yang straying outward). Thus, I would consider prescribing formulas that correspond with these patterns such as Xiao Chai Hu Tang, Si Ni San, Xiao Yao San, Chai Hu Jia Long Gu Mu Li Tang, Ban Xia Tian Ma Bai Zhu San, Zhi Bo Di Huang Tang, Wen Dan Tang, Gan Mai Da Zao Combining Ban Xia Hou Po Tang, or Jian Ling Tang.

For the puffy swelling (浮腫 fú zhong), this can likely be identified as damp-heat with water amassment (蓄水 xù shui) pattern, thus make sure to include Cang Zhu, Fu Ling, Ze Xie, Zhi Zi, and Huang Bo in your formula. For the chronic knee and lumbar pain, you can add Niu Xi and Du Zhong; and for the dry stool, you can add Tao Ren and Bo Zi Ren, and if necessary Da Huang. You should also advise the patient to exercise regularly (go for walks!), eat plenty of fruits, grains and vegetables, and get outside to enjoy some sunshine.

Remember! Patients with symptoms of psychogenic or psychosomatic origin can be *very* difficult to treat. You will have to be *very* patient and try to work towards resolution of both the physical symptoms and their potentially psychological origins.

Case Study #17: Vexing Heat in the Five Hearts – Autonomic Response to Stress and Anxiety

Q: A 40 y/o female patient explained that over the past 10 years she has had heat in the heart of the palms and soles, tidal heat, cold in the abdomen, an aversion to cold, palpitations on and off with varying degrees of severity and frequency, and gets a headache when she overeats.

I am not sure how to approach this case because there seems to be a stark overlap in contradictory pattern types involved. How would you treat this patient?

A: Vexing heat in the five hearts can be identified as Shao Yang heat pattern, cold in the abdomen and aversion to cold can be identified as Shao Yin pattern, and headache after overeating can be identified as Yang Ming stomach heat pattern.

In a nutshell, for the vast majority of patients who present with these types of "lingering" symptoms involving the gamut of pathomechanisms and patterns that seem to wax and wane over time the underlying etiology is of psychosomatic origin. Oh, these symptoms, or the "feeling" of these symptoms, may indeed exist, but are likely rooted in autonomic responses induced by stress and anxiety.

This condition can be identified as liver qi depression pattern, requiring administration of a spleen- and stomach-supplementing, phlegm-damp-transforming, and blood-nourishing wind-stabilizing formula such as Ban Xia Tian Ma Bai Zhu San, Xiao Yao San, Jia Wei Xiao Yao San, or Si Ni San. Just make sure to include The Sweets (boost qi and supplement the spleen and heart and nourish the blood and calm the spirit), Qing Hao, Zhi Mu, and Di Gu Pi (enrich yin and downbear fire, cool the blood and clear vacuity heat, and eliminate steaming bone), and Yu Sheng Wan (quiets the spirit and calms the nerves, promotes cerebral collateral circulation, and recalibrates autoregulation in the brain).

Remember! Advise the patient to get into a regular cardiovascular exercise routine (e.g., simply going for walks under the sun's mild rays may be the best!), eat a well-balanced diet, and get at least 8 hours of sleep every night.

Case Study #18: Diarrhea and Abdominal Urgency and Rectal Heaviness – Psychogenic Roots

Q: A 43 y/o female patient explained that she has been susceptible to bouts of abdominal pain ever since she was a child. And recently, over the past month, she has been suffering from right-sided rib-side distention and pain and severe diarrhea (up to 17 to 20 times per day!) that is occasionally accompanied by bloody stool with bright red blood.

Antidiarrheal medication prescribed by her gastroenterologist has been helpful in reducing the diarrhea down to about 7 to 8 stools per day. She has no fever or other signs or symptoms of external contraction and has already undergone a thorough medical examination (e.g., endoscopy, lab tests), but no abnormalities have been found.

Do you think this type of severe diarrhea could be of psychogenic etiology?

A: Typically, for patients presenting with this general history and spectrum of symptoms, once other organic diseases (e.g., inflammatory bowel disease (IBD)) have been ruled out, gastroenterologists will typically go ahead and diagnose the patient with irritable bowel syndrome (IBS). The pathophysiology of IBS is unknown, but there appears to be distinct psychogenic elements involved. So to answer your question, yes, I think you could approach this as a psychogenic disorder.

As for the blood in the stool, I would attribute this to abdominal urgency and rectal heaviness (tenesmus), and the simple fact she has to spend a lot of time on the toilet making sure it all gets out and waiting there for the next procession, which makes her more susceptible to developing anal fissures. Bloody stool (便血 biàn xi□) and descent (precipitation) of blood (下血 xià xuè) are umbrella terms that are *not* etiology specific. The etiology of the bleeding can be identified by the color, consistency, and amount of blood.

In this case, the patient has bright red blood, which may be visible on the toilet paper she wipes with, or possibly dripping out into the stool after sitting on the toilet for long periods, regardless of whether or not any feces has been excreted. This makes a differential diagnosis of red and white draining precipitation (瀉下赤白 xiè xià chì bái), which may present in IBD, and tarry stool with dried dark blood clots, which may present in intestinal bleeding, easily distinguishable!

Case Study #19: Suicidal Thoughts – Get Help Quickly!

Q: A 39 y/o male patient was brought in to see me accompanied by his family members. They explained that the patient had several episodes in which he "freaked out" at work, lambasting colleagues and screaming that he wanted to kill himself. After the third episode this year, the patient stopped going to the office and stayed at home, watching TV and fiddling around on the computer at home all day.

During his visit, the patient never made eye contact with me and looked away from me when he spoke (murmured). Besides the suicidal thoughts, anger issues, and reclusive behavior, he also has ungratifying defecation, poor appetite, and bad breath. In general, he said that his mind just feels "muddled" and he doesn't feel like talking. I observed a flushed face, a dark red tongue, and a rapid, stringlike pulse. I prescribed Wen Dan Tang combining Huang Lian Jie Du Tang. What is your impression of this patient? How would you treat this patient?

A: Oh!...Trying to provide care for people with suicidal thoughts or behavior is a deeply sensitive and complex task that involves the unique personal history and dynamics of each patient. Usually, the mental and emotional factors driving suicidal thoughts are depression and the desperation to escape the distraught feeling of futility in existence. Depending on the degree of risk, the family must take steps to monitor and protect their loved one; and in cases of imminent risk, the patient may even need to be hospitalized against his own will. Treatment should include psychological counseling and possibly administration of antidepressants (e.g., SSRIs) or antimanics (e.g., lithium).

As for TCM treatment, if the patient is open to taking medicinals, then I typically apply the following two-tiered pattern approach based on the patients mannerisms (e.g., tone of voice), demeanor (e.g., body language, facial expression), and pulse:

- For repletion heat pattern—presenting with noticeably agitated demeanor and rapid, slippery, long pulse, etc.—I would prescribe either Wen Dan Tang (clears Shao Yang depressed heat and transforms phlegm turbidity harassing the inner body), Chai Hu Jia Long Gu Mu Li Tang (harmonizes Shao Yang, settles fright, and quiets the spirit), or Zhi Bo Di Huang Tang (enriches yin, downbears fire, and eliminates steaming).
- For qi, blood, or yang vacuity pattern—presenting with reticence, melancholy, eyes diverted, pale complexion, etc.—I would prescribe a qi-, blood-, and kidney yang-supplementing formula such as Shi Quan Da Bu Tang, Ren Shen Yang Rong Tang, Gui Pi Tang, You Gui Yin, or Shen Qi Wan. And if constipation presents, then make sure to add Da Huang (drains and precipitates and frees the intestines).

Remember! For patients with mental and emotional disorders, regardless if the condition presents as repletion or vacuity pattern, make sure to include large doses of The Sweets—Gan Cao (at least 5 qian), Da Zao (from 10 up to as many as 50 pieces), and Long Yan Rou (from 8 qian up to 1.5 or even 2 liang). The Sweets boost qi and supplement the spleen and heart, nourish the blood and calm the spirit, and harmonize (moderate) the nature of medicinals.

Case Study #20: Emotional Trauma and Necrophobia – Damage by the Seven Affects

Q: Three weeks ago, a 38 y/o male patient visited a traditional wake of a close friend held by the family at the home of the deceased. At the ceremony, he began feeling heaviness and oppression in the chest; and ever since then, whenever he is under pressure and stress, a feeling of soreness and stiffness pervades his whole body, that same "oppression" comes back in the chest, and his mind feels "muddled and disoriented."

The history and onset of symptoms suggest mind-body disharmony (心身不合 x□n sh□n bù hé), a type of psychosomatic disorder. Thus, I prescribed a 2-week regimen of Gan Mai Da Zao Combining Ban Xia Hou Po Tang and will see him again next week on a follow-up visit.

Do you think this formula is the right approach?

A: Yes, it definitely sounds like you are on the right track. This patient likely suffers from emotional trauma from the loss of a close friend or possibly the fear of attending the funeral ceremony (necrophobia). This can be classified as a type of hysteria (癔症 yì zhèng), mind-body-spirit disharmony, or damage by the seven affects (e.g., seven-affect ill-being, seven-affect qi bind, seven-affect binding depression).

Oftentimes, people upholding devout religious and spiritual beliefs (regardless of the affiliation) will benefit from consultation, guidance, or rituals provided by a religious figure of his/her affiliation. For initiates, this positive spiritual direction will often give the person an optimistic outlook on life and help in getting the person back on the path towards healing and resolution (absolution, if you will) of the emotional trauma, whether it be the loss of a close friend, the fear of dead bodies (attending the funeral ceremony), or the fear of death in general.

As for TCM treatment, you will have to identify the pattern based on the presenting signs and symptoms. Typically, the pattern types that most commonly present are the following: spleen and stomach vacuity, phlegm-damp obstruction, kidney yang vacuity, center disharmony and disquieted heart spirit, and vacuity taxation with dual vacuity of yin and yang. Thus, depending on the pattern, you could consider prescribing formulas such as Xiang Sha Liu Jun Zi Tang, Ban Xia Tian Ma Bai Zhu San, Shen Qi Wan, You Gui Yin, Gan Mai Da Zao Combining Ban Xia Hou Po Tang, or Gui Zhi Jia Long Gu Mu Li Tang. Just make sure to add Yu Sheng Wan (quiets the spirit and calms the nerves, promotes cerebral collateral circulation, and recalibrates autoregulation in the brain).

Remember! At the onset, when pronounced agitation and/or disquieted heart spirit (心神不安 x□n shén bù □n) present, you should also make sure to include Chao Long Gu and Chao Mu Li* (calm the liver and subdue yang, quiet the spirit, and astringe and secure) in your formula. And since Long Gu and Mu Li have a tendency to cause indigestion in some patients, you may need to consider adding combinations of The Digestants (Cang Zhu, Shan Zha, Gu Ya, Mai Ya, Ji Nei Jin, and Shen Qu) to disperse food, arouse and fortify the spleen, open and harmonize the stomach, and promote digestion.

*Note: Dr. Lee explains that the use of Sheng (生 sh□ng = raw—minimally processed, but not submitted to heat!) Long Gu and Mu Li preserves the full potency and actions of the calcium (Ca) constituents (e.g., subdue yang and quiet the spirit), whereas the Chao (炒 chao = stir-fried) processing method magnifies the actions of the magnesium (Mg) constituents (e.g., astringes and secures) in these medicinals.

Case Study #21: Exam Study Burnout – Get Enough Sleep, Eat Healthy, and Exercise

Q: Every year when it comes around to exam time, teens and young adults are faced with the arduous task of exam preparation. This can take its toll on many who push themselves to the limit and end up getting study burnout. Parents bring their exhausted, jaded kids in asking me if there is anything I can prescribe to help maintain high energy and peak levels of concentration.

Do you ever have these kinds of patients? How would you handle these kinds of patients?

A: Fatigue may manifest in various pattern types depending on the individual body constitution and circumstances. However, taking medicine is *not* nearly as important as getting enough sleep, eating healthy, regularly exercising, drinking plenty of water, doing deep breathing exercises, and spending some time in the sunshine.

If the patient and/or parents really want you to prescribe medicinals, then I would consider one of the following formulas based on pattern identification as the basis for treatment:

- Shao Yang depressed heat with phlegm turbidity harassing the inner body pattern—Wen Dan Tang
- Shao Yang vacuity heat with hyperactivity of liver yang pattern—Chai Hu Jia Long Gu Mu Li Tang
- Spleen and stomach vacuity, phlegm-damp obstruction,

and vacuity wind harassing the upper body pattern—Ban Xia Tian Ma Bai Zhu San

- Qi and blood vacuity with insufficiency of kidney yang pattern—Shi Quan Da Bu Tang
- Dual qi and blood vacuity pattern—Bu Yang Huan Wu Tang
- Yin vacuity fire effulgence pattern—Zhi Bo Di Huang Tang
- Vacuity taxation with yin and yang vacuity pattern—Gui Zhi Jia Long Gu Mu Li Tang
- Kidney yang insufficiency pattern—Shen Qi Wan or You Gui Yin

Case Study #22: Pesticide Poisoning – Failed Suicide Attempt

Q: This 33 y/o male patient is still unmarried and currently unemployed. He has taken the bar exam in hopes of becoming a lawyer for the past 10 years, but has not been able to pass. Distraught, dejected, and feeling that there was no use living anymore, he attempted suicide by ingesting pesticide.

Though he was fortunate enough to be rescued and resuscitated, he incurred complete failure of the left lung and has only 50% of right lung function remaining. His doctors said that he only has 2 to 3 months left to live, but despite having difficulty breathing, he can still walk around the house independently and his urine and stool are normal.

Can TCM medicinals be prescribed to help this patient?

A: Attempted suicide by ingestion of a pesticide (organophosphates) causes bronchospasms and respiratory failure. Obviously, in the acute stage following ingestion, the focus of treatment should be on resuscitating the patient and maintaining vital signs under the emergency care provided at a hospital.

Once the patient's condition has stabilized, such as in this patient's case, then I would consider prescribing either a qi-boosting spleen-fortifying and qi-moving phlegm-transforming formula, such as Asthma Formula, or a blood-quickening stasis-transforming, blood-cooling, and qi-supplementing formula, such as Bu Yang Huan Wu Tang adding Ma Huang, Xing Ren, Di Long, and Lai Fu Zi.

If edema presents, then change the formula to either a kidney yang-warming qi transformation-promoting and bland-percolating dampness- and water-disinhibiting formula, such as Wu Ling San (Nephritis Formula), or a heat-clearing phlegm-damp-transforming, water-disinhibiting, qi-moving blood-quickening, and pain-relieving formula, such as Chai Ling Tang adding Ma Huang, Xing Ren, Di Long, Ren Shen/Chuan Qi Powder, and Huang Qi.

If frog rale in the throat (喉中有水雞聲 hóu zh□ ng you shui j□ sh□ ng) presents, then prescribe Asthma Formula adding Zi Wan, Kuan Dong Hua, and if necessary, The Three Great Yang-Supplementers.

Remember the saying from the classic novel *Journey to the West*: "Better to save one life than build a seven-storied pagoda."

Case Study #23: Two Hours to Eat a Bowl of Rice – Six Depressions

Q: A 44 y/o male patient visited me explaining that it usually takes about two hours for him to eat a light meal with a bowl of rice. If he eats at a quicker pace, he says that he will have abdominal pain. I asked where the pain was and he just motioned with his hand all around the abdomen. He usually has 1 stool per day, but sometimes feels abdominal urgency and rectal heaviness (tenesmus), and also said that he has been sleeping poorly recently (awakens easily).

This has been going on for the past half year now and the patient is wondering if I can prescribe something to help. What do you think about this case?

A: As in all cases, you must rule the possibility of organic illness. However, this sounds like a stereotypical case of depression, which can be classified as the six depressions (六鬱 liù yù) or damage by the seven affects (七情所傷 q□ qíng suo sh□ ng) and identified as liver qi depression or liver depression and qi stagnation pattern.

You could prescribe any number of formulas, including a qi-moving depression-resolving formula, such as Liu Yu Tang or Yue Ju Wan, and a liver-coursing depression-resolving formula, such as Si Ni San or Xiao Yao San. Personally, I like to prescribe the spleen- and stomach-supplementing, phlegm-damp-transforming, and blood-nourishing wind-stabilizing formula Ban Xia Tian Ma Bai Zhu San.

Whichever formula you choose, just make sure to include The Sweets (boost qi and supplement the spleen and heart and nourish the blood and calm the spirit) and Yu Sheng Wan (quiets the spirit and calms the nerves, promotes cerebral collateral circulation, and recalibrates autoregulation in the brain).

This approach should be able to resolve the depression, make eating pain free again, and get the patient back into good spirits.

Case Study #24: Carbon Monoxide Poisoning – Barbecue Smoke Exposure

Q: Every year when it gets to be winter time, I always read in the news about cases of people getting carbon monoxide poisoning from exposure at barbecues. It is that time of year again. Recently, two patients visited me saying that they were having barbecues over the weekend and began coming down with noticeable symptoms of carbon monoxide poisoning.

One patient is a 43 y/o male who said he developed a dull headache while at the barbecue, but felt all right again over the next couple days afterwards. Then, about 3 days later, he started feeling dizzy again with fatigue, inability to concentrate, and mild leg weakness.

The other patient is a 45 y/o male who began feeling a dull headache, groggy, lightheaded, forgetful, and unable to concentrate later on that same evening after the barbecue.

I administered a 1-week prescription of Ban Xia Tian Ma Bai Zhu San for both of them and am awaiting their return for a follow-up visit next week. How would you treat these types of patients?

A: There are many types of medicinals that can be prescribed for the treatment of carbon monoxide poisoning.

In the *acute* stage, you can prescribe a lung-diffusing exterior-resolving formula, such as Ma Huang Fu Zi Xi Xin Tang, Huan Hun Tang, or San Ao Tang; or even a blood-quickening stasis-transforming, blood-cooling, and qi-supplementing formula, such as Bu Yang Huan Wu Tang adding Ma Huang, Fu Zi, and Xi Xin. If night sweating presents, then add Qing Hao, Zhi Mu, and Di Gu Pi;

and if profuse phlegm presents, then add Lai Fu Zi, Sang Bai Pi, Sheng Shi Gao, and Huang Qin.

In the *post-acute* stage, if the patient no longer presents with the initial autonomic reflexes (e.g., headache, nausea, sweating, dizziness), then I would proceed directly to Bu Yang Huan Wu Tang. This formula will effectively improve blood perfusion throughout the body, mitigate the severity of the cardiovascular and metabolic manifestations, and reduce the potential for myocardial injury.

If autonomic reflexes still present, then you can consider adding Qing Hao, Zhi Mu, and Di Gu Pi (enrich yin and downbear fire, cool the blood and clear vacuity heat, and eliminate steaming bone). Or, you could also consider changing to a Shao Yang depressed heat-clearing phlegm turbidity harassing the inner body-dispelling formula, such as Wen Dan Tang adding Qing Hao, Zhi Mu, and Di Gu Pi; or even a spleen- and stomach-supplementing, phlegm-damp-transforming, and blood-nourishing wind-stabilizing formula, such as Ban Xia Tian Ma Bai Zhu San. Just make sure to include Ma Huang, Xi Xin, Shi Chang Pu, Chuan Xiong, Chi Shao, Yin Xin Ye, and a large dose of Huang Qi.

Section 2: Insomnia

Case Study #1: Can SARIs Help Patients with Insomnia?

Q: I have many patients with sleeping problems, especially women going through menopausal transition and the elderly. I have heard that serotonin antagonist and reuptake inhibitors (SARIs) (e.g., trazodone) can provide effective treatment for insomnia. What are your thoughts on this?

A: Patients commonly try over-the-counter sleep aids first, which will likely include an antihistamine (e.g., diphenhydramine, doxylamine) for its sedative actions. If this does*n't* work, then they may get an appointment to see their doctor for prescription drugs—SARIs (e.g., trazodone), benzodiazepines (e.g., triazolam), non-benzodiazpine sedatives (e.g., zolpidem, zaleplon), tricyclic antidepressants (e.g., amitriptyline), or atypical antidepressants (e.g., mirtazapine).

Initially, these drugs may provide relief for some patients, but this usually is temporary. Patients taking antidepressants and benzodiazepines easily develop drug tolerance, requiring higher doses for efficacy, face troubling side effects (especially if the drug(s) are taken in high doses and over long durations), and may incur withdrawal symptoms once they stop taking the medication.

TCM medicinals may provide an effective alternative for many patients with insomnia. Generally, for all types of insomnia—difficulty falling asleep (sleep onset insomnia), frequently awakening from sleep, awakening in the middle of the night (sleep maintenance insomnia), or awakening too early in the morning and can't get back to sleep again (sleep offset insomnia)—I like to prescribe the liver-settling wind-extinguishing and yin-enriching yang-subduing formula Jian Ling Tang (including Gan Cao) adding Long Yan Rou. For women going through menopausal transition, I would consider adding Qing Hao, Zhi Mu, Di Gu Pi, Huang Bo, Yu Sheng Wan, or possibly even Zi He Che (especially for female patients!). For patients with pronounced yang hyperactivity, I would consider adding The Three Yellows, Qing Hao, Zhi Mu, Di Gu Pi, Yu Sheng Wan, and Zi He Che.

Acupuncture may be effective for some patients as well. For the treatment of insomnia, I would choose combinations of the following acupoints: body—Shen Men (HT7), Tai Chong (LV3), San Yin Jiao (SP6), Xuan Zhong (GB39), Di Wu Hui (GB 42), and Nei Guan (P6); and auricular—Shen Men, Jiao Gan (sympathetic), and Xin (heart).

Case Study #2: Melatonin Deficiency

Q: A 38 y/o female patient visited me with a chief complaint of sleeping problems for the past 3 years. She can usually fall asleep without much difficulty, but often wakes up in the middle of the night and ca*n't* get back to sleep again after that. Occasionally, she also has the feeling of stuffiness and oppression in the chest.

She tried taking over-the-counter sleep medication, but these were *not* helpful, prompting her to go see a doctor who performed a lab workup that showed low melatonin levels. What would you prescribe for this patient?

A: Regardless if a patient has a melatonin deficiency or not, for sleep maintenance insomnia (*able* to fall asleep, but awakens in the middle of the night and ca*n't* get back to sleep) like this patient, I would consider prescribing either a gallbladder- and stomach-harmonizing and inner body harassment phlegm turbidity-dispelling formula, such as Wen Dan Tang, or a liver-settling wind-extinguishing and yin-enriching yang-subduing formula, such as Jian Ling Tang (including Gan Cao). Just make sure to add Long Yan Rou, Yu Sheng Wan, and possibly The Three Yellows.

Case Study #3: Mood Stabilizers, Anxiolytics, and Hypnotics – Withdrawal Symptoms

Q: Six months ago, a 47 y/o male patient was going through some tough times with his family, and not long after that, he began feeling restless with anxiety and irritability, which rapidly progressed to delirium. His family worried that he had "gone crazy" (either a severe manic episode or psychosis), so they managed to get him admitted into a psychiatric ward, where he was administered large doses of mood stabilizers (antipsychotics and tranquilizers). He showed major improvement and was eventually released from the psychiatric ward 5 months later.

However, he now feels fatigue and suffers from insomnia. The patient said that he has tried drinking a small amount of soju at night before bed, but this seems to have more of a stimulating effect; and when he drinks a large amount, he can get to sleep, but *only* for about 5 hours. Naturally, I advised him against relying on excess alcohol intake as a way to get to sleep!

My idea is that the fatigue results from the lack of sleep, so my focus is on treating the insomnia. I identified this condition as yang hyperactivity pattern and prescribed Jian Ling Tang variant, but it has not been effective. Do you have any advice or suggestions for treating this patient?

A: Insomnia, anxiety, irritability and fatigue are all potential withdrawal symptoms from the administration of mood stabilizers (lithium, anticonvulsants, and antipsychotics), hypnotics, and anxiolytics (antidepressants, benzodiazepines).

The most effective formula I have found for treating insomnia is still Jian Ling Tang (settles the liver and extinguishes wind and enriches yin and subdues yang). Just make sure to include Gan Cao (5 qian), Long Yan Rou (8 qian–1.5 liang), The Three Yellows (8 qian each), and if available Yu Sheng Wan. This formula functions as a potent suppressant of yang hyperactivity capable of regulating neurotransmitter levels and their reuptake to provide effective resolution of insomnia.

Alcohol in small amounts acts as a stimulant by sensitizing NMDA (N-methyl-D-aspartate) receptors in the brain, making them more responsive to the excitatory neurotransmitter glutamate, thus boosting brain activity. Alcohol in larger amounts acts as a depressant by desensitizing the same receptors, while also activating the inhibitory GABA system. That's what Li Bai (701–762 CE), the famous poet from the Tang dynasty extensively explores and elaborates on with aesthetic delight!

Case Study #4: Weight Gain After Insomnia Cured

Q: A 48 y/o female patient visited me complaining of insomnia, a sensation of heat in the upper body, hoarseness, constipation (1 stool every 2–3 days), and periodic transient swelling in the face, hands and feet. I thought that some of these symptoms may be caused by either menopausal transition or possibly of psychosomatic origin as a result of stress and anxiety.

In the end, I decided to go ahead and try treating the main symptom—insomnia, prescribing Jian Ling Tang adding Fu Ling, Ze Xie, Da Huang, Da Zao, and Yu Sheng Wan. After taking this formula for 1 month, the patient has seen positive results in improving sleep and getting her bowels moving more regularly. However, the swelling issues have *not* improved at all though, and she said that she has gained 7 kg.

The strange thing is that I have other insomnia patients, especially female, who have said the exact same thing: once their condition improves, they begin gaining weight. Have you noticed this phenomenon? Why do you think this would happen? What can I do about it?

A: Yes, that is perfectly normal. This can be explained nicely by the classical TCM pathophysiological theories explicated in *The Yellow Emperor's Inner Canon*, Plain Questions 5, Great Treatise on the Correspondences and Manifestations of Yin and Yang. It goes something like this: "*Vigorous* fire induces qi "expiry" [and] *lesser* fire produces "invigorating" qi; *vigorous* fire consumes qi [while] qi nurtures *lesser* fire; and *vigorous* fire dissipates qi [while] *lesser* fire engenders qi."

This can be interpreted as follows: The physiological function of yang qi in the body is "fire," also known as "*lesser* fire" (少火 shao huo). The hyperactivity of yang qi results in fire-heat engendering in the body, which is pathological "fire," also known as "*vigorous* fire" (壮火 zhuàng huo). Pathological fire accelerates the exhaustion of nutrients in the body and results in damage to yin and dissipation of qi, which is what the phrase "*vigorous* fire consumes qi" refers to. Now that pathological ("*vigorous*") fire has been extinguished and physiological ("*lesser*") fire is able to function normally, these patients will naturally regain vitality and put on a little weight. Over time, the body will once again regain its capacity of regulating the constitution.

Now that the insomnia has improved, you can go ahead and subtract Gan Cao and Da Zao, and add Huang Bo instead. This approach will continue providing effective treatment until the condition has completely resolved; plus, the patient will be able to take off the extra kilos more quickly and reach her desired weight.

Case Study #5: Antidepressants and Sedatives – Risk of Side Effects, Dependency, and Withdrawal Complications

Q: There seem to be so many different drugs now on the market that act on GABA (□-aminobutyric acid) neuroreceptors and provide effective relief for insomnia and anxiety. What is your impression of these drugs? And would you recommend patients to take these drugs?

A: I don't necessarily agree with that assertion. Drugs that either directly or indirectly regulate the neurotransmitters GABA, serotonin, norepinephrine, dopamine, and acetylcholine all have an inhibitory effect on neuronal activity, and thus cause central nervous system depression!

Long-term administration of these types of sedative-hypnotics and antidepressants may provide some temporary relief, but also present the risks of dependency, side effects, and withdrawal complications. Common side effects include confusion, drowsiness, impaired motor coordination, brain atrophy, and dementia. And in cases where patients take multiple medications, the severity of these negative side effects can be compounded into a toxic montage of iatrogenic illness.

So in the long run, Chinese medicine will provide a more comprehensive therapeutic approach that may include medicinals and/or acupuncture (body or auricular), without the undesirable side effects!

Remember! The best "therapeutic" approach for the patient is to cultivate good sleeping habits (e.g., stimulants, food intake, or strenuous exercise right before bed), maintain a regular sleep time and wake up schedule, exercise regularly (e.g., aerobics, walking, biking, swimming, deep breathing, yoga, qi gong, tai chi), and get lots of sunshine. And for some patients with chronic insomnia, cognitive behavioral therapy provides another option, which is much better than getting caught up in the vicious cycle of drug dependency, side effects, and withdrawal complications.

Case Study #6: Insomnia After Recovering from Respiratory Infection

Q: A 78 y/o woman with a history of chronic asthma caught a bad cold about 3 months ago, which lingered on and exacerbated her existing asthma. She received Western medical treatment and eventually recovered from the respiratory infection, and seemed to be back to relatively normal. The strange thing is that since recovering from her cold she has been suffering from insomnia.

I decided to prescribe Jian Ling Tang (including Gan Cao) adding The Three Yellows, Da Zao, Sang Bai Pi, Qing Hao, Di Gu Pi, and Yu Sheng Wan. She has taken this formula for about 1 1/2 months now with*out* any noticeable effect. Do you think this could have been caused by the medication she was taking for her cold? She also said that the sleeping pills (GABA agonist) her doctor prescribed has been helping her get to sleep for about 3 or 4 hours before awakening again.

A: Mmh…this chronic asthma patient who caught a cold would likely have been prescribed a bronchodilator containing ephedrine (or pseudoephedrine) and inhaled and/or oral corticosteroids, all of which may cause sleep problems in some patients. For this type of insomnia, you should consider these five pattern types:

- Shao Yang residual (or depressed) heat pattern—Prescribe Chai Hu Jia Long Gu Mu Li Tang or Wen Dan Tang. If asthma is pronounced, then add Ma Huang Gen (enters the lung channel and mildly resolves the exterior), Xing Ren, Bai Guo, Wu Wei Zi, and Shan Yao. And if yin vacuity cough presents, then also add Zi Wan, Kuan Dong Hua, and Xi Xin.
- Hyperactivity of yang due to kidney yin vacuity pattern—Prescribe Zhi Bo Di Huang Tang, Ba Xian Chang Shou Wan, Bai He Gu Jin Tang, or Da Zao Wan. Just make sure to include asthma-stabilizing medicinals such as Ma Huang Gen, Xing Ren, Bai Guo, Wu Wei Zi, Shan Yao, Zi Wan, Kuan Dong Hua, and Xi Xin.
- Disquieted heart spirit (心神不寧 x□n shén bù níng), disharmony of the heart spirit (心神不合 x□n shén bù hé), or dual vacuity of the heart and spleen pattern—Prescribe Gan Mai Da Zao Tang Combining Ban Xia Hou Po Tang adding Long Yan Rou (8 qian–1.5 liang) and Da Zao (20–30 pieces). Remember! Sweet foods (preferably natural!) boost qi

and supplement the spleen and heart and nourish the blood and calm the spirit, and are especially effective for children, the elderly, and overmedicated patients.

- Yang straying outward pattern—Prescribe Jian Ling Tang (including a large dose of Gan Cao) adding large doses of Long Yan Rou and Da Zao.
- Lung qi failing to downbear (肺氣不降 fèi qì bù jiàng) and stomach qi ascending counterflow (胃氣上逆 wèi qì shàng nì) pattern—In mild cases, prescribe either Gui Zhi Jia Hou Po Xing Ren Tang adding Bo Zi Ren and Suan Zao Ren, or Bo Zi Ren Wan adding Xing Ren, Hou Po, Zi Wan, and Kuan Dong Hua. In more severe cases, prescribe Xuan Fu Dai Zhe Tang adding Xing Ren, Hou Po, Zi Wan, and Kuan Dong Hua.

Remember! Astringents such as Wu Wei Zi, Bai Guo, and Jin Ying Zi (constrain the lung and sweat, check discharge and diarrhea, engender liquid and astringe essence, and quiet the heart and calm the spirit) inhibit all types of abnormal body fluid from being excreted, including mucous (lungs), feces (intestines), and urine (kidneys), as well as restraining the heart spirit and calming the mind for a quiet sleep.

Most Western medicine insomnia drugs are directed at increasing GABA or serotonin levels, either directly or indirectly, which functions to promote sleep. This may be effective at first because it can tap into the sleep-wake control center of the brain, but the sleep it induces tends to be non-REM sleep, and tolerance tends to build up that leads to dependency, ineffectiveness and withdrawal symptoms. So in the long run, it is still best to regulate the constitution with Chinese medicine for the resolution of insomnia.

XI. RARE DISORDERS

Case Study #1: Tetralogy of Fallot

Q: This 23 y/o male was born with tetralogy of Fallot, a congenital heart defect, and underwent a successful surgical repair at the age of 7 y/o. He had been living a normal, symptom-free life up until last summer when he went through a period of heavy "partying" that included excessive alcohol intake and smoking a lot of cigarettes. Since then, he began noticing the gradual development of abdominal fullness and mild ascites, edema in the lower extremities (mild pitting), shortness of breath, and irregular pulse rhythm with alternating strong and weak beats (pulsus alternans).

He went in for a thorough examination, which revealed an enlarged heart (cardiomegaly) that is pressing down on the liver and lungs and the tell-tale reduced cardiac output of congestive heart failure (CHF). His cardiologist suspects that the congenital heart disorder is the cause and prescribed drugs which have *not* been effective in treating the condition; in fact, the symptoms have gotten worse!

I prescribed Wu Ling San (Nephritis Formula) (including large doses of Fu Ling, Zhu Ling, and Ze Xie (1 liang each)) adding Ting Li Zi, Fang Ji, Ma Huang, Xing Ren, Pu Gong Ying, and Jin Ying Zi. Please offer your advice and guidance on this patient.

A: I like your formula variant, but I don't see why you would need to add Pu Gong Ying and Jin Ying Zi, and I would also make sure to add large doses of Huang Qi (2 liang) and Ting Li Zi (8 qian–1 liang). Or, you could also consider prescribing Bu Yang Huan Wu Tang (quickens the blood and transforms stasis, cools the blood, and supplements qi) combining Wu Ling San (Nephritis Formula) (warms kidney yang and promotes qi transformation and disinhibits dampness and water by bland percolation). And if pronounced edema and shortness of breath present, then incrementally increase the doses of Fu Ling and Ze Xie (up to 1.5 liang each, if necessary) and begin adding The Three Great Yang-Supplementers (incrementally increasing the doses over time up to 5–8 qian each).

If the swelling continues to worsen in the beginning, don't get overanxious and overly concerned about it. Just continue to prescribe your formula and you will gradually see positive results. Remember! You must also be on the lookout for edema that results from hyponatremia, hypokalemia, and hypoproteinemia. As for the Western medicine drugs, you can recommend that he gradually begin to wean away from the diuretics and digoxin (a cardiac glycoside that increases cardiac output) by substituting these drugs with large doses of Fu Ling and Ze Xie (8 qian–1 liang each) and Ren Shen/Chuan Qi Powder (starting out at 10 g/3x/day and then gradually increasing the dose of Ren Shen up to 20 g/3x/day).

His cardiologist will have to make further determination based on imaging studies and the status of his condition as to whether or not it is necessary to surgically repair any valves that may have sprung a leak since the initial repair in his childhood.

Case Study #2: Cerebellar Syndrome

Q: A 37 y/o female visited me with symptoms of dizziness, unsteady gait, slow speech (dysarthia), weakness in the lower limbs, and reduced visual acuity. These symptoms first started appearing when she was 33 y/o and have gotten progressively worse since then.

Other people in her immediate family have fallen ill with similar symptoms—her mother passed away at the age of 45 y/o, her older brother started having symptoms when he was 38 y/o and is now bedridden, and her younger brother started having symptoms when he was 10 y/o, but can still take care of himself.

She said that she has had imaging studies and blood tests performed and nothing abnormal was found, but she did say that the MRI findings of her older brother confirmed cerebellar atrophy.

I prescribed Ban Xia Tian Ma Bai Zhu San (including a large dose of Huang Qi and Tian Ma (8 qian) adding Yin Xing Ye, Ren Shen, and Chuan Qi. Do you think this patient could have multiple sclerosis (MS)? How would you treat this patient?

A: This must be some type of cerebellar syndrome, which is a broad term that describes any acute (e.g., virus, infarction, head trauma, drug-induced) or subacute/chronic (e.g., brain tumor, alcoholism, vitamin deficiency, autoimmune response, genetic disorder) condition that includes symptoms of ataxia, imbalance, uncoordinated movements (dysmetria), dysarthria, and oculomotor disorders (e.g., nystagmus).

In your patient's case, this must be a hereditary ataxia, most likely spinocerebellar ataxia (SCA). This inherited pathocondition may present with the clinical features of ataxia, optic atrophy, blindness, dementia, and extrapyramidal symptoms (e.g., bradykinesia, rigidity, dystonia, athetosis, chorea, tics, tremors). The specific manifestations and prognosis depends on the specific type of autosomal dominant spinocerebellar ataxia (ADSA).

As for the formula variant you prescribed, yes, I think that is a good choice. Just make sure to gradually increase the dose of Ren Shen (promotes an increase in the transport of oxygen and nutrients in the blood and protects cells by slowing down the rate of apoptosis) up to about 5–6 qian and add Yu Sheng Wan (promotes cerebral collateral circulation and recalibrates autoregulation in the brain), which is effective for improving conditions such as cerebrovascular disorders, brain tumors, and depression.

Case Study #3: Hodgkin Lymphoma

Q: I have never had a patient with Hodgkin lymphoma. I was reading up on it the other day and am curious how you would treat this condition with Chinese medicine.

A: Hodgkin lymphoma (HL) and non-Hodgkin lymphoma (NHL) can both be identified as steaming bone and Shao Yang depressed heat pattern. Thus, for this type of cancer I would prescribe an yin-enriching fire-downbearing and steaming bone-eliminating formula such as Zhi Bo Di Huang Tang (including a large dose of Zhi Mu) adding large doses of Qing Hao and Di Gu Pi (enrich yin and downbear fire, cool the blood and clear vacuity heat, and eliminate steaming bone), and possibly Zhi Zi (drains fire and eliminates vexation, clears heat and disinhibits dampness, cools the blood and resolves toxin, and disperses swelling and relieves pain). Make sure to closely monitor HL and NHL patients' complete blood count, especially WBC, WBC DC (differential count), RBC, and PLT, so you can modify your formula as needed.

Case Study #4: Mitochondrial Disease

Q: A 15 y/o male visited me explaining that he began having periodic episodes of seizures with spasms of the arms and legs since the age of 7 y/o. Subsequently, he developed a succession of neuropathies as follows: right-sided facial palsy, occasional limb spasticity upon extension, and sensory deficits in his hands and feet. Recently, he has had cold hands and feet, generalized weakness, and occasional urinary incontinence.

He was put through the gamut of medical tests and examinations, which eventually led to the diagnosis of mitochondrial disease. How would you treat this condition with Chinese medicine?

A: Mitochondria are tiny organelles commonly known as the "power plants of the cell" and appear in higher numbers in cells that require higher amounts of energy (e.g., brain, heart, liver, eyes, ears, kidney, GI tract). Mitochondria even have their own DNA (mtDNA) that is different from the nuclear DNA (nDNA).

Mitochondrial disease is a chronic, genetic disorder that occurs when the mitochondria of cells fail to produce adequate energy for cell or organ function. It can be present at birth or develop later in life, and can manifest in a variety of muscular and neurological symptoms including muscle weakness, exercise intolerance, trouble with balance and coordination, heart defects, dementia, movement disorders, stroke-like episodes, deafness, blindness, and seizures. The prognosis varies from patient to patient and ranges from progressive weakness to death from heart and respiratory failure. Western medicine currently has no specific treatment and can only provide palliative care.

Based on the etiology and presenting symptoms, for a patient like this I would try prescribing either Wen Dan Tang (clears Shao Yang depressed heat and dispels phlegm turbidity harassing the inner body) or Ban Xia Tian Ma Bai Zhu San (supplements the spleen and stomach, transforms phlegm-damp, and nourishes the blood and stabilizes wind). Just make sure to combine Bu Yang Huan Wu Tang (quickens the blood and transforms stasis, cools the blood, and supplements qi) and include Ren Shen/Chuan Qi Powder, Lai Fu Zi, Ji Nei Jin, Mai Ya, Gu Ya, and large doses of Tian Ma, Wu Zhu Yu, and Chuan Xiong. If seizures present, then add Zhu Ru, Mu Dan Pi, Chi Shao, The Three Insects, and Yu Sheng Wan.

You can follow up by monitoring the patient's serum lactate and pyruvate over time and modify your formula accordingly.

APPENDIX

DR. LEE'S MEDICINALS

This section introduces the medicinals Dr. Lee most commonly prescribes and includes details on processing, properties, actions, indications, dosage, and pharmacodynamics. The vast majority of medicinals prescribed in this text are decocting pieces of mostly raw plants, some crude minerals and shells, and rarely animal products. There are a few exceptions of pulverized medicinals that can be administered orally, either directly ingested or made into pills, or topically applied in the form of rub-on powders, ointments, washes, infusions, and suppositories.

References from TCM classical texts are included, mostly from *The Essential Herbal Foundation* (本草備要 *Ben Cao Bei Yao*), to provide insights into the foundations of Dr. Lee's medicinal applications. Contemporary sources that present commonly acknowledged medicinal attributes (e.g., flavor, nature, and channel entry) and experimental findings are also included to provide examples of evidence-based biomedical support of clinical efficacy. The primary source texts for the contemporary medicinal attributes and experimental findings are *Chinese Materia Medica Grand Dictionary* (新編中藥大辭典 *Xin Bian Zhong Yao Da Ci Dian*) and *Clinical Applications of Traditional Chinese Medicine* (中藥臨牀應用 *Zhong Yao Lin Chuang Ying Yong*).

Frequently administered medicinal pairs and combinations are introduced both as single medicinals and together with their counterparts. It is important to reiterate that these profiles are intended to highlight and clarify some of the distinctive features and applications of Dr. Lee's commonly prescribed medicinals, and not an attempt to present a complete listing of every medicinal Dr. Lee utilizes in clinical practice.

*__Disclaimer__: The medicinals provided in Dr. Lee's commonly prescribed medicinals listed below and throughout this entire three-volume series are *for reference purposes only* and are *not* intended for indiscriminate administration by other individuals or parties. Prescription of these medicinals should only be administered by a licensed traditional Chinese medicine (TCM) physician or practitioner who has carefully evaluated the patient's history, signs, and symptoms, and conducted pattern identification as the basis for determining treatment. Licensed TCM practitioners must be aware that these medicinals are *for reference purposes only* and solely intended for administration by Dr. Lee in his own clinical practice.

Bai Guo Ye – refer to **Yin Xing Ye**

Bai Ji Li – refer to **Ci Ji Li**

Bai Jiang Can (白僵蠶/Bombyx Batryticatus/Silkworm/aka **Jiang Can)**

In classical literature on pharmacopoeia, it is described as follows: "[**Bai**] **Jiang** [**Can**] doesn't rot and obtains clearing and transforming qi, thus is able to treat wind and transform phlegm, and dissipate binds and move the channels...."

In contemporary texts, it is described as having a salty and acrid flavor and a balanced nature; entering the liver and lung channels; and having wind-extinguishing tetany-checking, wind-dispelling pain-relieving, and phlegm-transforming bind-dissipating actions. It is recognized as being particularly effective for treating pathoconditions involving fright-wind and epilepsy with phlegm-heat.

Traditionally, **Bai Jiang Can** is combined with medicinals such as **Quan Xie**, **Tian Ma**, and **Huang Lian** (i.e., Qian Jin San) for the treatment of infantile phlegm-heat acute fright; **Quan Xie** and **Wu Gong** (i.e., She Feng San) for the treatment of tetanus, spasm, and convulsion with arched-back rigidity; and **Quan Xie** and **Bai Fu Zi** (i.e., Qian Zheng San) for the treatment of wind striking the channels and network vessels and deviated eyes and mouth.

*For more details, refer to **The Three Insects** profile.

Bai Shao – refer to **Chi Shao**

Bai Zhi (白芷/Radix Angelicae Dahuricae/Dahurian Angelica Root/Fang Xiang)

Bai Zhi was first introduced in *The Divine Husbandman's Herbal Foundation Canon* (神農本草經 *Shen Nong Ben Cao Jing*) as a middle grade medicinal with the alternative name of **Fang Xiang** (芳香 f□ ng xi□ ng), literally meaning "aromatic."

In classical literature on pharmacopoeia, it is described as follows: "Acrid [in flavor] dissipates wind, warm [in nature] eliminates dampness, [and] aromatic [in qi] opens the orifices," "[**Bai Zhi**] moves [through] the hand and foot Yang Ming [channels], enters the hand Tai Yang [channel], and is a chief Yang Ming medicinal," and "Treats Yang Ming clouded head and vision with headache and eye pain (頭目昏痛 tóu mù h□ n tòng), eyebrow bone pain, toothache, deep-source nasal congestion (鼻淵 bí yu□ n), itchy eyes, snivel, dark facial complexion, blemishes, dry itchy skin, wind-heat [pattern] disease in the three channels, flooding and blood block, intestinal wind and hemorrhoids and fistulas, welling-abscesses, flat-abscesses and sores, and damp-heat [pattern] disease in the three channels. [**Bai Zhi**] quickens the blood and expels pus, engenders flesh and relieves pain, and resolves arsenic [poisoning] and snake venom...."

In contemporary texts, it is described as having an acrid flavor and warm nature; entering the lung and stomach channels; and having exterior-resolving wind-dissipating, orifice-freeing, pain-relieving, dampness-drying vaginal discharge-checking, and swelling-dispersing pus-expelling actions.

Traditionally, it is prescribed for the treatment of external contraction wind-cold, headache, and nasal congestion; Yang Ming headache, toothache, deep-source nasal congestion (sinusitis) (鼻淵 bí yu□ n), and wind-damp impediment pain; excessive vaginal discharge (leukorrhea); and swelling and toxin of sores and welling-abscesses.

Dr. Lee uses **Bai Zhi** as a conductor medicinal for the nose, mouth, face, and lower gastrointestinal tract (i.e., colon, rectum, and anus) in the treatment of a broad spectrum of pathoconditions from the common cold, rhinitis, anal fissures and hemorrhoids to Bell's palsy, nasopharyngeal carcinoma (NPC) and colorectal cancer. And the medicinal pair **Bai Zhi** and **Fang Feng** is also included in Xian Fang Huo Ming Yin for the treatment of dermatological pathoconditions.

Dr. Lee also commonly prescribes the medicinal pair **Bai Zhi** and **Fang Feng** (resolves the exterior, dissipates wind, and frees the orifices) for gastrointestinal pathoconditions presenting as Yang Ming heat with exterior pattern (e.g., Crohn's disease), Yang Ming channel pattern (e.g., common cold), and Tai Yang and Yang Ming combination disease (e.g., wind evil assailing the outer body (風邪外襲 f□ ng xié wài xí) manifesting as Bell's palsy).

Bai Zhu (白朮/Rhizoma Atractylodis Macrocephalae/White Atractylodes Rhizome)

In classical literature on pharmacopoeia, it is described as follows: "**Bai Zhu** is an essential medicinal for fortifying the spleen and stomach, expelling dampness, eliminating impediment, and dispersing food. [For] vacuous and unfortified spleen, [**Bai**] **Zhu** can supplement; and [for] stomach vacuity failing to absorb, [**Bai**] **Zhu** can assist."

In contemporary texts, it is described as having a bitter and sweet flavor and a warm nature; entering the spleen and stomach channels; and having qi-supplementing spleen-fortifying, dampness-drying water-disinhibiting, sweat-checking, and fetus-quieting actions.

This medicinal contains the primary constituent atractylone as well as esters and carbohydrates (e.g., mannose, fructose) that strengthen the constitution (promote absorption of nutrients by the spleen), disinhibit urine, lower blood sugar levels, and provide anticoagulant, antimicrobial, and anti-inflammatory actions.

Ban Xia (半夏/Rhizoma Pinelliae Ternatae/Pinellia Tuber)

In classical literature on pharmacopoeia, it is described as follows: "Mobile and dissipates and dries and moistens. Harmonizes the stomach and fortifies the spleen, supplements the liver and moistens the lung, eliminates dampness and transforms phlegm, and effuses the exterior and opens depression. Precipitates counterflow qi, checks vomiting and vexation, promotes the voice, disinhibits the waterways, and rescues sudden collapse. Treats cough and counterflow dizzy head, reversal phlegm headache, brow ridge bone pain, sore throat, chest distention, cold damage cold and heat, phlegm malaria sleeplessness, and stomach reflux vomiting; and dissipates impediment, eliminates goiter, disperses swelling, and checks sweating."

In contemporary texts, it is described as having an acrid flavor, warm nature, and toxicity; entering the spleen, stomach, and lung channels; and having dampness-drying phlegm-transforming, counterflow-downbearing vomit-checking, and glomus-dispersing bind-dissipating actions. Ban Xia is recognized as an essential medicinal for drying dampness and transforming phlegm, warming and transforming cold phlegm, and checking vomiting.

Dr. Lee includes the medicinal combination comprising the essential medicinals of Er Chen Tang—**Ban Xia**, **Chen Pi**, **Fu Ling**, and **Gan Cao**—in the formulas Ban Xia Tian Ma Bai Zhu San, Wen Dan Tang, Xiang Sha Liu Jun Zi Tang, Atopic Dermatitis Formula, Tearing on Exposure to Wind Formula, and Asthma Formula; and the medicinal combination **Ban Xia**, **Hou Po**, **Fu Ling**, and **Gan Cao** in Ban Xia Hou Po Tang. Additionally, Dr. Lee commonly adds the medicinal combination **Ban Xia**, **Jie Geng**, and **Gan Cao** into formulas for the treatment of upper respiratory tract (especially the throat) pathoconditions.

Cang Zhu (蒼朮/Rhizoma Atractylodis/Black Atractylodes Rhizome/Chi Zhu)

In classical literature on pharmacopoeia, it is described as follows: "Dries the stomach and strengthens the spleen, promotes sweating and eliminates dampness, and upbears and effuses yang qi in the stomach…an essential medicinal for dissipating wind-cold-damp in the treatment of wilting [pattern]. And [**Cang Zhu**] can also resolve the six depressions: phlegm, fire, qi, blood, dampness, and food."

In contemporary texts, it is described as having an acrid and bitter flavor and warm nature; entering the spleen and stomach channels; and having spleen-fortifying dampness-drying and wind-damp-dispelling sweat-promoting actions.

Cang Zhu has the spleen-fortifying action of **Bai Zhu**, along with the advantages of stomach dampness-drying and antimicrobial actions for the treatment of gastrointestinal disorders (e.g., sloppy stool, diarrhea, dysentery) and other infectious diseases. Thus, this medicinal is ideal for Taiwan's humid subtropical climate.

Dr. Lee includes **Cang Zhu** in many Yu Sheng formulas, either added into the formula or substituted in place of **Bai Zhu** (unless the patient presents with qi vacuity!). Dr. Lee commonly adds the medicinal pair **Cang Zhu** and **Shan Zha**, and sometimes **Ji Nei Jin**, into formulas containing large doses of medicinals (e.g., heat-clearing toxin-resolving, yin-nourishing blood-supplementing, blood-quickening stasis-transforming, yin-enriching yang-subduing) that may impair digestion and cause sloppy stools in some patients. Dr. Lee also prescribes **Cang Zhu** for the treatment of damp-heat pattern myasthenia gravis, which can be classified as wilting pattern.

The physiological mechanism of its dampness-drying action primarily involves its capacity to promote increased interstitial permeability of water between membranes throughout the body.

*For more details, refer to **The Digestants** and **The Four Lings** profiles.

Chai Hu (柴胡/Radix Bupleuri/Bupleurum Root)

In classical literature on pharmacopoeia, it is described as follows: "Bitter [in flavor] and balanced and slightly cold [in nature], and weak flavor (味薄 wèi báo) and qi upbearing are yang," "Governs yang qi fall, conducts clear qi upward, and thus calms evil heat in the Shao Yang and Jue Yin [channels]. [**Chai Hu**] perfuses and disinhibits qi and blood and dissipates binds and regulates menstruation, and thus is [classified as] a foot Shao Yang exterior medicinal. Treats cold damage evil heat, phlegm-heat repletion binds, vacuity damage flesh heat, retching and vomiting and heart vexation, all [types of] malarial heat (fever) and [aversion to] cold, dizzy head and red eyes, chest impediment and rib-side pain, bitterness of mouth and deafness, heat entering the blood chamber in women, all [types of] antepartum and postpartum heat, pox sores in children, and five (visceral) gan (五疳 wu g□n) surplus heat. [It] dissipates sores and flat-abscesses of the twelve channels and congeals blood and gathers qi, just like the action of **Lian Qiao**," "Treats binding qi in the heart [region], abdomen, stomach and intestines, dietary accumulations and gatherings, alternating heat (fever) and cold (chills) evil qi [e.g., evil lying depressed in Shao Yang, evil heat depressed internally, liver channel depressed heat], and removes the old and institutes the new (推陳之新 tu□ chén zh□ x□n)," and "In summary, **Chai Hu** is indicated for only two conditions, one is repletion heat [pattern], for patients with external evil half-interior half-exterior, [it] conducts outward [and] thus enables external evil to naturally effuse from the exterior; and another is right vacuity (正虛 zhèng x□) [pattern], for patients with clear qi falling into the yin aspect, [it] lifts and raises and returns to its residence [and] thus enables qi in the stomach to naturally revitalize."

In contemporary texts, it is described as having a bitter and acrid flavor and slightly cold nature; entering the liver and gallbladder channels; and having heat-clearing and -dissipating, liver-coursing depression-resolving, and yang-upbearing fall-raising actions.

Chai Hu is recognized as a Shao Yang pattern essential medicinal that courses and dissipates Shao Yang half-exterior half-interior evil for the treatment of evil in the Shao Yang channel presenting with symptoms of alternating cold and heat, fullness in the chest and rib-side, bitter taste in the mouth, and dry throat.

Dr. Lee includes the medicinal pair **Chai Hu** and **Huang Qin** in the formulas Xiao Chai Hu Tang, Chai Ling Tang, and Long Dan Xie Gan Tang.

Chan Tui (蟬蛻/Periostracum Cicadae/Cicada Molt)

In classical literature on pharmacopoeia, it is described as follows: "Salty and sweet [in flavor], cold [in nature], and no toxicity," "Slightly sweet and slightly salty in flavor and slightly cool in nature," and "**Chan** embodies the transformation of earth and wood excess qi and [it] drinks wind dew, thus does not intake food. Its qi is clear and vacuous and sweet [in flavor] and cold [in nature], thus eliminates wind-heat. Its body is light and floating, thus effuses pox sores. Its nature excels at molting, thus abates eye screen and hastens delivery and aborts the fetus. Its **molt** is an exoskeleton, thus treats skin sores and dormant papules, and its sound is clear and resonant, thus treats wind strike with loss of voice. Also, [it] rings in the day and rests at night, thus checks night crying in infants."

In contemporary texts, it is described as having a sweet flavor and cold nature; entering the lung and liver channels; and having wind-coursing heat-dissipating, papule-outthrusting itch-relieving, eye-brightening screen-abating, and fright-checking actions.

Dr. Lee classifies **Chan Tui** as an exterior membrane (i.e., eyes and skin) conductor based on its innate substance as slough (shed epithelial tissue) and its inherent capacity to *peel off* the agglutinated protein build-up on the membranous surfaces of the eyes. This is an example of the classical TCM treatment method of "resembling forms treat respective body parts and resembling organs treat respective organs (以形治形、以臟治臟 yi xíng zhì xíng, yi zàng zhì zàng)."

Dr. Lee typically prescribes the medicinal pair **Chan Tui** and **She Tui** (dispels wind, disperses swelling, kills worms, abates screens, and stabilizes fright) for the treatment of ophthalmological pathoconditions, such as lens opacities (e.g., cataract) and corneal opacities (e.g., eye screen (目翳 mù yì), scarring), and for dermatological pathoconditions presenting with intense pruritis.

*For more details, refer to **The Eye Brighteners** and **The Itch Relievers** profiles.

Chi Shao (赤芍/Radix Paeoniae Rubra/Red Peony Root)

In classical literature on pharmacopoeia, the attributes of **Chi Shao** and **Bai Shao** (白芍) are described as follows: "**Bai Shao** supplements and contracts and **Chi Shao** drains and dissipates. **Bai** [**Shao**] benefits the spleen and drains water from earth [spleen]; **Chi** [**Shao**] dissipates evil and moves stagnation in the blood."

In contemporary texts, **Chi Shao** is described as having a bitter flavor and slightly cold nature; entering the liver channel; and having heat-clearing blood-cooling and stasis-dissipating pain-relieving actions. **Bai Shao** is described as having a bitter, sour, and sweet flavor and slightly cold nature; entering the liver and spleen channel; and having yin-nourishing menstruation-regulating, liver-calming pain-relieving, and yin-consolidating sweat-checking actions.

A contemporary comparison of these two medicinals is as follows: "**Chi Shao** excels at quickening the blood and dissipating stasis and **Bai Shao** is better at tranquilizing and relieving pain; both have supplementing actions with **Bai Shao** superior at supplementing blood and nourishing yin, and **Chi Shao** superior at cooling the blood and expelling stasis."

Dr. Lee explains that most traditional formulas designed in times of antiquity originally included **Bai Shao** because the clinical presentation of dual qi and blood vacuity was far more prevalent back then, thus necessitating the emphasis of this medicinal's blood-nourishing actions. Our modern lifestyle, diet, and living environs have altered people's body constitutions, with blood stasis and stagnation and a predilection towards blood heat more predominant nowadays. The blood-cooling stasis-expelling actions of **Chi Shao** are more suitable for patients of today—this is the reasoning for **Chi Shao** replacing **Bai Shao** in Yu Sheng formula compositions and variants. Additionally, Dr. Lee also adds large doses of this medicinal into formulas during certain stages of cancer treatment to inhibit tumor angiogenesis (neovascularization).

Chuan Qi (川七/Radix Notoginseng/Notoginseng Root/aka **San Qi** and **Shan Qi)**

In classical literature on pharmacopoeia, it is described as follows: "Dissipates blood and settles pain. Treats blood ejection and spontaneous external bleeding, blood dysentery and flooding, red eyes and swollen welling-abscesses, and is an essential medicinal for knife, club, and incised wounds" and "**Chuan Qi**...excels at transforming static blood, [it] also excels at stanching the frenetic movement of blood, is an essential medicinal for blood ejection and spontaneous external bleeding, and following [treatment] and recovery no static blood is left behind in the channels and network vessels…and [it] transforms blood stasis without compromising the engendering of new blood, making it a superb blood-rectifying medicinal."

In contemporary texts, it is described as having a sweet and slightly bitter flavor and a warm nature; entering the liver and stomach channels; and having stasis-transforming blood-stanching and blood-quickening pain-settling actions.

This medicinal is clinically recognized as a blood-stanching and stasis-transforming essential medicinal that improves the viscoelasticity of vascular walls and promotes blood flow in the microvasculature. It can be prescribed for the treatment of a wide range of blood stasis pattern pathoconditions, such as compromised blood perfusion (e.g., cardiovascular disease (CVD), cerebrovascular disease (CVA), peripheral artery disease (PAD), peripheral vascular disease (PVD)) and all types of bleeding and hemorrhage.

Chuan Qi is an expensive medicinal and the process of decoction diminishes potency, thus Dr. Lee typically administers it as a pulverized powder to minimize cost and maximize efficacy. This powder is either added directly into a formula after the decoction has cooled or ingested separately. Since Dr. Lee prescribes this medicinal in pulverized powder form, it is omitted from Yu Sheng formula composition listings, which are decocting pieces only. **Chuan Qi** is often paired with **Ren Shen** (powder) (greatly supplements original qi and stems vacuity desertion, supplements the spleen and boosts the lung, engenders liquid, and quiets the spirit) to form **Ren Shen/Chuan Qi Powder**, one of the pillars of Dr. Lee's therapeutic approaches.

*For more details, refer to the **Ren Shen/Chuan Qi Powder** profile.

Ci Ji Li (刺蒺藜/Fructus Tribuli/Caltrop Fruit/aka Ji Li Zi and Bai Ji Li)

In classical literature on pharmacopoeia, it is described as follows: "Bitter and acrid [in flavor] and warm [in nature]," "Enters the lung, liver, and kidney channels," and "Supplements the kidney with bitterness and warmth, drains lung qi with acridity and warmth, and also dissipates liver wind, and boosts essence and brightens the eyes.

Treats vacuity taxation lumbar pain, seminal emission and vaginal discharge, cough counterflow and lung wilting, milk block and concretions and conglomerations, hemorrhoids and fistulas and yin depletion, diseases of the liver, kidney, and lung channels, and hastens delivery and aborts the fetus."

In contemporary texts, it is described as having a bitter and acrid flavor and balanced nature; entering the liver, kidney, and lung channels; and having liver-calming liver-coursing and wind-dispelling eye-brightening actions.

Traditionally, **Ci Ji Li** is prescribed in combination with **Chan Tui** and **Fang Feng** for the treatment of exterior wind-heat, damp-heat, and blood desiccation pattern skin pathoconditions presenting with itchy papules (e.g., urticaria, eczema (damp papules), neurodermatitis); and with **Zao Jiao Ci** and **Chan Tui** to promote the dispersion and rupture of welling-abscesses and sores and relieve itching.

Dr. Lee typically adds the medicinal pair **Ci Ji Li** and **Zao Jiao Ci** (quickens the blood and disperses swelling and expels pus and frees milk) into formula variants for the treatment of exterior wind-heat pattern ophthalmological pathoconditions affecting the tear ducts (e.g., epidemic keratoconjunctivitis ("pinkeye")) and damp-heat pattern dermatological pathoconditions (e.g., lipomas, flat warts).

Dr. Lee further classifies **Ci Ji Li**, **Zao Jiao Ci**, and **Lu Lu Tong** (expels wind and frees the network vessels and disinhibits water and eliminates dampness) as pore conductors with their capacity to regulate—*opening* and *closing* (開闔 k□i hé)—the pores and promote dermal circulation. Thus, he also adds this medicinal combination into formula variants for exterior wind-heat (or wind-heat-damp) and blood desiccation with exterior wind-heat (or wind-heat-damp) pattern skin pathoconditions that present with pruritic papules and maculopapular and vesicular eruptions (e.g., dyshidrotic eczema (pompholyx), palmoplantar pustulosis (PPP), wind papules (urticaria), acute stage atopic dermatitis).

Dr. Lee explains that blood-quickening stasis-transforming medicinals (e.g., **Dang Gui**, **Chuan Xiong**, **Ru Xiang**, **Mo Yao**) promote an increase of angiogenic proteins, the precursors necessary for angiogenesis, while the medicinal pair **Zao Jiao Ci** and **Ci Ji Li** has the capacity to open up pathways in the granulation tissue and collagen deposition formed during the wound healing process. The prescription of these mutually complementary medicinals reestablishes patent vasculature and perfusion at the site of the fibrous tissue (i.e., scar) formation, restores the natural skin coloration, and shrinks the size of the scar, thus improving the cosmetic appearance of both hypertrophic and keloid scars.

*For more details, refer to **The Eye Brighteners** and **The Itch Relievers** profiles.

Ci Shi (磁石/Magnetitum/Magnetite)

This medicinal is the naturally occurring rock mineral ferrous ferric oxide (Fe3O4), which contains 31% ferrous oxide (FeO) (aka wüstite) and 69% ferric oxide (Fe2O3) (aka hematite), along with other trace minerals such as magnesium oxide (MgO), aluminum oxide (Al2O3), manganese ion (Mn+2), calcium ion Ca+2, and silicate (SiO3).

In classical literature on pharmacopoeia, it is described as follows: "Cold [in nature] and black in color belongs to water," "[**Ci Shi**] can conduct lung-metal qi into the kidney, supplement the kidney and boost the essence, eliminate vexation and heat, and sharpen the hearing and brighten the eyes. Treats emaciation and weakness (羸弱 léi ruò) and generalized impediment, joint aching pain, fright epilepsy and phlegm node, accidental swallowing of iron, and stanches bleeding from incised wounds."

In contemporary texts, it is described as having a salty flavor and cold nature; entering the heart, liver, and kidney channels; and having fright-settling spirit-quieting, liver-calming yang-subduing, hearing-sharpening eye-brightening, and qi absorption-promoting panting-stabilizing actions.

Ci Shi is commonly prescribed together with other heavy settling yang-subduing medicinals—**Zhu Sha** and **Sheng Mu Li**—for the treatment of disquieted heart spirit, fright palpitations, insomnia, epileptic seizures, and ascendant hyperactivity of liver yang. It is also combined with kidney-enriching medicinals—**Shou Di Huang**, **Shan Zhu Yu**, and **Wu Wei Zi**—and liver- and kidney-supplementing eye-brightening medicinals—**Ju Hua**, **Gou Ji Zi**, and **Nu Zhen Zi**—for the treatment of dim vision.

Dr. Lee includes the medicinal combination **Ci Shi**, **Dai Zhe Shi**, and **Sheng Mu Li**—calm the liver and subdue yang—in Jian Ling Tang, one of his most commonly prescribed formulas for the treatment of all types of ascendant hyperactivity of liver yang (肝陽上亢 g□n yáng shàng kàng) pattern and yin vacuity with yang hyperactivity (陰虛陽亢 y□n x□ yáng kàng) pattern pathoconditions (e.g., diabetes, hypertension, hyperthyroidism, other overactive endocrine disorders).

Cu Lu Rong – refer to **Lu Rong**

Da Huang (大黃/Radix et Rhizoma Rhei/Rhubarb Root)

This medicinal is processed in Dr. Lee's in-house processing facility. Purchased **raw** (生 sh□ng = **Sheng**), it is first **wine-steeped** (酒浸泡 jiu jìn pào = **Jiu Jin Pao**)—steeped in rice wine over a period of 10 days (in warm weather) to 2 weeks (in cold weather) until thoroughly saturated, oven-dried (烘乾 h□ng g□n) at low temperature, and then cut for use as decocting pieces or pulverized into a powder for topical application. **Sheng Da Huang** has accumulation-attacking stagnation-abducting, precipitation-draining, and fire-draining blood-cooling actions. Steeping Da Huang in rice wine moderates the cold precipitation actions and conducts the medicinal strength upwards to provide heart fire-draining and liver fire-draining actions for the treatment of heat pattern pathoconditions. Thus, unless specified differently, whenever **Da Huang** is used throughout this text, it refers to **Wine-Steeped Da Huang**.

In classical literature on pharmacopoeia, it is described as follows: "Great bitter [in flavor] and great cold [in nature]," "Enters the foot Tai Yin [channel] and hand and foot Yang Ming and Jue Yin [channels] blood aspect," and "Its nature is upbearing and thus does not sink, and its action is mobile and thus is not static. If steeped in wine [it] can also conduct upwards, [for] application in flushing the stomach and intestines and precipitating dryness-bind to eliminate static heat. It treats cold damage seasonal disease (傷寒時疾 sh□ng hán shí jí), heat effusion (fever) with delirious speech, warm-heat miasmic malaria (瘴瘧 zhàng nüè), red and white dysentery, abdominal pain and urgency, jaundice and water-swelling (edema), concretions, conglomerations, accumulations and gatherings, lodged rheum and abiding food (留飲宿食 liú yin sù shí), distention and fullness in the heart [region] and abdomen, fecal and urinary stoppage, blood ejection and spontaneous external bleeding, blood block and blood desiccation, blood accumulation due to damage, and all [types of] repletion heat and latent heat in the blood (血分伏熱 xuè f□n fú rè). Moves water and eliminates phlegm, erodes pus and disperses swelling, and can remove the old and institute the new."

In contemporary texts, it is described as having a bitter flavor and cold nature; entering the spleen, stomach, large intestine, liver, and heart channels; and having draining and precipitating, accumulation-attacking, heat-clearing toxin-resolving, fire-draining, blood-quickening stasis-transforming, and blood-stanching actions.

This medicinal is administered for patients with a wide range of pathoconditions from gastrointestinal disorders (e.g., constipation, gallstones) to elevated intracranial pressure. Its heat-clearing draining precipitation, fire-draining, accumulation-attacking, and blood-quickening stasis-transforming actions promote the removal of metabolic waste byproducts resulting from nerve cell damage and static blood; break down bile; reduce pressure of the portal vein and relax the diaphragm muscles; stimulate intestinal motility; and eliminate endothelial hyperplasia (e.g., inflammation from autoimmune disease, viral infection).

For the treatment of increased intracranial pressure (ICP), initially small amounts are prescribed, increasing incrementally in 5 fen doses up to 7–8 qian until the desired draining precipitation action is achieved, which is typically 2–3 stools per day (sometimes as much as 5 stools per day depending on the pathocondition).

In addition to oral administration, **Da Huang** powder can be topically applied on open sores for its antimicrobial and blood-stanching actions. It dries and forms a protective barrier that prevents infectious agents from entering the wound and simultaneously fights infection within the lesion. For these reasons, Da Huang is often applied topically in Dr. Lee's clinic following bloodletting therapy. Da Huang can also be blended into either a petrolatum or an emulsifying hydrophilic ointment base for the treatment of inflammatory skin pathoconditions (e.g., streptococcal, staphylococcal).

Da Zao (大棗/Fructus Jujubae/Jujube/aka **Hong Zao)**

In classical literature on pharmacopoeia, it is described as follows: "[**Da Zao**] is a spleen channel blood aspect medicinal" and "[It] supplements earth and boosts qi, enriches spleen-earth, moistens the heart and lungs, harmonizes construction and defense, moderates yin and blood, engenders liquid and humor (fluids), pleases the complexion, frees the nine orifices, aids the twelve channels, and harmonizes the hundred medicinals. Add into cold damage and supplementing formulas to promote the upbearing of [clear] qi by the spleen and stomach."

In contemporary texts, it is described as having a sweet flavor and warm nature; entering the spleen and stomach channels; and having center-supplementing qi-boosting, yin-nourishing spirit-quieting, and medicinal nature-moderating actions.

Traditionally, it is eaten both as a foodstuff and administered as a medicinal. For the treatment of blood vacuity withered-yellow [complexion], visceral agitation, and disquieted spirit-mind, it is commonly combined with **Gan Cao** and **Xiao Mai** (e.g., Gan Mai Da Zao Tang). **Da Zao** and **Sheng Jiang** form one of most commonly prescribed medicinal pairs in the Chinese medicine pharmacopoeia—added into exterior-resolving formulas, the pair harmonizes construction and defense, and added into supplementing and boosting formulas, the pair regulates and supplements the spleen and stomach. Plus, in large doses, it can be added to harsh formulas (e.g., Shi Zao Tang) to mitigate toxicity, safeguard the spleen and stomach, and nourish right qi.

Dr. Lee commonly prescribes the medicinal combination **Da Zao**, **Long Yan Rou**, and **Gan Cao**—boost qi and supplement the spleen and heart and nourish the blood and calm the spirit—for the treatment of stress, anxiety, depression, poor nutrition, and psychosomatic or psychogenic pathoconditions.

Da Zao's bioactive constituents include alkaloids (e.g., stepharine), triterpenes (e.g., betulonic acid, oleanoic acid), saponins (e.g., ziziphussaponin I, II, III and jujuboside B), cyclic adenosine monophosphate (cAMP), cyclic guanosine monophosphate (cGMP), glucose, fructose, sucrose, vitamins (e.g., thiamine (B1), riboflavin (B2), vitamin C), and minerals.

*For more details, refer to **The Sweets** profile.

Dai Zhe Shi (代赭石/Haematitum/Hematite)

This medicinal is the naturally occurring rock mineral ferric oxide (Fe_2O_3) (hematite), which contains moderate amounts of silicic acid and aluminide and small amounts of other trace minerals such as magnesium, manganese, and calcium.

In classical literature on pharmacopoeia, it is described as follows: "[**Dai Zhe Shi**] nourishes blood and qi and calms blood heat. Enters the liver and pericardium [channels], and specializes in the treatment of blood aspect diseases of these two channels, blood ejection and spontaneous external bleeding and flooding and vaginal discharge, stirring fetus and difficult delivery, chronic fright in children, and engenders flesh of incised wounds."

In contemporary texts, it is described as having a bitter flavor and cold nature; entering the liver and heart channels; and having liver-calming yang-subduing, heavy settling counterflow-downbearing, and blood-cooling blood-stanching actions.

Dr. Lee includes the medicinal combination **Dai Zhe Shi**, **Ci Shi**, and **Sheng Mu Li**—calm the liver and subdue yang—in Jian Ling Tang, one of his most commonly prescribed formulas for the treatment of all types of ascendant hyperactivity of liver yang (肝陽上亢 g□n yáng shàng kàng) pattern and yin vacuity with yang hyperactivity (陰虛陽亢 y□n x□ yáng kàng) pattern pathoconditions (e.g., diabetes, hypertension, hyperthyroidism, other overactive endocrine disorders). Additionally, Dr. Lee will also add combinations of **Dai Zhe Shi**, **Sheng Mu Li**, **Chuan Qi**, and **Zhu Sha** into formulas for the treatment of profuse menstruation (e.g., menorrhagia, hypermenorrhea).

Dan Pi – refer to **Mu Dan Pi**

Dan Shen (丹參/Radix Salviae Miltiorrhizae/Salvia Root)

In classical literature on pharmacopoeia, it is described as follows: "**Dan Shen** is bitter in flavor, engenders the new and dispels evil, breaks accumulations and regulates menstruation, and disperses welling- and flat-abscesses" and "…[its] actions are equivalent to Si Wu [Tang], and is an essential gynecological medicinal."

In contemporary texts, it is described as having a bitter flavor and slightly cold nature; entering the heart and liver channels; and having blood-quickening menstruation-regulating, blood-cooling welling abscess-dispersing, and spirit-quieting actions. Traditionally, it is recognized as an essential blood-quickening stasis-resolving medicinal and one of the most commonly used medicinals for gynecological and obstetric pathoconditions.

Dr. Lee commonly includes **Dan Shen** decocting pieces in qi-supplementing, blood-supplementing, and stasis-dispelling formulas to improve cerebrovascular, cardiovascular, and peripheral vascular circulation and diffuse depressed heat. This is founded in the TCM classical theory of enduring illness results in stasis, which applies to many of Dr. Lee's patients who seek treatment for their chronic pathoconditions. Depending on the presenting signs, symptoms, and pattern, Dr. Lee may prescribe **Ren Shen** (powder) (or **Ren Shen/Chuan Qi Powder**) and **Dan Shen** together, with their respective qi- and blood-supplementing actions forming a complementary medicinal combination that adheres to the TCM classical theory of qi is the commander of blood and blood is the mother of qi (氣為血之帥、血為氣之母 qì wèi xuè zh□ shuài, xi□ wéi qì zh□ mu).

Dang Gui (當歸/Radix Angelicae Sinensis/Chinese Angelica Root)

This medicinal is processed in-house in Dr. Lee's own medicinal processing and decoction facility. **Dang Gui** (head, body, and tail) is first washed and cleaned, and then placed in barrels, where it is **wine-steeped** (酒浸泡 jiu jìn pào = **Jiu Jin Pao**)—steeped in rice wine over a period of 10 days (in warm weather) to 2 weeks (in cold weather) until thoroughly saturated, oven-dried (烘乾 h□ ng g□ n) at low temperature, and then cut to preserve freshness and ensure longer storage life. Steeping **Dang Gui** in rice wine also enhances its blood-supplementing actions. Thus, unless specified differently, whenever **Dang Gui** is used throughout this text, it refers to **Wine-Steeped Dang Gui**.

In classical literature on pharmacopoeia, it is described as follows: "Supplements the blood, moistens dryness, and lubricates the intestines," "**Dang Gui** is sweet [in flavor] and warm [in nature], engenders blood and supplements the heart, supports vacuity and boosts detriment, and expels stasis and engenders the new," and "**Dang Gui** is sweet in flavor and heavy, thus specializes in supplementing blood; it is acrid [in flavor] and its qi is light, thus it also moves blood. Movement in supplementation and supplementation in movement, indeed, it is a qi-in-blood medicinal (血中氣藥 xuè zhòng qì yào) and an in-blood sage medicinal."

In contemporary texts, it is described as having a sweet and acrid flavor and a warm nature; entering the liver, heart, and spleen channels; and having blood-supplementing blood-harmonizing, menstruation-regulating pain-checking, and dryness-moistening intestine-lubricating actions. Prescribed in small doses (≤ 2 qian), it nourishes blood; and in large doses (3–4 qian), it has blood-quickening stasis-transforming actions.

Dang Shen (黨參/Radix Codonopsis/Codonopsis Root)

In classical literature on pharmacopoeia, it is described as follows: "Enters the hand and foot Tai Yin channel qi aspect" and "Supplements the center and boosts qi, harmonizes the spleen and stomach, and eliminates vexation-heat. [For] slight vacuity of center qi, use [**Dang Shen**] to regulate and supplement, it's the most appropriate."

In contemporary texts, this medicinal is described as having a sweet flavor and a slightly warm nature; entering the spleen and lung channels; and having center-supplementing qi-boosting, spleen-fortifying lung-boosting, and liquid-engendering actions.

Considering the comparatively high cost of **Ren Shen**, for mild cases of center qi vacuity, many TCM physicians will prescribe **Dang Shen** instead. However, for the types of severe acute diseases and chronic disorders that Dr. Lee commonly treats, presenting with pronounced blood stasis and qi vacuity, **Dang Shen** is generally *not* a viable substitute. Instead, Dr. Lee will prescribe **Dan Shen** (quickens the blood, transforms stasis, and cools the blood) decocting pieces in place of **Dang Shen**, and separately add either **Ren Shen** (powder) (greatly supplements original qi and stems vacuity desertion, supplements the spleen and boosts the lung, engenders liquid, and quiets the spirit) or **Ren Shen/Chuan Qi Powder** (supplements original qi, engenders liquid, stems vacuity desertion, quickens the blood and transforms stasis, and stanches bleeding).

Dr. Lee *does* include **Dang Shen** in formulas, such as Gui Zhi Jia Long Gu Mu Li Tang, Pu Xiao Dang Bao Tang, and Sheng Hua Tang, to improve the flavor of the formula, supplement qi, fortify the stomach, and promote digestion.

Di Gu Pi (地骨皮/Cortex Lycii/Chinese Wolfberry Root Bark)

Di Gu Pi is the root bark of either *Lycium chinensis* Mill. or *Lycium barbarum* L., of which the ripe fruit of the latter is **Gou Qi Zi** (enriches yin, moistens the lung, supplements the liver, and brightens the eyes).

In classical literature on pharmacopoeia, it is described as follows: "Downbears latent fire in the lung and drains liver and kidney vacuity heat. Cools the blood and supplements right qi, thus treats evil heat of the five [organs] internally, blood ejection (吐血 tù xi□) and bloody urine, and cough and dispersion-thirst (消渴 xi□o k□).... Treats exterior unfixed location wind evil and corpse transmission (consumption) (傳戶 chuán hù) steaming bone with sweating."

In contemporary texts, it is described as having a sweet and bland flavor and cold nature; entering the lung, liver, and kidney channels; and having blood-cooling steam-eliminating and lung-clearing fire-downbearing actions. It is recognized as among the best medicinals for abating vacuity heat and taxation heat and treating steaming bone qi aspect pathoconditions.

Dr. Lee includes the medicinal pair **Di Gu Pi** and **Mu Dan Pi** (a steaming bone blood aspect medicinal) in the formula Di Gu Pi Yin, and the medicinal combination **Di Gu Pi**, **Qing Hao** (clears vacuity heat, eliminates steaming bone, resolves summerheat, and interrupts malaria), and **Zhi Mu** (clears heat and drains fir and enriches yin and moistens dryness) in Hyperactive Immune Formula. Additionally, he commonly adds the medicinal combination **Qing Hao**, **Di Gu Pi**, and **Zhi Mu**—enrich yin and downbear fire, cool the blood and clear vacuity heat, and eliminate steaming bone—into formula variants for the treatment of all types of pathoconditions that present with symptoms such as include intermittent fever, enduring heat, enduring cough, and yin vacuity dryness.

Di Huang – refer to **Sheng Di Huang**

Di Long (地龍/Lumbricus/Earthworm/aka **Qiu Yin)**

In classical literature on pharmacopoeia, it is described as follows: "Cold in nature, but descending [in movement]—cold in nature, thus can resolve all types of heat diseases, [and] descending [in movement], thus can disinhibit urine—for the treatment of lower extremity diseases and freeing the channels and network vessels. Indicated for cold damage malaria, great heat mania and vexation, urinary stoppage in adults and children, acute and chronic fright wind (**急慢憬風** jí màn jing f□ng), and joint-running wind pain (歷節風痛 lì jié f□ng tòng)."

In contemporary texts, it is described as having a salty flavor and cold nature; entering the liver, spleen, and urinary bladder channel; and having heat-clearing wind-extinguishing, channel-freeing network vessel-quickening, panting-calming, and urine-disinhibiting actions.

Dr. Lee prescribes the medicinal pair **Di Long** and **Ma Huang** (opens the nine orifices and stimulates the nervous system)—serve as nervous system conductors—for pathoconditions affecting the respiratory and vasomotor centers in the brainstem (e.g., cerebrovascular accident (CVA), trauma, microbial infection, enduring illness) and for the treatment of wind-cold-damp impediment.

Ding Shu Xiu (丁豎朽/Scaber Elephantopus/Elephant's Foot)

In contemporary texts, it is described as having an acrid flavor and cool nature; entering the liver, kidney, stomach, and small intestine; and having urine-disinhibiting swelling-dispersing, blood-cooling toxin-resolving, phlegm-dispelling, and pain-relieving actions.

In Dr. Lee's pharmacopoeia, it is an essential medicinal for inhibiting the synthesis of blood urea nitrogen (BUN) and serum creatinine (Cr) in the treatment of pathological conditions that result from hypoperfusion of blood through functionally normal kidneys (prerenal), structural damage to the renal parenchyma (intrinsic renal), and urinary tract obstruction (postrenal).

Dr. Lee commonly adds the medicinal pair **Ding Shu Xiu** and **Ren Dong Teng** (clears heat, resolves toxin, and frees the network vessels) into Wu Ling San (Nephritis Formula), Chai Ling Tang, and other formula variants based on presenting signs, symptoms, and patterns.

Du Zhong (杜仲/Cortex Eucommiae/Eucommia Bark)

In classical literature on pharmacopoeia, it is described as follows: "For all [types of] vacuity in the lower burner, without **Du Zhong** [one] cannot supplement; [for] dampness in the lower burner, without **Du Zhong** [one] cannot disinhibit; [for] aching in the legs, without **Du Zhong** [one] cannot eliminate, and [for] pain in the lumbus and knees, without **Du Zhong** [one] cannot eliminate.... [For] supplementing the liver and boosting the kidney, [it] is indeed an essential medicinal," "Treats lumbar spine pain, supplements the center and boosts qi, hardens the sinew and bone, strengthens the mind, and eliminates genital damp itch and dribble after voiding," and "Sweet [in flavor] and warm [in nature], [it] can supplement; and mildly acrid [in flavor], [it] can moisten. The color purple enters the liver channel qi aspect, moistens liver dryness, and supplements liver vacuity. The child makes the mother replete, thus [it] also supplements the kidney. When the liver is full, the sinews are fortified and when the kidney is full, the bones are strengthened, thus enabling sinew and bone to fix together [attach]. Treats aching lumbus and knees, genital damp itch, dribble after voiding, and fetal spotting and miscarriage."

In contemporary texts, it is described as having a sweet flavor and warm nature; entering the liver and kidney channels; and having liver and kidney-supplementing, sinew- and bone-strengthening, and fetus-quieting actions.

Dr. Lee commonly pairs **Du Zhong** and **Niu Xi** (quickens the blood and frees the channels, supplements the liver and kidney, strengthens sinew and bone, disinhibits water and frees strangury, and conducts fire (blood) downward)—serve as lumbus (spine) and lower limb conductors—in the formulas You Gui Yin, Tong Jing Fang, Paralysis Formula #1, Paralysis Formula #3, and Zuo Gui Yin. Dr. Lee also pairs **Du Zhong** and **Xu Duan** (supplements the liver and kidney, strengthens sinew and bone, and stanches bleeding and quiets the fetus)—serve as lumbus (spine) and lower limb conductors—in the formula Dang Gui San.

Duan Long Gu (Calcined Dragon Bone) – refer to **Long Gu**

Duan Mu Li (Calcined Oyster Shell) – refer to **Mu Li**

Duan Shi Gao (Calcined Gypsum) – refer to **Shi Gao**

Fang Feng (防風/Radix Saposhnikoviae/Saposhnikovia Root)

In classical literature on pharmacopoeia, it is described as follows: "Acrid and bitter [in flavor] and upfloating are yang" and "Tracks the liver and drains the lung, dissipates stagnant qi in the head and eyes, and abides dampness in the channels and network vessels. Indicated for blood in the upper part of the body, upper burner wind evil, headache and dizzy vision, pain in the spine and rigidity of the neck, generalized pain, and Tai Yang channel pattern [pathoconditions]. [**Fang Feng**] also moves [through] the spleen and stomach channel [and] is a wind-dispelling dampness-overcoming essential medicinal. [It] dissipates red eyes and sores.

Li Shi-Zhen (李時珍), author of *Herbal Foundation Compendium* (本草綱目 *Ben Cao Gang Mu*) written during the Ming dynasty in 1590 CE, described **Fang Feng** as a "wind medicinal with moistening actions."

In contemporary texts, it is described as having an acrid and sweet flavor and slightly warm nature; entering the urinary bladder, liver, and spleen channels; and having exterior-effusing wind-dissipating, dampness-overcoming pain-relieving, and tetany-checking actions.

Fang Feng is warmer in nature than **Jing Jie** and can overcome dampness, thus it is also prescribed for the treatment of wind-damp impediment pain. Traditionally, the medicinal pair **Fang Feng** and **Jing Jie** is commonly prescribed for the treatment of exterior wind-heat pattern pathoconditions, itchy wind papules, and sores in the acute stage that present with exterior pattern.

Dr. Lee includes the medicinal pair **Fang Feng** and **Jing Jie** (effuses the exterior and dissipates wind, outthrusts papules and heals sores, and rectifies the blood) in Wan Ling Dan for the treatment of a wide range of pathoconditions (e.g., from intractable skin conditions and parasitic infections to benign tumors and cancer). This medicinal pair is also added into formulas for the treatment of exterior wind-heat pattern dermatological and ophthalmological conditions (e.g., conjunctivitis, keratitis).

Fang Feng and **Bai Zhi** (resolves the exterior, dissipates wind, and frees the orifices) are included in Xian Fang Huo Ming Yin, to which Dr. Lee commonly will add **Jing Jie**, for the treatment of dermatological pathoconditions. And Dr. Lee commonly prescribes the medicinal pair **Fang Feng** and **Bai Zhi** for gastrointestinal pathoconditions presenting with Yang Ming heat with exterior pattern (e.g., Crohn's disease), Yang Ming channel pattern (e.g., common cold), and Tai Yang and Yang Ming combination disease (e.g., wind evil assailing the outer body (風邪外襲 f□ng xié wài xí) manifesting as Bell's palsy).

Fu Ling (茯苓/Sclerotium Poriae Cocos/Poria)

In classical literature on pharmacopoeia, it is described as follows: "**Fu Ling** is sweet [in flavor] and warm [in nature], engenders liquid and checks thirst, abates heat and quiets the fetus, and boosts the spleen and aides yang" and "...percolates dampness and disinhibits the orifices and eliminates dampness...."

In contemporary texts, it is described as having a sweet and bland flavor and balanced nature; entering the heart, spleen, and kidney channels; and having water-disinhibiting dampness-percolating, and spleen-fortifying spirit-quieting actions. It is experimentally proven to increase the urinary excretion of electrolytes (e.g., potassium, sodium, chloride), lower blood sugar levels, and provide sedative actions.

As a general rule, for patients presenting with pronounced water amassment or water-rheum collecting internally (e.g., generalized edema, ascites, pericardial effusion, pleural effusion, increased intracranial pressure (ICP)), Dr. Lee will prescribe the medicinal pair **Fu Ling** and **Ze Xie** in equivalently large doses (≥ 8 qian) for their mutually accentuating water-disinhibiting actions.

*For more details, refer to **The Four Lings** profile.

Fu Zi (附子/Radix Aconiti Lateralis Carmichaeli Praeparata/Aconite)

The medicinal referred to as **Fu Zi** is actually **Tian Xiong (天雄)**, which is the root tuber of this plant without the daughter (accessory) roots. The processing of this medicinal entails steeping in a solution of magnesium chloride (MgCl2), sodium chloride (NaCl), and water, and then it is dried and sliced into small pieces.

In classical literature on pharmacopoeia, it is described as follows: "The mother [root] is **Wu Tou (烏頭)**, the [peripheral] accessory roots are **Fu Zi**, the [peripheral] extensions [of the accessory roots] are **Ce Zi (側子)**, and the long slender part [extending from the mother root] is **Tian Xiong**," "…great drying and yang returning, kidney- and life fire-supplementing, and wind-cold-damp-expelling [actions]," and "…frees the twelve channels [with] no limits beyond its reach."

In contemporary texts, it is described as having an acrid and sweet flavor, hot nature, and toxicity; entering the heart, kidney, and spleen channels; and having yang-returning counterflow-stemming, yang-reinforcing fire-supplementing, and cold-dissipating pain-relieving actions.

*For more details, refer to **The Three Great Yang-Supplementers** profile.

Gan Cao (甘草/Radix Glycyrrhizae/Licorice Root/aka **Guo Lao)**

Dr. Lee stocks only **Sheng Gan Cao (生甘草/Raw Licorice Root)** in his in-house dispensary, which is processed by culling and washing to get rid of the impurities, soaked in water, and then the moistened root is sliced into pieces and dried. Thus, unless specified differently, whenever **Gan Cao** is used throughout this text, it refers to **Sheng Gan Cao**.

In classical literature on pharmacopoeia, it is described as follows: "Prescribed raw (生 sh□ ng) [its] qi is balanced, [and it] supplements spleen and stomach insufficiency, and drains heart fire. Prescribed mix-fried (炙 zhì) [its] qi is warm, [and it] supplements triple burner original qi and disperses exterior cold. Added to harmonizing formulas

[it] supplements and boosts, added to sweat-promoting (effusing) formulas [it] resolves flesh, added to cooling formulas [it] drains evil heat, added to drastic precipitating formulas [it] moderates right qi, and added to moistening formulas [it] nourishes yin-blood. [It] moderates all medicinals to ensure no struggle (negative interactions), engenders flesh and relieves pain, frees the twelve channels, and resolves the toxicity of the hundred medicinals, therefore it is known as **Guo Lao** [Nationally Revered] (國老 guó lao)."

In contemporary texts, it is described as having a sweet flavor and balanced nature; entering the heart, lung, spleen, and stomach channels; and having qi-boosting center-supplementing, heat-clearing toxin-resolving, phlegm-dispelling cough-suppressing, tension-relaxing pain-relieving, and medicinal nature-harmonizing actions.

Gan Cao's bioactive constituents include glycyrrhizin (a triterpenoid saponin that is hydrolized into glycyrrhetic acid and glycuronic acid), flavonones (e.g., liquiritin, liquiritigenin, glycerol), mannite, glucose, sucrose, betulinic acid, asparagine, nicotinic acid (vitamin B3), and biotin (vitamin H). It is experimentally and clinically proven to have mineralocorticoid and glucocorticoid (i.e., inhibits histamine-induced gastric acid secretions, neutralizes stomach acidity, and relieves gastrointestinal smooth muscle spasm), antitussive and expectorant, anti-inflammatory and antiallergic (i.e., relieves inflammation of the respiratory tract mucosa), and detoxifying (e.g., strychnine) actions.

Dr. Lee fully utilizes **Gan Cao**'s wide array of actions and indications, adding it into formulas for supplementing spleen and heart qi (e.g., palpitations, fatigue, anxiety, stress, depression, visceral agitation), dispelling phlegm and suppressing cough, relaxing tension and relieving pain (e.g., hypertonicity and spasm of the stomach duct, abdomen and extremities), moderating and harmonizing the nature of draining precipitation medicinals, and mitigating the potential for the toxicity of other medicinals.

Dr. Lee commonly prescribes the medicinal combination **Gan Cao**, **Da Zao**, and **Long Yan Rou** for the treatment of disquieted heart spirit (心神不寧 x□n shén bù níng) and dual vacuity of the heart and spleen pattern pathoconditions, as well as stress and anxiety-induced symptoms (i.e., psychosomatic or psychogenic) that manifest in other disease patterns.

*For more details, refer to **The Sweets** profile.

Gan Di Huang – refer to **Sheng Di Huang**

Gan Jiang (乾薑/Rhizoma Zingiberis Officianalis/Dried Ginger)

This medicinal is processed by steaming **Sheng Jiang** with sulfur.

In classical literature on pharmacopoeia, it is described as having "drying, yang-returning, diffusing, and vessel-freeing [actions]" and the complementary relationship between **Gan Jiang** and **Fu Zi** is expressed as follows: "**Fu Zi** is mobile [extends throughout body] and **Gan Jiang** is both mobile and static [long-lasting effect]."

In contemporary texts, it is described as having a bitter and astringent flavor and a warm nature, entering the spleen and liver channels, and having center-warming cold-expelling, yang-returning vessel-freeing, and dampness-drying phlegm-dispersing actions.

*For more details, refer to **The Three Great Yang-Supplementers** profile.

Ge Gen (葛根/Radix Puerariae/Kudzu Root)

In classical literature on pharmacopoeia, it is described as follows: "Acrid and sweet [in flavor] and balanced [in nature] and light [and] buoyant [so it] upbears and effuses," "[**Ge Gen**] enters Yang Ming channel, thus can move stomach qi upwards, engender liquid and check thirst; and also enters the spleen channel, thus opens the interstices and promotes sweating and resolves flesh and abates heat. [It] is a sage medicinal for treating spleen and stomach vacuity diarrhea. Treats cold damage and wind strike, Yang Ming headache, blood dysentery and warm malaria, and intestinal wind and pox sores (痘瘡 dòu chu□ ng). [It] can also raise yin wind, dissipate bind fire, resolve liquor toxicity, disinhibit stool and urine, and kill the toxin of the hundred medicinals."

In contemporary texts, it is described as having a sweet and acrid flavor and cool (or balanced) nature; entering the spleen and stomach channels; and having flesh-resolving heat-abating, measles- and papules-outthrusting, liquid-engendering thirst-allaying, and yang-upbearing diarrhea-checking actions.

The main constituents of **Ge Gen** are daidzein, puerarin and other isoflavones, which function as signal carriers and defense responses to pathogenic attacks; and it also contains phytoestrogens with antioxidant properties. This medicinal has been experimentally proven to increase coronary and cerebral blood flow, reduce myocardial oxygen consumption and increase oxygen supply, directly dilate blood vessels, and inhibit platelet aggregation.

Gen Gen is the sovereign medicinal in Ge Gen Tang, which Dr. Lee commonly prescribes for pathoconditions such as externally contracted wind-cold, crick in the neck (落枕 lào zh□ n) and painful stiff nape (頭項強痛 tóu xiàng qiáng tòng). Dr. Lee also combines this medicinal with **Huang Qin** and **Huang Lian** to form a variant of Ge Gen Qin Lian Tang for the treatment of exterior (evil) not yet resolved and evil heat entering the interior with heat diarrhea (or heat dysentery).

Gou Qi Zi (枸杞子/Fructus Lycii/Wolfberry Fruit)

In classical literature on pharmacopoeia, it is described as follows: "[**Gou Qi Zi**] moistens the lung and clears the liver, enriches the kidney and boosts qi, engenders essence and assists yang, supplements vacuity taxation, strengthens sinew and bone, dispels wind and brightens the eyes, and disinhibits the large and small intestines. Treats dry throat and dispersion-thirst (消渴 xi□ o k□)." "Enriches the kidney, moistens the lung, and brightens the eyes."

In contemporary texts, it is described as having a sweet flavor and balanced nature, entering the liver and kidney channels, and having liver- and kidney-supplementing and eye-brightening actions.

This medicinal contains the bioactive constituents betaine, polysaccharides, crude fat, crude protein, thiamine (vitamin B1), riboflavin (vitamin B2), carotene, ascorbic acid (vitamin C), niacin (vitamin B3), zeaxanthin, calcium, phosphorus, iron, zinc, copper, and other trace minerals.

This little berry packs a powerful punch! In addition to its nutritional benefits as an energy source full of fibers and fats, it contains antioxidants, carotenoids, and trace minerals that make it a sight to behold "for the eyes!" **Gou Qi Zi** can be administered in combination with other medicinals (e.g., **Ju Hua**, **Jue Ming Zi**, **Huang Qi**) to help protect the surface of the cornea, keep the eyes lubricated, prevent corneal ulcers and opacities, improve peripheral vision and night vision, prolong vision in people with retinitis pigmentosa, and decrease the risk of vision loss from age-related macular degeneration (AMD). You can also add **Gou Qi Zi** into Si Shen Tang (nourishes the heart and quiets the spirit, fortifies the spleen, secures essence, and boosts the immune system) to enhance the flavor and add another dimension to its wholesome actions.

*For more details, refer to **The Sweets** profile.

Gu Sui Bu (骨碎補/Rhizoma Drynariae/Boneknit Root)

In classical literature on pharmacopoeia, it is described as follows: "Bitterness and warmth supplement the kidney, thus [it] treats tinnitus and kidney vacuity enduring diarrhea. [Since] the kidney governs bone, [it] treats fractures and toothache. [**Gu Sui Bu**] also enters Jue Yin [channel] and can break blood and stanch bleeding."

In contemporary texts, it is described as having a bitter flavor and warm nature; entering the liver and kidney channels; and having blood-quickening injury-mending and kidney-supplementing bone-strengthening actions.

Dr. Lee commonly adds the medicinal pair **Gu Sui Bu** and **Xu Duan** (quickens the blood, joins sinew and bone, supplements the liver and kidney, and quiets the fetus)—serve as a hard tissue conductors—into formula variants for the treatment of skeletal bone, marrow, and dental pathoconditions (e.g., fractures, osteoporosis, periodontitis). The medicinal pair is also included among the essential medicinals in the medicinal paste Diao Fen Gao (Suspension Powder Paste).

The medicinal combination **Gu Sui Bu**, **Xu Duan** and **Niu Xi** (quickens the blood and frees the channels, supplements the liver and kidney, strengthens sinew and bone, disinhibits water and frees strangury, and conducts fire (blood) downward)—serve as lumbus (spine) and lower limb and hard tissue conductors—comprises the essential medicinals of the formula Tong Jing Fang, which Dr. Lee commonly prescribes for the treatment of pathoconditions involving bone, marrow, striated muscle, the female reproductive system, and both benign and malignant tumors.

Gu Ya (穀芽/Fructus Oryzae Germinatus/Rice Sprouts/aka **Dao Ya)**

In classical literature on pharmacopoeia, it is described as follows: "[**Gu Ya**] opens the stomach and disinhibits the spleen, descends qi and harmonizes the center, and disperses food and transforms accumulations.

In contemporary texts, it is described as having a sweet flavor and balanced nature, entering the spleen and stomach channels, and having food-dispersing stomach-fortifying actions.

Traditionally, it is prescribed for the treatment of food stagnation caused by starchy foods—cereal (e.g., rice, wheat, rye, oats, corn, barley, sorghum), Dioscorea tubers (e.g., cassava, yam, potato), and taro—and spleen vacuity with low food intake. **Gu Ya** is often prescribed paired or in combination with other food-dispersing medicinals in a mutual need (相須 xi□ ng x□) or empowering (相使 xi□ ng shi) relationship to accentuate or enhance respective actions. For the treatment of food stagnation caused by starchy foods, it can be paired with **Mai Ya**, which has superior food-dispersing stomach-fortifying actions; for food stagnation with distention in the stomach duct and abdomen, it can be combined with **Shan Zha**, **Shen Qu**, and **Qing Pi**; and for spleen vacuity with low food intake, it can be paired with **Dang Shen**, **Bai Zhu**, and **Chen Pi**.

The bioactive constituents of this medicinal include protein, fatty oils, starch, amylase, maltose, adenine (one of the four nucleobases in the nucleic acid of DNA), choline (an essential nutrient with an amino acid-like metabolism), and a total of 18 amino acids (e.g., aspartic acid, □ -aminobutyric acid).

*For more details, refer to **The Digestants** profile.

Gui Zhi – refer to **Rou Gui**

He Shou Wu (何首烏/Radix Polygoni Multiflori/Fleeceflower Root)

Dr. Lee stocks only **Zhi Shou Wu** (製 zhì = **processed**) in his in-house dispensary. Thus, unless specified differently, whenever **He Shou Wu** is used throughout this text, it refers to **Zhi Shou Wu**.

In classical literature on pharmacopoeia, it is described as follows: "Bitterness consolidates the kidney, warmth supplements the liver, sweetness boosts blood, and acridity astringes essential qi. [**He Shou Wu**] replenishes essence and boosts the marrow, nourishes blood and dispels wind, strengthens sinew and bone, darkens the moustache and hair, enables a person to have offspring (promotes fertility), and [thus] is considered an exceptional nourishing and supplementing medicinal...."

In contemporary texts, it is described as having a bitter, sweet, and acrid flavor and slightly warm nature; entering the liver, heart, and kidney channels; and having liver- and kidney-supplementing, essence-blood-boosting, sinew- and bone-strengthening, kidney-securing, and beard- and hair-blackening actions.

Zhi Shou Wu has superior liver- and kidney-supplementing and essence-blood-boosting actions, whereas **Sheng Shou Wu** (生 sh□ ng = **raw**) has superior intestine-lubricating, precipitation-draining, and anti-inflammatory actions. Compared to **Di Huang** (cools the blood and clears heat and nourishes yin and engenders liquid), **He Shou Wu** has superior liver-supplementing actions, whereas **Di Huang** has superior kidney-supplementing actions. Based on clinical consensus, **He Shou Wu** is superior for supplementing heart blood and promoting cerebral blood flow and perfusion, whereas **Di Huang** is superior for promoting peripheral blood flow and perfusion.

Dr. Lee includes the medicinal pair **He Shou Wu** and **Dang Gui** along with the medicinal pair **Tu Si Zi** and **Sha Yuan Zi** in Blood Desiccation Formula, a commonly prescribed formula for a wide variety of yin and blood vacuity and blood desiccation pattern pathoconditions (e.g., dermatology, gynecology, hepatology). **He Shou Wu** is also included in Atopic Dermatitis Formula and Wan Ling Dan.

Hong Zao – refer to **Da Zao**

Huang Bai – refer to **Huang Bo**

Huang Bo (黃柏/Cortex Phellodendri/Phellodendron Bark/aka **Huang Bai)**

In classical literature on pharmacopoeia, it is described as follows: "Drains ministerial fire and supplements kidney water," "**Huang Bo** is bitter [in flavor] and cold [in nature], drains fire and nourishes yin, and can be used [to treat] steaming bone with damp-heat and precipitation of blood," "[It is a] foot Tai Yang channel conductor medicinal," and "Combined with **Cang Zhu** [this pair] is called Er Miao Wan (二妙丸) (aka Mysterious Two Powder), [with its] heat-clearing dampness-disinhibiting actions forming an essential medicinal [pair] for treating wilting [pattern]."

In contemporary texts, this medicinal is described as having a bitter flavor and cold nature; entering the kidney, urinary bladder, and large intestine channels; and having heat-clearing dampness-drying, fire-draining toxin-resolving, and heat-abating steam-eliminating actions.

*For more details, refer to **The Three Yellows** profile.

Huang Lian (黃連/Rhizoma Coptidis/Coptis Rhizome)

In classical literature on pharmacopoeia, it is described as follows: "**Huang Lian** is bitter in flavor, drains the heart and eliminates impediment, drains heat and resolves toxin, and thickens the intestines and checks diarrhea" and "It has six actions: one, drains heart fire; two, eliminates middle burner heat; three, is indispensable for [treating] all sores; four, eliminates wind-damp; five, treats fulminant fire eye (暴發火眼 bao f□ huo yan); and six, checks blood in the stool."

In contemporary texts, it is described as having a cold nature and bitter flavor; entering the heart, liver, stomach, and large intestine channels; and having heat-clearing dampness-drying and fire-draining toxin-resolving actions.

The market price of this medicinal frequently fluctuates and is considerably more expensive than **Huang Qin** and **Huang Bo**. Thus, due to cost considerations, Dr. Lee has a tendency to either prescribe smaller doses of this medicinal, substitute it altogether using **Huang Qin** and/or **Huang Bo** instead, or prescribe a combination of all three (aka **The Three Yellows**), depending on the pattern and pathocondition being treated. Typically, larger doses of **Huang Lian** are reserved for severe heat patterns or specific pathoconditions such as vasculitis, gastrointestinal ulcers, and inflammatory autoimmune disorders.

*For more details, refer to **The Three Yellows** profile.

Huang Qi (黃耆/Radix Astragali/Astragalus Root)

Dr. Lee only administers premium quality raw northern **Huang Qi**, which is distinguishable by the reddish phloem that encircles the xylem of the vascular tissue.

In classical literature on pharmacopoeia, it is described as follows: "**Raw** [**Huang Qi**] secures the exterior, effuses in the absence of sweating, checks in the presence of sweating, warms the seam of the flesh (肉分 ròu f□n), fortifies the interstices of the flesh, drains yin fire, and resolves flesh heat. **Mix-fried** [**Huang Qi**] supplements the center and boosts original qi, warms the triple burner, strengthens the spleen and stomach, engenders blood and flesh, expels pus and internally draws, and is a sore and welling-abscess sage medicinal."

In contemporary texts, it is described as having a sweet flavor and a slightly warm nature; entering the spleen and lung channels; and having qi-supplementing yang-upbearing, water-disinhibiting swelling-dispersing, and sore-expressing flesh-engendering actions.

For the treatment of qi vacuity pattern pathoconditions, Dr. Lee typically starts out with a dose of 1 liang, increasing incrementally by 5 qian every 1–2 weeks, depending on the patient's presenting signs and symptoms, and eventually peaking at a maximum dose of 2.5 liang. Excessive doses beyond 3–5 liang may cause compromised blood vessels to rupture or paroxysmal increases in intracranial pressure in the presence of arteriosclerosis, atherosclerosis, hematoma, or adhesions in the subarachnoid space of the meninges.

Dr. Lee explains that **Huang Qi** promotes accelerated exchanges across membranes throughout the body and regulates the permeability of the glomerular membrane to inhibit protein loss. This medicinal has been experimentally and clinically proven to eliminate nephritic proteinuria, increase myocardial contractility, contain estrogen-like effects, and provide broad-spectrum antimicrobial efficacy.

Among its bioactive constituents, astragalus saponins lower blood pressure, promote erythrocyte membrane stability, increase c-AMP concentration of blood plasma and tissues, boost immune function, and promote the regeneration of liver DNA synthesis; and astragalus polysaccharides enhance immune function, regulate blood sugar levels, protect the cardiovascular system, and accelerate regeneration of tissue growth in patients suffering from radiotherapy complications.

Huang Qin (黃芩/Radix Scutellariae/Scutellaria Root)

In classical literature on pharmacopoeia, it is described as follows: "Bitter [in flavor] enters the heart, cold [in nature] overcomes heat, drains the middle burner fire [and] eliminates spleen domain damp-heat.... Stir-fried with wine [**Huang Qin**] ascends, drains lung fire, [and] disinhibits qi in the chest for the treatment of wind-heat and damp-heat in the upper burner...." and [Zhu (朱)] Dan Xi (丹溪) states: "**Huang Qin** is an upper and middle burner medicinal...phlegm is moved by fire, so [to move phlegm] first downbear fire."

In contemporary texts, it is described as having a cold nature and bitter flavor; entering the lung, stomach, gallbladder, and large intestine channels; and having heat-clearing dampness-drying, fire-draining toxin-resolving, blood-cooling blood-stanching, and heat eliminating fetus-quieting actions.

*For more details, refer to **The Three Yellows** profile.

Ji Nei Jin (雞內金/Endothelium Corneum Gigeriae Galli/Chicken Gizzard/aka **Ji Zhun Pi)**

This medicinal derives from the chicken gizzard inner lining of the black-bone silky fowl (*Gallus gallus domesticus* Brisson). Accessibility of this medicinal has declined over the years and the reduced supply has driven its price up. Thus, sometimes the decision of whether or not to add this medicinal is based *not* on efficacy, but on cost, and also considerations for those who prefer *not* to intake animal products.

In classical literature on pharmacopoeia, it is described as follows: "Sweet and balanced [in flavor] and astringent in nature" and "Disperses grain and water, eliminates heat and relieves vexation, and frees the small intestine and urinary bladder. Treats diarrhea and dysentery and frequent defecation, enuresis and bloody urine, flooding and vaginal discharge and intestinal wind, diaphragm dispersion and stomach reflux, and food malaria in children."

In contemporary texts, it is described as having a sweet flavor and neutral nature; entering the spleen, stomach, small intestine, and urinary bladder channels; and having food-dispersing stomach-fortifying and essence-astringing (seminal) emission- and enuresis-checking actions.

Dr. Lee may include **Ji Nei Jin** together with the more commonly prescribed medicinal pair **Cang Zhu** (dries dampness and fortifies the spleen and dispels wind-damp) and **Shan Zha** (disperses food and transforms accumulations, moves qi and dissipates stasis, and expels tapeworm) in formulas containing large doses of medicinals (e.g., heat-clearing toxin-resolving, yin-nourishing blood-supplementing, blood-quickening stasis-transforming, yin-enriching yang-subduing) that may impair digestion and cause sloppy stools in some patients. The medicinal pair **Ji Nei Jin** and **Shan Zha** is also added into formula variants for the treatment of hyperlipidemia and hypertrigliceridemia.

The main bioactive constituents of this medicinal are gastrin, keratin, amino acids, and small concentrations of the digestive enzymes pepsin and amylase.

*For more details, refer to **The Digestants** profile.

Ji Li Zi – refer to **Ci Ji Li**

Jiang Can – refer to **Bai Jiang Can**

Jie Geng (桔梗/Radix Platycodi/Platycodon Root)

In classical literature on pharmacopoeia, it is described as follows: "White in color and belongs to metal, enters the lung and drains heat. [**Jie Geng**] also enters the hand Shao Yin heart and the foot Yang Ming stomach channels" and "Opens and raises qi and blood, resolves exterior cold evil, clears and disinhibits the head, eyes and throat, and opens stagnant qi in the chest and diaphragm. [Treats] all [types of] phlegm congestion and hasty panting, nasal congestion, and red eyes, throat impediment and sore throat, toothache and mouth sores, pulmonary welling-abscesses, and dry cough.... [It] is a boat medicinal (舟楫之藥 zh□u jí zh□ yào) that carries all medicinals upwards and conducts bitter discharging and drastic precipitating medicinals [downwards]...."

In contemporary texts, it is described as having a bitter and acrid flavor and balanced nature; entering the lung channel; and having lung-diffusing phlegm-transforming, throat-disinhibiting, and pus-expelling actions. Its balanced nature makes this medicinal suitable for use in both cold and heat pattern pathoconditions.

Dr. Lee commonly adds the medicinal combination **Jie Geng**, **Ban Xia**, and **Gan Cao** into formulas for the treatment of upper respiratory tract (especially the throat) pathoconditions.

Jing Jie (荊芥/Herba Schizonepetae/Schizonepeta Stem and Bud)

In classical literature on pharmacopoeia, it is described as follows: "Acrid and bitter [in flavor] and warm [in nature] and fragrant and dissipating," "Enters the liver channel qi aspect and also moves the blood aspect," and "Its nature is upfloating [thus] can promote sweating, dissipate wind-damp, clear the head and eyes, and disinhibit the throat [for the] treatment of cold damage headache, wind strike (stroke) clenched jaw, stiffness of the body and rigidity of the neck, deviated face and mouth, and black flowers in the vision (目中黑花 mù zh□ng h□i hu□).... [**Jing Jie**] is a wind disease, blood disease, and sore domain (瘡家 chu□ng ji□) sage medicinal."

Li Zhong-Zi (李中梓) (Style: Li Shi-Cai (李士材), Ming dynasty, 1588–1655 CE) explained that "For wind inside the skin but outside the membrane [interstices] (皮裡膜外 pí li mó wài), **Jing Jie** is superior, unlike **Fang Feng**, which enters the flesh and bone."

In contemporary texts, it is described as having an acrid flavor and slightly warm nature; entering the lung and liver channels; and having exterior-effusing wind-dissipating, papule-outthrusting sore-healing, and blood-rectifying actions. Traditionally, the medicinal pair **Jing Jie** and **Fang Feng** is commonly prescribed for the treatment of externally contracted exterior pattern pathoconditions (e.g., microbial infections of the respiratory tract) and exterior wind-heat pattern dermatological pathoconditions (e.g., itchy wind papules, sores, boils, welling-abscesses).

Dr. Lee includes both **Jing Jie** and **Fang Feng** (effuses the exterior and dissipates wind, overcomes dampness and relieves pain, and checks tetany) in Wan Ling Dan for the treatment of a wide range of pathoconditions (e.g., from intractable skin conditions and parasitic infections to benign tumors and cancer). Typically, he will add **Jing Jie** into Xian Fang Huo Ming Yin, which already includes **Fang Feng** and **Bai Zhi** (resolves the exterior, dissipates wind, and frees the orifices) in its composition, for the treatment of dermatological pathoconditions. Dr. Lee also adds the medicinal pair **Jing Jie** and **Fang Feng** into formulas for the treatment of exterior wind-heat pattern dermatological and ophthalmological conditions (e.g., conjunctivitis, keratitis).

However, due to **Jing Jie**'s relatively weak qi (氣薄 qì bó)—volatile oils that readily degrade during decoction—and its lightness in substance (質輕 zhì q□ng), requiring large bulk quantities to achieve efficacy, Dr. Lee typically prescribes **Ma Huang**, with its relatively hardy qi (氣厚 qì hòu) and heaviness in substance (質重 zhì zhòng), instead.

Ju He (橘核/Semen Citri Reticulatae/Tangerine Seed)

In classical literature on pharmacopoeia, it is described as follows: "Bitter [in flavor], balanced [in nature], and no toxicity," "Enters foot Jue Yin [channel]," "Enters the kidney and urinary bladder [channels]," and "**Ju He** is bitter [in flavor] and warm [in nature], so it can enter the kidney and urinary bladder [channels], and in addition to diseases resulting from yin cold, [it] is commonly included in formulas [for treating] mounting qi (hernia)."

In contemporary texts, it is described as having a bitter flavor and balanced nature; entering the liver and kidney channels; and having qi-moving bind-dissipating and pain-relieving actions for the treatment of mounting qi (hernia), painful swollen testicles, mammary welling-abscesses (乳癰 ru y□ng), lumbar pain, and urinary bladder qi pain. It is commonly prescribed in combination with **Li Zhi He**, **Xiao**

Hui Xiang, and **Chuan Lian Zi** for the treatment of stomach pain and mounting qi (hernia) pain.

Due to **Ju He**'s lightness in substance and relative bulkiness, Dr. Lee typically prefers to add **Li Zhe He** and **Long Yan He** into a main formula instead. However, since tangerines are grown locally, inexpensive and easily accessible, he simply advises the patient to eat the seeds of this medicinal as dietary therapy.

*For more details, refer to **The Seeds** profile.

Li Zhi He (荔枝核/Semen Litchi/Litchi Seed)

In classical literature on pharmacopoeia, it is described as follows: "Sweet and slightly astringent [in flavor] and warm [in nature]," "Enters the liver and kidney [channels]," and "Dissipates stagnant qi and repels cold evil. Treats stomach duct pain and women's blood qi pain. Its fruit [grows] double bound and the seed resembles gonads, and thus treats bulging mounting (㿗疝 tuí shàn) and swollen testicles based on its similarity of appearance. The **shell** [殼 ké] promotes eruption of pox sores (痘瘡 dòu chu□ ng)."

In contemporary texts, it is described as having a sweet and slightly bitter flavor and warm nature; entering the liver and kidney channels; and having qi-moving bind-dissipating, cold-dissipating pain-relieving, and liver-coursing qi-rectifying actions. It is commonly prescribed in combination with **Xiao Hui Xiang**, **Ju He**, and **Chuan Lian Zi** for the treatment of stomach pain and mounting qi (hernia) pain.

Early on in Dr. Lee's clinical practice he would also prescribe **Xiao Hui Xiang** and **Chuan Lian Zi**, but nowadays prescribes **Mu Xiang** and **Yuan Hu Suo** instead. In fact, this exemplifies a general pattern that has occurred over the years: as Dr. Lee gains clinical experience, he has gradually discontinued the usage of many medicinals with narrowly defined actions, in preference for medicinals with a broader therapeutic spectrum.

*For more details, refer to **The Seeds** profile.

Long Dan Cao (龍膽草/Radix Gentianae/Chinese Gentian Root)

In classical literature on pharmacopoeia, it is described as follows: "Great bitterness [in flavor] and great cold [in nature]" and "Abates liver channel heat evil, eliminates swelling of lower burner damp-heat, and drains urinary bladder fire."

In contemporary texts, it is described as having a bitter flavor and cold nature; entering the liver, gallbladder, and urinary bladder channels; and having liver and gallbladder repletion heat-draining and lower burner damp-heat-clearing and -eliminating actions.

Traditionally, **Long Dan Cao** is prescribed for the treatment of damp-heat pouring downward pattern, liver and gallbladder repletion fire pattern, and lower burner damp-heat pattern pathoconditions.

Long Dan Cao is the sovereign medicinal in Long Dan Xie Gan Tang, a formula Dr. Lee commonly prescribes for the treatment of microbial infections of the genitourinary system, gout, and herpes zoster (shingles). He also includes this medicinal in his Antimicrobial Wash used as an immersion and wash therapy for infections of the skin and mucous membranes (i.e., lips, vulva and vaginal opening).

Long Gu (龍骨/Os Draconis/Dragon Bone)

The sources of this medicinal are the fossilized skeletal bones of mammals, such as mammoths, hipparions (an extinct genus of horse), rhinoceros, elephant, deer, and bovine. The primary constituents of **Long Gu** are calcium carbonate (CaCO3) and calcium phosphate (Ca3(PO4)2), along with small amounts of iron (Fe), magnesium (Mg), aluminum (Al), potassium (K), sodium (Na), chlorine (Cl), and sulfate (SO4).

In classical literature on pharmacopoeia, it is described as follows: "Sweet and astringent [in flavor] and slightly cold [in nature]," "Enters the hand Shao Yin and Yang Ming and foot Jue Yin channels," and "Promotes contraction of floating away right qi (浮越之正氣 fú yuè zh□ zhèng qì) and astringes the intestines and boosts the kidney, quiets the soul and settles fright, and repels evil and resolves toxin. Treats profuse confused dreaming, fright epilepsy and malarial dysentery; blood ejection and spontaneous external bleeding; and seminal emission and prolapse of the rectum [anal desertion]. Disinhibits the small and large intestines, secures essence and checks sweating, stabilizes panting and closes sores, and astringes, checks, and stems [all types of] desertion (脫 tu□)."

In contemporary texts, it is described as having a sweet and astringent flavor and balanced nature and entering the heart, liver and kidney channels. **Sheng Long Gu (生龍骨/Crude Dragon Bone)** subdues yang and quiets the spirit for the treatment of yin vacuity with yang hyperactivity, vexation, agitation and irascibility, palpitations and insomnia, dizzy head and vision, mania, withdrawal, and fright. **Duan**

Long Gu (煅龍骨/Calcined Dragon Bone) astringes and secures for the treatment of seminal emission and premature ejaculation, vaginal discharge and flooding and spotting, vacuity sweating and enduring diarrhea, damp sores and itchy papules, sores that fail to close, and bleeding due to external injury. Traditionally, **Duan Long Gu** is ground into powder for use as a topical application in the treatment of damp sores with discharge (i.e., transudation, exudation) that fail to heal over a prolonged period of time.

Despite its superior astringing and wound-healing efficacy, **Duan Long Gu** also causes *intense* skin and tissue irritation (e.g., stinging pain) lasting up to an hour after topical application. Based on clinical experience, Dr. Lee believes **Sheng Long Gu** provides adequate astringing efficacy, with the potential for only *mild*, *if any*, skin irritation, so he prescribes the crude form for both internal and external administration. Thus, unless specified differently, whenever **Long Gu** is used throughout this text, it refers to **Sheng Long Gu**.

*For more details, refer to the **Long Gu and Mu Li** medicinal pair profile.

Long Gu and Mu Li

This is one of Dr. Lee's commonly prescribed medicinal pairs. **Long Gu** has a sweet and astringent flavor and balanced nature, predominantly enters the *liver* channel, and thus excels at settling fright and quieting the spirit. **Mu Li** has a salty and astringent flavor and cold nature, predominantly enters the *kidney* channel, and thus excels at securing the lower orifices and clearing heat to preserve yin and check diarrhea. Both **Long Gu** and **Mu Li** have astringent properties and spirit-quieting stirring palpitation-checking actions. **Mu Li** also *has* hardness-softening bind-dissipating actions, whereas **Long Gu** does *not*.

This medicinal pair has liver-calming yang-subduing, fright-settling spirit-quieting, and yin-constraining and -astringing actions for the treatment of disquieted heart and spirit, fright palpitations, forgetfulness, vacuity sweating and seminal emission, vacuity efflux desertion (滑脱 huá tu□), enduring dysentery and enduring diarrhea, flooding and spotting and vaginal discharge, clouded head and flowery vision resulting from vacuity yang straying upward (上越 shàng yuè), rib-side distention and pain, and persistent coughing of blood and blood ejection (吐衄 tu nu).

Dr. Lee utilizes the actions of **Long Gu and Mu Li** in Jian Ling Tang, Gui Zhi Jia Long Gu Mu Li Tang, and Chai Hu Jia Long Gu Mu Li Tang. Plus, he also commonly adds this medicinal pair into other formula variants for the treatment of presenting signs and symptoms whose cause can be identified as either yin and yang vacuity (or Shao Yang vacuity heat) with hyperactivity of liver yang pattern. This medicinal pair is also included in Body Soothing Powder, a topical application for the treatment of exterior damp-heat pattern skin pathoconditions that present with *intense itch* and/or *excessive perspiration.*

Long Yan He (龍眼核 / Semen Longan/Longan Seed)

In classical literature on pharmacopoeia, it is described as follows: "Treats mounting qi (疝氣 shàn qì) [taken orally] and sores and lichen applied topically, and also stanches bleeding from incised wounds" and "For the treatment of foxy smell [armpit odor], grind six **Long Yan He** and 27 pepper kernels together, and apply [topically] when perspiration presents."

In contemporary texts, it is described as having a slightly bitter and astringent flavor and balanced nature; entering the liver, spleen, and urinary bladder channels; and having qi-moving bind-dissipating, dampness-drying diarrhea-checking, blood-stanching, and pain-relieving actions.

Taken orally, it is commonly prescribed for the treatment of stomach pain and mounting qi (hernia) pain (i.e., in combination with **Li Zhe He** and **Xiao Hui Xiang**); and applied topically it can treat bleeding from wounds, burns, arm pit odor, scabs and lichen, and damp sores. It is also possible to crush the entire fruit, including the **shell** (殼 ké), **flesh** (肉 ròu), **pit** (核 hé), and **seed** (子 zi), for decoction.

*For more details, refer to **The Seeds** profile.

Long Yan Rou (龍眼肉 /Arillus Longan/Dried Longan Pulp/aka Yi Zhi)

Longan is one of the most commonly cultivated fruits in Southern China and Southeast Asia. After the fresh fruit is harvested in autumn, the fruit is shelled, the seed removed, and the flesh is dried until it is no longer viscous on the outside, but still moist on the inside. This dried pulp turns a dark burgundy-brown color, a moist chewy texture, and a rich chocolaty flavor.

In classical literature on pharmacopoeia, it is described as follows: "Boosts the spleen and promotes wisdom [and] nourishes the heart and supplements blood, thus is used in Gui Pi Tang. Treats [excessive] thought and preoccupation and taxation damage of the heart and spleen, and intestinal wind bleeding."

In contemporary texts, it is described as having a sweet flavor and warm nature, entering the heart and spleen channels, and having heart and spleen-supplementing and blood-nourishing spirit-quieting actions. For the treatment of heart and spleen vacuity detriment and insufficiency of qi and blood that manifests in symptoms such as palpitations, insomnia, and forgetfulness, **Long Yan Rou** is recognized as a balanced and harmonizing medicinal with exceptional enriching and supplementing efficacy. It can be prescribed as a single medicinal or together with other supplementing medicinals, such as **Huang Qi**, **Ren Shen**, and **Dang Gui** (e.g., Gui Pi Tang).

Dr. Lee commonly prescribes the medicinal combination known as **The Sweets—Long Yan Rou**, **Da Zao** and **Gan Cao**—harmonize (moderate) the nature of medicinals, boost qi and supplement the spleen and heart, and nourish the blood and calm the spirit—for the treatment of stress, anxiety, depression, poor nutrition, and psychosomatic or psychogenic pathoconditions. Plus, if you keep a box of dried **Long Yan Rou** in the refrigerator, it is a convenient and tasty "dizzy" needle prophylactic snack to give patients who have *not* eaten prior to receiving acupuncture treatment. A little bit of **Long Yan Rou** can save you and your patient the trouble of going through a stressful case of needle sickness.

Long Yan Rou's bioactive constituents include an abundance of carbohydrates (e.g., glucose, sucrose), fatty acids (e.g., leucocic acid), nucleic acids (e.g., adenine), proteins (e.g., leucine, valine, glycine), vitamins (e.g., vitamin C), and minerals (e.g., potassium).

*For more details, refer to **The Sweets** profile.

Lu Jiao – refer to **Lu Rong**

Lu Jiao Shuang – refer to **Lu Rong**

Lu Lu Tong (路路通/Fructus Liquidamberis/Sweetgum Fruit/aka **Feng Qiu** and **Feng Guo)**

In classical literature on pharmacopoeia, it is described as follows: "Frees the twelve channels" and "Repels miasma and eliminates scourge (辟瘴却瘟 pì zhàng què w□n), brightens the eyes, eliminates dampness, soothes hypertonicity of the sinew network vessels (筋絡拘攣 j□n luò j□ luán), [relieves] whole body impediment pain [and] limb and lumbar pain, and the smell of its smoke upon burning will cure all."

In contemporary texts, it is described as having a bitter flavor and balanced nature; entering the liver and kidney channels; and having wind-expelling network vessel-freeing and water-disinhibiting dampness-eliminating actions.

It is traditionally prescribed for the treatment of impediment pain in the limbs and hypertonicity of the extremities, water swelling (edema), distention and fullness, scant breast milk and menstrual block, and welling- and flat-abscesses, scab, lichen, and eczema (damp papules).

Dr. Lee further classifies **Lu Lu Tong**, **Ci Ji Li** (calms and courses the liver and dispels wind and brightens the eyes), and **Zao Jiao Ci** (quickens the blood and disperses swelling and expels pus and frees milk) as pore conductors with their capacity to regulate—*opening* and *closing* (開闔 k□i hé)—the pores and promote dermal circulation. Thus, he adds this medicinal combination into formula variants for the treatment of exterior wind-heat (or wind-heat-damp) and blood desiccation with exterior wind-heat (or exterior wind-heat-damp) pattern skin pathoconditions that present with pruritic papules and maculopapular and vesicular eruptions (e.g., dyshidrotic eczema (pompholyx), palmoplantar pustulosis (PPP), wind papules (urticaria), acute stage atopic dermatitis).

*For more details, refer to **The Eye Brighteners** and **The Itch Relievers** profiles.

Lu Rong (鹿茸/Cornu Cervi Pantotrichum/Deer Antler)

In classical literature on pharmacopoeia, it is described as follows: "Sweet [in flavor], warm [in nature], and pure yang" and "Engenders essence and supplements marrow, nourishes blood and assists yang, and strengthens the sinews and fortifies bone. Treats lumbar and kidney vacuity cold, aching and pain in the extremities, dizzy head and eye blackening (眼黑 yan h□i) [spots in visual field], flooding and vaginal discharge and seminal emission, and all [types of] vacuity-detriment taxation damage. Suitable for patients with a fine sunken pulse and debilitation of the ministerial fire."

In contemporary texts, it is described as having a sweet and salty flavor and warm nature; entering the kidney and liver channels; and having yang-invigorating, blood essence-supplementing, sinew- and bone-strengthening, thoroughfare and controlling vessel-harmonizing, and toxin- and sore-expressing actions.

Lu Rong is the whole cartilaginous antler in a pre-calcified stage, with hair that looks and feels like velvet. It contains many growth factors (e.g., NT-3, NGF, IGF) and has been experimentally and clinically proven to increase hormone levels (e.g., testosterone, luteinizing hormone), stimulate adrenal cortical function, and promote hematopoiesis.

In his clinical practice, Dr. Lee prescribes either **Cu Lu Rong** or **Xi Lu Rong**, depending on the pathocondition and presenting signs, symptoms, and pattern.

Cu Lu Rong (粗鹿茸/Coarse-Haired Deer Antler)

This is a type of **Lu Rong** that is fully developed, but *not* yet completely calcified (thus having low hormone levels), for which Dr. Lee identifies as **Cu Lu Rong**, with the "coarse" (粗 c□) antler hairs describing its texture and appearance. This medicinal is less expensive than **Xi Lu Rong** and requires larger doses (typically, 8 qian/3x/day) to achieve efficacy, thus Dr. Lee administers this medicinal in decocting piece form rather than powder.

Cu Lu Rong is *inferior* to **Xi Lu Rong** at increasing hormone levels and promoting hematopoiesis, but *superior* to **Lu Jiao** at quickening the blood and transforming stasis. **Cu Lu Rong** has been experimentally and clinically proven to inhibit tumor vasculature from generating hormones and thus functioning to inhibit tumor angiogenesis and tumerogenesis.

Dr. Lee typically prescribes this medicinal for cancer patients at high risk of bone metastasis or with existing metastasis, and for bone cancers, spinal cord tumors, and fractures that fail to heal properly (i.e., delayed union and nonunion).

Xi Lu Rong (細鹿茸/Fine-Haired Deer Antler)

This is a premium quality **Lu Rong** that has reached 60% to 70% growth (thus at peak hormone levels), for which Dr. Lee identifies as **Xi Lu Rong**, with the "fine" (細 xì) velvet sheen of the antler describing its texture and appearance. This medicinal is a precious natural resource, very expensive, and typically only requires small doses (typically, 5 fen/3x/day) to achieve efficacy, thus Dr. Lee administers this medicinal in pulverized powder form rather than decocting pieces.

Xi Lu Rong is *superior* to **Cu Lu Rong** and **Lu Jiao** at increasing hormone levels and promoting hematopoiesis. Dr. Lee prescribes **Xi Lu Rong** for severe cases of thrombocytopenia (low platelet count), whether it is caused by *impaired platelet production* resulting from bone marrow failure (e.g., aplastic anemia), bone marrow suppression (e.g., chemotherapy, radiotherapy, immunotherapy), infection (e.g., cytomegalovirus (CMV), Epstein-Barr virus (EBV), hepatitis C virus (HCV), HIV), or malignancy (e.g., leukemia, lymphoma, myelodysplastic syndrome); *increased platelet turnover* resulting from autoimmune diseases (e.g., immune thrombocytopenia (ITP), systemic lupus erythematosus (SLE), rheumatoid arthritis (RA)), drug-induced side effects (e.g., heparin, quinine, sulfa drugs, NSAIDS, anticonvulsants), pregnancy, or infection; or *redistribution and dilution* (e.g., liver disease, splenomegaly, gestational, post-transfusion).

Lu Jiao (鹿角/Cervi Cornu/Mature Deer Antler)

Lu Jiao is the completely calcified antler, with its coarse hairs having already shed, and it contains high calcium phosphate content.

In classical literature on pharmacopoeia, it is described as follows: "Salty [in flavor] and warm [in nature]. …dissipates heat and moves blood, disperses swelling and repels evil…."

In contemporary texts, it is described as having a salty flavor and a warm nature; entering the liver and kidney channels; and having blood-quickening stasis-transforming actions. Traditionally, it is prescribed for the treatment of all types of vacuity taxation and offers exceptional efficacy for flat-abscesses and cold-type pus sores.

Lu Jiao can be processed into **Lu Jiao Shuang (Cervi Cornu Degelatinatum/Degelatinated Deer Antler)**, which Dr. Lee uses in powder form combined with **Fu Zi**, **Gan Jiang**, and **Sheng Shi Gao**—Antler Aconite Ginger Gypsum Powder—for the treatment of chronic, nonhealing and noninfectious (dry) skin ulcerations (e.g., stasis ulcers, diabetic ulcers).

Lu Jiao can also be processed into **Lu Jiao Jiao (Cervi Cornus Gelatinum/Deer Antler Glue)** and combined with **Gui Ban Jiao (Tortoise Plastron Glue)** to make Gui Lu Er Xian Jiao (Tortoise Shell and Deerhorn Two Immortals Glue), which Dr. Lee typically includes in formulas for the treatment of true origin vacuity detriment pattern and extreme exhaustion of essence pattern pathoconditions that manifest in symptoms such as extreme exhaustion of bone (e.g., osteoporosis), emaciation and shortage of qi, and dim vision (e.g., presbyopia). **Lu Jiao Jiao** can also be administered in small doses and eaten like candy (it's soft and chewy!) as a method of regulating the constitution for the elderly.

Ma Huang (麻黃/Herba Ephedrae/Ephedra Stem)

In classical literature on pharmacopoeia, it is described as follows: "Enters Tai Yang [channel] along with hand Shao Yin [and] Yang Ming [channels], and is a lung domain (家 ji□) chief medicinal" and "Promotes sweating and resolves flesh, and dispels cold evil at the construction [level] and wind-heat at the defense [level]. It regulates blood vessels, frees the nine orifices, and opens the pores; treats wind strike and cold damage, headache and warm malaria, cough and counterflow qi ascent, phlegm wheezing and panting, red and black macule toxin, toxic wind papules (measles) impediment (毒風疹痹 dú f□ng zh□n bì), skin insensitivity, sore red swollen eyes, and water swelling and wind swelling."

In contemporary texts, it is described as having an acrid and slightly bitter flavor and a warm nature; entering the lung and urinary bladder channels; and having sweat-promoting exterior-resolving, lung-diffusing panting-calming, water-disinhibiting swelling-dispersing, nasal orifice-freeing, papule-outthrusting, and itch-relieving actions.

However, this medicinal takes on an even broader role in Dr. Lee's pharmacopoeia. Dr. Lee interprets **Ma Huang**'s action of opening the pores (開竅 k□i qiào) broadly to mean it can "open up" and transport other medicinals across all membranes of the body at the cellular level, which makes it an effective "systemic" conductor for treating all types of diseases (e.g., pulmonology, dermatology, rheumatology, cardiology, neurology). Of course, Dr. Lee utilizes **Ma Huang**'s revered bronchodilation action for the treatment of respiratory tract pathoconditions (e.g., sinusitis, bronchitis, COPD, pneumonia) as well.

Dr. Lee also interprets **Ma Huang**'s action of "opening the nine orifices" as innervating the nervous system (CNS, PNS, and ANS), prompting its application for neurological disorders of the brain and nervous system. Dr. Lee prescribes the medicinal pair **Ma Huang** and **Di Long** (clears heat and checks tetany, calms the liver and subdues yang, frees the channels and quickens the network vessels, and calms panting and disinhits urine)—serve as nervous system conductors—for pathoconditions affecting the respiratory and vasomotor centers in the brainstem (e.g., cerebrovascular accident (CVA), trauma, microbial infection, enduring illness) and for the treatment of wind-cold-damp impediment.

As for dosage, it depends on the patient's condition, constitution, and the particular season. Start out with a small dose of anywhere from 5 fen to 1.5 qian, incrementally increasing in 5 fen doses up until the patient notices difficulty sleeping, and then adjust the dose back down a bit to the optimal dose where efficacy is maximized and sleep is unaffected. A typical dose is 1.5 qian to 3 qian.

Mai Men Dong (麥門冬/Radix Ophiopogonis/Ophiopogon Tuber/aka **Mai Dong)**

In classical literature on pharmacopoeia, it is described as follows: "[**Mai Men Dong**] clears the heart and moistens the lung, strengthens yin and boosts essence, drains heat and eliminates vexation, disperses phlegm and suppresses cough, and moves water and engenders liquid. Treats retching and vomiting, wilting and hobbling, visiting qi and vacuity taxation, expired pulse and shortness of breath, lung wilting and spitting up of pus, frenetic blood heat, dry menses and breast [milk] block, and brightens the eyes and pleases the complexion."

In contemporary texts, it is described as having a sweet flavor and slightly bitter nature; entering the heart, lung, and stomach channels; and having yin-nourishing lung-moistening, stomach-boosting liquid-engendering, and heart-clearing vexation-eliminating actions.

Mai Men Dong and **Tian Men Dong** (nourishes yin, moistens dryness, clears fire, and engenders liquid) are members of the lily family (Liliaceae) and share similar flavors, natures, actions, and indications. However, **Mai Men Dong** provides *superior* efficacy at clearing and moistening lung dryness, whereas **Tian Men Dong** provides *superior* efficacy at nourishing and supplementing the lung and kidney.

Dr. Lee includes **Mai Men Dong** as the sovereign medicinal in Mai Men Dong Tang for the treatment of yin vacuity dryness pattern manifesting on the mucous membranes (e.g., lungs, eyes, gastrointestinal tract, skin). Additionally, he commonly adds either the medicinal pair **Mai Men Dong** and **Tian Men Dong**, or combinations that include other yin-nourishing dryness-moistening medicinals, such as **Yuan Shen**, **Sha Shen**, and **Bai He** (also a member of the Liliaceae family!), for the treatment of yin vacuity dryness pattern pathoconditions (e.g., yin vacuity cough, pulmonary tuberculosis, Sjogren's syndrome, caustic damage of the mucous membranes caused by radiotherapy).

Mai Ya (麥芽/Fructus Hordei Germinatus/Barley Sprouts/aka **Da Mai Ya)**

In classical literature on pharmacopoeia, it is described as follows: "Aids in the ascendance of stomach [and] thus supports movement and transformation, supplements the spleen and loosens the intestines, harmonizes the center and descends qi, disperses food and eliminates distention, dissipates binds and dispels phlegm, promotes digestion of all types of rice, wheat, and fruit, and frees milk and aborts the fetus."

In contemporary texts, it is described as having a sweet flavor and balanced nature; entering the spleen, stomach, and liver channels; and having food-dispersing stomach-fortifying and lactation-terminating distention-dispersing actions.

The main bioactive constituents of this medicinal are □- and □-amylase, catalyticase, and peroxidisomerase, and it also contains hordenine, hordatine A and B, adenine, choline, protein, amino acids, and the vitamins D, E, and C.

*For more details, refer to **The Digestants** profile.

Mang Xiao (芒硝/Mirabilitum/Glauber's Salt)

The primary constituent of this medicinal is sodium sulfate decahydrate ($Na_2SO_4 \cdot 10H_2O$). However, depending on availability and physician preference, **Mang Xiao** may be substituted with **Epsom salt** (**Magnesium Sulfate**). In the past, a distinction was made establishing different grades of processed crude mirabilite based on the level of purity, with **Po Xiao (朴消)** classified as having the most *impurities*, **Mang Xiao** as a *purer* form, and **Xuan Ming Fen (玄明粉)** as the *purest* form. Nowadays, there is no such distinction made, and if *less refined* medicinals are used, it is standard practice to denote these medicinals as **Po Xiao** in the prescription.

In classical literature on pharmacopoeia, it is described as follows: "**Po Xiao** settles at the bottom, the crystals are coarse, and turbid and heavy in substance. **Mang Xiao** and **Ya Xiao (牙消)** form [float] on the top, the crystals are refined, and clear and light in substance…, "**Mang Xiao** is salty [in flavor] and cold [in nature], can eliminate abiding grime, transform accumulations and disperse phlegm, and abate all [types of] heat," and "Acridity can moisten dryness, saltiness can soften hardness, bitterness can precipitate diarrhea, and great cold can eliminate heat.... [It] can flush away triple burner and gastrointestinal repletion heat, and remove the old and institute the new...."

In contemporary texts, it is described as having a salty, bitter flavor and a cold nature; entering the stomach and large intestine channels; and having heat-draining stool-freeing, dryness-moistening hardness-softening, and fire-clearing swelling-dispersing actions.

This medicinal has the action of inhibiting the large intestine's capacity to absorb water and thus promotes the excretion of large amounts of water. It must be prescribed prudently in small doses to prevent excessive watery diarrhea that may lead to malabsorption. Dr. Lee only prescribes this medicinal in cases where large doses (5–7 qian) of **Da Huang** have already been administered for a period of time without efficacy to promote defecation and maintain 2–3 stools per day.

Mi Meng Hua (密濛花/Flos Buddlejae/Pale Butterfly Bush Flower)

In classical literature on pharmacopoeia, it is described as follows: "Treats clear-eye blindness [glaucoma] (青盲 q□ng máng) and floating screens [corneal opacities] (浮翳 fú yì), red and dry eyes and copious eye discharge and tearing, and disperses red vessels in the eyes, and bran and legumes (麸豆 f□ dòu) and gan qi (疳氣 g□n qì) attacking the eyes in children."

In contemporary texts, it is described as having a sweet flavor and slightly cold nature; entering the liver channel; and having liver-clearing eye-brightening and blood-cooling screen-abating actions.

Mi Meng Hua is an essential ophthalmological medicinal traditionally prescribed for blood vacuity liver heat pattern and liver channel repletion heat pattern pathoconditions of the eyes that present with sore, red, swollen and itchy eyes; copious tearing and eye discharge; red vessels in the eyes; clouded vision; and aversion to light (e.g., acute and chronic conjunctivitis, uveitis, retinitis, clouded vision, night blindness, eye screen (目中翳障 mù zh□ng yì zhàng), wind ulceration of the eyelid rim (風弦赤爛 f□ng xián chì làn), gan accumulation (疳積 g□n j□) in children).

Dr. Lee commonly prescribes the medicinal pair **Mi Meng Hua** and **Qian Li Guang** (clears heat and resolves toxin, abates screens and brightens eyes, and kills worms and relieves itch)— serve as eye orifice conductors—for the treatment of all types of heat (e.g., exterior wind-heat, residual heat, liver channel repletion heat, liver channel vacuity heat, blood stasis heat, blood desiccation with heat, and yin vacuity heat) pattern ophthalmological pathoconditions that present with sore, red, swollen and itchy eyes (e.g., acute and chronic conjunctivitis, uveitis, retinitis, ocular hypertension).

*For more details, refer to **The Eye Brighteners** profile.

Mo Yao (沒藥/Myrrha/Myrrh)

In classical literature on pharmacopoeia, it is described as follows: "Enters the twelve channels" and "Dissipates qi bind, frees stagnant blood, disperses swelling, stabilizes pain, and engenders flesh. Supplements heart and gallbladder vacuity and liver blood insufficiency. Treats incised wound and club injuries, malign sores and hemorrhoids, nebulous eye screen (雲翳 yún yì) and red eye, postpartum qi and blood pain, and breaks accumulations and aborts the fetus."

In contemporary texts, it is described as having a bitter and acrid flavor and balanced nature; entering the heart, liver, and spleen channels; and having blood-quickening pain-relieving and swelling-dispersing flesh-engendering actions.

This medicinal has been experimentally and clinically proven to have inhibitory effects on pathogenic mycoses (fungi). And laboratory experiments have shown hypolipidemic effects in male rabbits with hypercholesterolemia, as well as the capacity to prevent plaque formation.

*For more details, refer to the **Ru Xiang and Mo Yao** medicinal pair profile.

Mu Dan Pi (牡丹皮/Cortex Moutan/Tree Peony Root Bark)

In classical literature on pharmacopoeia, it is described as follows: "**Mu Dan Pi** is cold [in nature], breaks blood and frees the channels, and [treats] heat in the blood aspect and steaming bone without sweating," "[It] is acrid and sweet [in flavor] and slightly cold [in nature] and enters the hand and foot Shao Yin and Jue Yin [channels]," and "Drains latent heat in the blood and harmonizes and cools the blood, thus engenders the blood, breaks blood accumulations, frees the channels and vessels, and is an essential medicinal for blood ejection and spontaneous external bleeding. Treats wind strike [stroke] and five taxations, and fright epilepsy and tugging and slackening [clonic spasm]. Eliminates vexation heat, treats welling-abscesses and sores, aborts the fetus and placenta, and abates steaming bone without sweating."

In contemporary texts, it is described as having a bitter and acrid flavor and slightly cold nature; entering the heart, liver, and kidney channels; and having heat-clearing blood-cooling and blood-quickening stasis-dissipating actions. It is recognized as among the best medicinals for eliminating yin aspect latent heat and treating steaming bone *blood* aspect pathoconditions.

Dr. Lee pairs this medicinal together with **Di Gu Pi** (a steaming bone *qi* aspect medicinal, cools the blood and abates steaming, and clears the lung and downbears fire) in the formula Di Gu Pi Yin, and with **Sheng Di Huang** (cools the blood and clears heat and nourishes yin and engenders liquid) in Zhi Bo Di Huang Tang. It is also one of the medicinals in Gui Zhi Fu Ling Wan, which is included in Po Xiao Dang Bao Tang.

Additionally, Dr. Lee commonly adds **Mu Dan Pi** into Ru Mo Si Wu Tang, forming a medicinal pair with **Chi Shao** (clears heat and cools the blood and dissipates stasis and relieves pain) to inhibit tumor angiogenesis; adds the medicinal pair **Mu Dan Pi** and **Zhi Zi** (drains fire and eliminates vexation, clears heat and disinhibits dampness, cools the blood and resolves toxin, and disperses swelling and relieves pain) into formulas to treat *acute* inflammation of vasculature walls (e.g., vasculitis, arteritis); and adds the medicinal pair **Mu Dan Pi** and **Sheng Di Huang** into formulas to treat *chronic* inflammation of vasculature walls (e.g., vasculitis, arteritis).

Mu Li (牡蠣/Concha Ostreae/Oyster Shell)

In classical literature on pharmacopoeia, it is described as follows: "Salty [in flavor], thus softens hardness and transforms phlegm and disperses scrofula and nodes and old blood and conglomeration-mounting (瘕疝 jia shàn). Astringent [in flavor], thus contracts desertion (脫 tu□) and treats seminal emission and flooding and vaginal discharge, suppresses cough and constrains sweat, and secures the small and large intestines. Slightly cold [in nature], thus [it] clears heat and supplements water [for the] treatment of vacuity taxation and vexation heat, warm malaria and red dysentery; and [it] serves as a liver and kidney blood aspect medicinal."

In contemporary texts, it is described as having a salty and astringent flavor and slightly cold nature; entering the liver and kidney channels; and having liver-calming yang-subduing, hardness-softening bind-dissipating, and astringing and securing actions.

Mu Li is a commonly prescribed medicinal for checking vacuity sweating and transforming phlegm and softening hardness. It contains 80 to 95% calcium carbonate (CaCO3), calcium phosphate (Ca3(PO4)2), and calcium sulfate (CaSO4), along with small amounts of magnesium (Mg), aluminum (Al), silicon (Si), iron oxide (Fe3O4), and organic matter. The calcium salts in **Mu Li** contain antacid properties and mild sedative (fright-settling) and anti-nflammatory actions. This medicinal has been experimentally and clinically proven to offer efficacy for the treatment of gastric and duodenal ulcers and boosting the immune system. Traditionally, **Duan Mu Li** is ground into powder for use as a topical application in the treatment of damp sores with discharge (i.e., transudation, exudation) that fail to heal over a prolonged period of time.

Despite the fact that **Duan Mu Li (煅牡蠣/Calcined Oyster Shell**) offers superior astringing efficacy for topical application, it also causes more *intense* skin and tissue irritation (e.g., stinging pain) lasting for up to an hour after topical application. Based on clinical experience, Dr. Lee believes **Sheng Mu Li (生牡蠣/Crude Oyster Shell**) provides adequate astringing efficacy, with only *mild, if any*, skin irritation, so he only prescribes the crude form for both internal and external administration. Thus, unless specified differently, whenever **Long Gu** is used throughout this text, it refers to **Sheng Long Gu**.

*For more details, refer to the **Long Gu and Mu Li** medicinal pair profile.

Niu Xi (牛膝/Radix Achyranthis Bidentatae/Oxknee Root/aka **Huai Niu Xi)**

Dr. Lee uses **Huai Niu Xi (懷牛膝/*Achyranthes bidentata* Bl.)** in his pharmacopoeia, which has superior liver- and kidney-supplementing and sinew-soothing bone-fortifying actions compared to **Chuan Niu Xi (川牛膝/*Cyathula officinalis* Kuan)**, which has superior blood-quickening stasis-dissipating and joint-perfusing actions.

In classical literature on pharmacopoeia, it is described as follows: "A foot Jue Yin channel and Shao Yin channel medicinal [that] conducts all other medicinals downwards. **Steamed with wine** (酒蒸 jiu zh□ ng = **Jiu Zheng**) it is sweet and sour [in flavor] and warm [in nature], boosts the liver and kidneys and strengthens sinew and bone, and treats pain in the lumbus, knees and bones, wilting of the legs and hypertonicity of the sinews (筋攣 j□ n luán), yin wilt [impotence] and incontinence, enduring malaria and dysentery, and scant qi during injury. Used **raw** (生 sh□ ng = **Sheng**) it dissipates evil blood, breaks accumulations and binds, and treats all [types of] pain in the heart [region] and abdomen, stranguric urination (淋痛 lín tòng) and bloody urine, menstrual block and difficult delivery, throat impediment and toothache, welling-abscess, swellings and evil sores, and incised wounds and fractures. Removes bamboo and wood [splinters]."

In contemporary texts, it is described as having a bitter, sweet, and sour flavor and balanced nature; entering the liver and kidney channels; and having blood-quickening channel-freeing, liver- and kidney-supplementing, sinew- and bone-strengthening, water-disinhibiting strangury-freeing, and fire (blood)-conducting downwards actions. **Niu Xi** is recognized as an essential medicinal for conducting medicinals downwards and for the treatment of strangury.

Dr. Lee includes the medicinal pair **Niu Xi** and **Du Zhong** (supplements the liver and kidney, strengthens sinew and bone, and quiets the fetus)—serve as lumbus (spine) and lower limb conductors—in the formulas You Gui Yin, Paralysis Formula #1, Paralysis Formula #3, and Zuo Gui Yin. He includes the medicinal combination **Niu Xi**, **Gu Sui Bu** (quickens the blood and transforms stasis, breaks blood, and treats injury and mends breakages), and **Xu Duan** (quickens the blood, joins sinew and bone, supplements the liver and kidney, and quiets the fetus)—serve as lumbus (spine) and lower limb and hard tissue conductors—in Tong Jing Fang. And he includes the medicinal combination **Niu Xi**, **Huang Bo**, and **Cang Zhu** (aka San Miao Wan)—clear heat and dry dampness and conduct medicinals downwards—in the formulas You Gui Yin and Zhi Bo Di Huang Tang.

Po Xiao – refer to **Mang Xiao**

Qian Li Guang (千里光/Herba Senecionis Scandens/Ragwort)

In classical literature on pharmacopoeia, it is described as follows: "Treats unclear vision, eliminates red-thread [bloodshot eyes] (紅絲 hóng s□) and white obstruction [cataract] (內障 nèi zhàng), and tearing on exposure to wind" and "Brightens the eyes and eliminates stars obstruction (星障 x□ ng zhàng)...."

In contemporary texts, it is described as having a bitter flavor and cold nature; entering the lung and liver channels; and having heat-clearing toxin-resolving, screen-abating eye-brightening, and worm-killing itch-relieving actions. Traditionally, this medicinal is prescribed for the treatment of all types of acute infections and inflammation involving the eyes, skin, and respiratory, digestive, and genitourinary systems.

Dr. Lee commonly prescribes the medicinal pair **Qian Li Guang** and **Mi Meng Hua** (clears heat and resolves toxin, abates screens and brightens eyes, and kills worms and relieves itch)—serve as eye orifice conductors—for the treatment of all types of heat (e.g., exterior wind-heat, residual heat, liver channel repletion heat, liver channel vacuity heat, blood stasis heat, blood desiccation with heat, and yin vacuity heat) pattern ophthalmological pathoconditions that present with sore, red, swollen and itchy eyes (e.g., acute and chronic conjunctivitis, uveitis, retinitis, ocular hypertension).

*For more details, refer to **The Eye Brighteners** profile.

Qing Hao (青蒿/Herba Artemisiae Annuae/Sweet Wormwood)

In classical literature on pharmacopoeia, it is described as follows: "[**Qing Hao**] is bitter [in flavor] and cold [in nature]," "Obtains Spring wood Shao Yang the earliest, thus enters Shao Yang and Jue Yin *blood* aspect," "Treats steaming bone taxation heat, childbirth taxation vacuity heat, wind toxin heat jaundice, enduring malaria and enduring diarrhea, scabies and malign sores, demonic qi and cadaverous infixation (鬼氣戶疰 gui qì hù zhù), and supplements the center and brightens the eyes," and "Treats malarial heat (fever) and [aversion to] cold."

In contemporary texts, it is described as having a bitter and acrid flavor and cold nature; entering the liver, gallbladder, and kidney channels; and having yin vacuity heat-clearing, steaming bone-eliminating, summerheat-resolving, and malaria-interrupting actions.

Qing Hao contains the active constituent artemisinin, which can inhibit the development of and directly kill malaria parasites. And because of its fragrant qi and flavor, unlike other cold bitter medicinals, it does *not* damage the spleen and stomach.

Dr. Lee includes the medicinal combination **Qing Hao**, **Di Gu Pi** (a steaming bone qi aspect medicinal, cools the blood and abates steaming, and clears the lung and downbears fire), and **Zhi Mu** (clears heat and drains fir and enriches yin and moistens dryness) in Hyperactive Immune Formula; and commonly adds the medicinal combination **Qing Hao**, **Di Gu Pi**, and **Zhi Mu**—enrich yin and downbear fire, cool the blood and clear vacuity heat, and eliminate steaming bone—into formula variants for the treatment of all types of pathoconditions that present with symptoms such as intermittent fever, enduring heat, enduring cough, and yin vacuity dryness.

Qiu Yin – refer to **Di Long**

Quan Xie (全蠍/Buthus Martensi/Scorpion/aka **Xie)**

In classical literature on pharmacopoeia, it is described as follows: "Green-blue is associated with wood, thus [**Quan Xie**] treats all [types of] wind with shaking and dizzy vision, fright epilepsy and pulling, deviated eyes and mouth, malarial wind sores, deafness, vaginal discharge, and hernia, and Jue Yin wind and wood diseases."

In contemporary texts, it is described as having an acrid flavor, balanced nature, and toxicity; entering the liver channel; and having wind-extinguishing tetany-checking, toxin-attacking bind-dispersing, and network vessel-freeing pain-relieving actions.

Traditionally, **Quan Xie** is combined with **Bai Jiang Can** and **Chan Tui** (i.e., Wu Hu Zhui Feng San) for the treatment of tetanus, spasm, and convulsion with arched-back rigidity; **Bai Jiang Can** and **Wu Gong** (i.e., She Feng San) for the treatment of tetanus, spasm, and convulsion with arched-back rigidity; and **Bai Jiang Can** and **Bai Fu Zi** (i.e., Qian Zheng San) for the treatment of wind striking the channels and network vessels, deviated eyes and mouth, and intractable headache (e.g., migraine, cluster headache).

*For more details, refer to **The Three Insects** profile.

Ren Dong Teng (忍冬藤/Caulis Lonicerae/Honeysuckle Stem)

In classical literature on pharmacopoeia, it is described as follows: "Sweet and bitter in flavor and slightly cold in nature," "Enters the heart and lung channels," and "Governs heat-toxin, blood dysentery, and water dysentery."

Traditionally, this medicinal is prescribed for its heat-clearing toxin-resolving and network vessel-freeing actions. In Dr. Lee's pharmacopoeia, it is an essential medicinal for inhibiting the synthesis of blood urea nitrogen (BUN) and serum creatinine (Cr) in the treatment of pathological conditions that result from hypoperfusion of blood through functionally normal kidneys (prerenal), structural damage to the renal parenchyma (intrinsic renal), and urinary tract obstruction (postrenal).

Dr. Lee commonly adds the medicinal pair **Ren Dong Teng** and **Ding Shu Xiu** (disinhibits urine and disperses swelling, cools the blood and resolves toxin, dispels phlegm, and relieves pain) into Wu Ling San (Nephritis Formula), Chai Ling Tang, and other formula variants based on presenting signs, symptoms, and patterns.

Ren Shen (人參/Radix Ginseng/Ginseng Root)

In classical literature on pharmacopoeia, it is described as follows: "**Ren Shen** is sweet [in flavor] and balanced [in nature], greatly supplements original qi, checks thirst and engenders fluid, and regulates construction and nourishes defense."

In contemporary texts, it is described as having a sweet and slightly bitter flavor and mildly warm nature; entering the heart, lung, and spleen channels; and having great original qi-supplementing vacuity desertion-stemming, spleen-supplementing lung-boosting, liquid-engendering, and spirit-quieting actions.

Ren Shen is an expensive medicinal and thermal degradation during decoction diminishes potency, thus Dr. Lee typically administers this medicinal as a pulverized powder to minimize cost and maximize efficacy. This powder is either added directly into a formula after the decoction has cooled or ingested separately. Since Dr. Lee prescribes **Ren Shen** in pulverized powder form, it is omitted from Yu Sheng formula composition listings, which are decocting pieces only. This medicinal is often paired with **Chuan Qi (powder)** to form **Ren Shen/Chuan Qi Powder**, one of the pillars of Dr. Lee's therapeutic approaches.

Dr. Lee explains in a more modern biomedical perspective: "As an adaptogenic medicinal, **Ren Shen** has the capacity to regulate cell metabolism throughout the entire body, down-regulating and up-regulating whenever it is necessary, and offers exceptional efficacy in repairing and maintaining physiological function of spinal nerves."

*For more details, refer to the **Ren Shen/Chuan Qi Powder** profile.

Ren Shen/Chuan Qi Powder (人參/川七粉)

This medicinal pair forms one of the pillars of Dr. Lee's therapeutic approaches. **Ren Shen** (greatly supplements original qi and stems vacuity desertion, supplements the spleen and boosts the lung, engenders liquid, and quiets the spirit) and **Chuan Qi** (transforms stasis and stanches bleeding and quickens the blood and settles pain). Together, this medicinal pair exemplifies the TCM classical theory of qi is the commander of blood and blood is the mother of qi (氣為血之帥、血為氣之母 qì wèi xuè zh□ shuài, xi□ wéi qì zh□ mu).

Ren Shen/Chuan Qi Powder can be prescribed for the treatment of a wide spectrum of pathoconditions that involve compromised vasculature, leading to insufficient blood perfusion, excessive blood loss or hemorrhage, and chronic diseases in which taxation and desertion present. Specific pathoconditions include cardiovascular disease (e.g., coronary heart disease (CHD), aortic aneurysm, peripheral artery disease (PAD), deep vein thrombosis (DVT)), cerebrovascular disease (e.g., stroke, transient ischemic attack (TIA), vascular dementia), neurodegenerative disorders (e.g., Parkinson's disease (PD)), autoimmune disorders (e.g., systemic lupus erythematosus (SLE), dermatomyositis), gynecological disorders (e.g., menorrhagia, hypermenorrhagia, spotting), and end-stage cancer patients among others.

For severe blood stasis, **Dan Shen** decocting pieces are commonly prescribed along with **Ren Shen/Chuan Qi Powder** to further enhance the blood-quickening stasis-transforming actions and complement the pair with blood-cooling actions. The administration of medicinals with blood-quickening stasis-transforming actions in chronic pathoconditions is based on the TCM classical theory of enduring illness results in stasis.

The pulverized powder of **Ren Shen** and **Chuan Qi** (aka **Ren Shen/Chuan Qi Powder**) are mixed together and placed in zip lock packets with a typical dosage of 7g/3x/day (a total of 21 g/day).

Rou Gui (肉桂/Cortex Cinnamoni Cassiae/Cinnamon Bark/aka **Yu Gui)**

In classical literature on pharmacopoeia, it is described as follows: "Acrid and sweet [in flavor] and great heat [in nature] and thick qi pure yang," "Enters the *blood* aspect of the liver and kidney [channels]," and "Supplements insufficiency of the life gate ministerial fire and boosts yang to disperse yin. Treats intractable cold and deep cold, promotes sweating, frees the blood vessels, and perfuses and conducts the hundred medicinals. Eliminates construction and defense wind-cold, exterior vacuity spontaneous sweating, cold pain in the abdomen, and cough and counterflow qi bind…."

In contemporary texts, it is described as having an acrid and sweet flavor and hot nature; entering the spleen, kidney, heart, and liver channels; and having fire-supplementing yang-assisting, cold-dissipating pain-relieving, and channel-warming vessel-freeing actions.

The majority of formulas Dr. Lee prescribes are variants of classical formulas derived from *Treatise on Cold Damage and Miscellaneous Diseases* (**傷寒雜病論** *Shang Han Za Bing Lun*) (which was subsequently compiled into two books called *On Cold Damage* (**傷寒論** *Shang Han Lun*) and *Essential Prescriptions of the Golden Coffer* (**金匱要略方論** *Jin Gui Yao Lue Fang Lun*)). In this classic text, the instructions to "remove the skin" from **Gui Zhi** (the twig), which can be interpreted as scrape away the thin layers of fungal growth on the surface of the bark, suggests that the bark (**Rou Gui**), with its higher volatile oil content, was in fact used instead of the twig (**Gui Zhi**). Also, due to logistical considerations during the Eastern Han dynasty (25–220 CE), it would have been much more viable to transport the relatively lighter bark (**Rou Gui**) up to northern China, where Zhang Zhong-Jing wrote his TCM classic, from its primary habitat and distribution in southern China (or Vietnam), where the cinnamon tree (*Cinnamomum cassia* Presl.) grows.

And from a practical perspective, it is also much simpler to decoct the entire formula composition together, instead of adding the medicinals containing volatile oils towards the end of decoction to mitigate the extent of thermal degradation. Since **Rou Gui** (the bark) contains a much higher volatile oil content than **Gui Zhi** (the twig), a higher potency of the bioactive constituents in these volatile oils will be retained during decoction. Thus, Dr. Lee predominantly prescribes **Rou Gui** in place of **Gui Zhi**, even in exterior-resolving formulas such as Gui Zhi Tang and Yang Dan Tang, and with the exception of **Chai Ling Tang**, the only other time he prescribes **Gui Zhi** is to serve as an upper extremity conductor medicinal. Amidst this dynamic, **Rou Gui**'s actions can be interpreted as encompassing those of **Gui**

Zhi—exterior-resolving, spleen-fortifying, pain-relieving, and antimicrobial—while also containing vasodilation actions that more effectively promote blood circulation.

*For more details, refer to **The Three Great Yang-Supplementers** profile.

Ru Xiang (乳香/Olibanum/Frankincense)

In classical literature on pharmacopoeia, it is described as follows: "Disperses welling-abscesses, flat-abscesses, and all toxins; internally expresses and safeguards the heart; quickens the blood, stabilizes pain, and extends sinews; and treats female difficult delivery and fractures" and "Fragrant [odor] penetrates and enters the heart [region], bitter [flavor] and warm [nature] supplement the kidney, [and] acrid [flavor] and warm [nature] free the twelve channels, [thus **Ru Xiang**] can dispel wind and extend sinews, quicken the blood and regulate qi, internally express and safeguard the heart, [and] engender flesh and relieve pain."

In contemporary texts, it is described as having a warm nature and acrid and bitter flavor; entering the liver, heart, and spleen channels; and having blood-quickening qi-moving, swelling-dispersing flesh-engendering, and pain-relieving actions. It is recognized as an external medicine and traumatology essential medicinal.

*For more details, refer to the **Ru Xiang and Mo Yao** medicinal pair profile.

Ru Xiang and Mo Yao

This is one of Dr. Lee's commonly prescribed medicinal pairs for the treatment of static blood pattern pathoconditions presenting in internal medicine (e.g., gynecology, ophthalmology, oncology), external medicine (e.g., dermatology), and traumatology (e.g., sprains, knocks and falls, pulling of the sinews and bone fractures).

In classical literature on pharmacopoeia, this medicinal pair is described as follows: "**Ru Xiang** quickens the blood, **Mo Yao** dissipates the blood, [and] both can relieve pain, disperse swelling and engender flesh, thus these two medicinals are often prescribed together" and "**Ru Xiang and Mo Yao** prescribed together are an essential organ- and viscera-perfusing and channel-freeing medicinal [pair] that can be prescribed for the treatment of all types of stomach, rib-side, abdomen, limb, and joint pain. The pair also treats abdominal pain during menstruation, postpartum static blood pain, and menstruation at irregular intervals [menstrual irregularities]. The capacity for freeing qi and quickening the blood makes the pair effective in the treatment of wind-cold-damp impediment, generalized numbness, paralysis [paresis] of the limbs, and all types of swollen and painful sores or hard sores without pain. For external application, pulverize [the decocting pieces] into powder and apply on sores to resolve toxin and disperse swelling and engender flesh and relieve pain. Despite having freeing actions, the pair will not damage qi and blood; indeed, it is a superb medicinal [pair]."

In contemporary texts, this medicinal pair is described as having similar mutually accentuating actions and indications, with **Ru Xiang** having more pronounced qi-moving sinew-extending actions and **Mo Yao** having more pronounced blood-dissipating stasis-transforming actions.

Ru Xiang and Mo Yao improve the viscoelasticity and functional patency of the vasculature, specifically the tunica intima (innermost layer of arteries and veins), which is made up of one layer of endothelial cells and supported by an internal elastic lamina. These endothelial cells are in direct contact with the blood flow and influence the secretion of inflammatory and clotting factors. Thus, **Ru Xiang and Mo Yao** provide exceptional anti-inflammatory actions and mild blood-stanching actions, with the overall effect of accelerating the healing process. **Ru Xiang and Mo Yao** serve as the principal medicinals in the Yu Sheng formulas Ru Mo Si Wu Tang, Xian Fang Huo Ming Yin, Diao Fen Gao (Suspension Powder Paste), and Huo Luo Dan.

San Qi – refer to **Chuan Qi**

Sang Bai Pi (桑白皮/Cortex Mori Albae Radicis/Mulberry Root Bark)

In classical literature on pharmacopoeia, it is described as follows: "Sweet and acrid [in flavor] and cold [in nature]," "Drains lung fire, disinhibits urine and stool, dissipates static blood, precipitates qi and moves water, and suppresses cough and clears phlegm. It treats lung heat panting and fullness, spitting of blood and heat thirst, and water swelling and cranium distention. Made into string it can [be used for] sewing incised wounds," and "Drains fire evil in the lung, but not lung qi. Fire and original qi are incompatible, and once fire is eliminated then qi will be calm."

In contemporary texts, it is described as having a sweet flavor and cold nature; entering the lung channel; and having lung-draining panting-calming and water-moving swelling-dispersing actions.

Dr. Lee describes this medicinal as having the capacity to "clean up the metabolic waste that clogs cell membranes throughout the entire body." Metabolic waste build-up may derive from normal metabolic processes or from inflammatory responses to disease, which may inhibit (or further exacerbate) the normal function of cellular mechanisms, disrupt homeostasis, and lead to heat pattern pathoconditions such as diabetes. For this reason, **Sang Bai Pi** is an essential medicinal for the treatment of diabetes and it is also prescribed for other heat pattern pathoconditions of the respiratory tract (e.g., acute bronchitis, emphysema) and skin (e.g., atopic dermatitis).

Sha Ren (砂仁/Fructus Amomi/Cardamom)

The TCM pharmacopoeia includes various species and subtypes of **Sha Ren**. Dr. Lee stocks only **Yang Chun Sha (陽春砂/*Amomum villosum* Lour.)** in his in-house dispensary, which is recognized as the best quality, containing the highest concentration of volatile oils that serve as its main bioactive constituents.

In classical literature on pharmacopoeia, it is described as follows: "Acrid [in flavor], warm [in nature], and aromatic [in qi] penetrates" and "[**Sha Ren**] supplements the lung and boosts the kidney, harmonizes the stomach and arouses the spleen, disinhibits qi and regulates the center, and frees binds and stagnation. Treats abdominal pain, glomus and distention, dysphagia-occlusion (噎膈 y□ gé) and retching and vomiting, ascendant qi cough, red and white diarrhea and dysentery, cholera cramps, and running-piglet and flooding and vaginal discharge. Dispels phlegm and expels cold, disperses food and dispels the effects of liquor, and relieves pain and quiets the fetus. Dissipates floating heat of the throat, mouth and teeth and transforms copper, iron, and fish bones." "[**Sha Ren**] enters the hand and foot Tai Yin, Yang Ming, and Tai Yang [channels] and the foot Shao Yin channel." "[**Sha Ren**] moistens the kidney, supplements the liver, supplements the life gate, harmonizes the spleen and stomach, and frees binding depression."

In contemporary texts, it is described as having an acrid flavor and warm nature; entering the spleen and stomach channels; and having dampness-transforming qi-moving, center-warming stomach-harmonizing, spleen-arousing, diarrhea-checking, and fetus-quieting actions.

Sha Ren is an essential medicinal in Xiang Sha Liu Jun Zi Tang, one of Dr. Lee's most commonly prescribed formulas for the treatment of dampness encumbering spleen-earth and spleen and stomach qi stagnation pattern pathoconditions. Dr. Lee will also add **Sha Ren** into kidney yang-supplementing formulas (e.g., You Gui Yin, Shen Qi Wan), which contain large doses of rich and greasy medicinals (i.e., **Di Huang**).

Sha Yuan Ji Li (沙苑蒺藜/Semen Astragali Complanati/Flattened Milkvetch Seed/aka **Sha Yuan Zi)**

This medicinal is processed in-house in Dr. Lee's own medicinal processing and decoction facility. **Sha Yuan Ji Li** is **plain stir-fried** (清炒 q□ng chao = **Qing Chao**) on low flame until faint crackling sounds can be heard, an aromatic scent arises, and the seeds turn a dark yellow to light brown color. The purpose for processing in this way is to crack open the seed coat, thus allowing the bioactive constituents to be easily extracted upon decoction. Thus, unless specified differently, whenever **Sha Yuan Ji Li** is used throughout this text, it refers to **Qing Chao Sha Yuan Ji Li**.

In classical literature on pharmacopoeia, it is described as follows: "Supplements the kidney, treats lumbar pain and seminal discharge and vacuity detriment and taxation" and "**Sha Yuan Ji Li** [is a] kidney-supplementing essence-astringing medicinal. ...[it] nourishes the liver and brightens the eyes and moistens the pupils, supplements the kidney and secures essence, strengthens yang [increases male libido] for bearing seeds [promotes fertility], [it's] neither harsh nor dry, checks dribble after voiding, and is a balanced and moderate moistening medicinal."

In contemporary texts, it is described as having a sweet flavor and warm nature; entering the liver and kidney channels; and having kidney-supplementing essence-securing and liver-nourishing eye-brightening actions. It is traditionally prescribed for the treatment of liver and kidney insufficiency, aching lumbus and knees, hemorrhoids and fistulas, clouded vision, seminal emission and premature ejaculation, enuresis, bloody urine (hematuria), and vaginal discharge.

Dr. Lee includes the medicinal pair **Sha Yuan Ji Li** and **Tu Si Zi** (supplements the kidney and secures essence, nourishes the liver and brightens the eyes, checks diarrhea, and quiets the fetus) in Atopic Dermatitis Formula and Blood Desiccation Formula. He also commonly adds this medicinal pair into formula variants for their balanced and moderate liver and kidney yin-nourishing actions. Together, these medicinals offer superior capacity for retaining moisture (cellular hydration) and maintaining cell metabolic activity.

Sha Yuan Zi – refer to **Sha Yuan Ji Li**

Shan Qi – refer to **Chuan Qi**

Shan Yao (山藥/Rhizoma Dioscoreae/Chinese Yam/aka **Huai Shan)**

In classical literature on pharmacopoeia, it is described as follows: "**Shan Yao** fortifies the spleen and supplements vacuity and enriches essence and secures the kidney, and treats all types of vacuity and the hundred injuries (百損 bai sun), and five taxations (五勞 wu láo) and seven damages (七傷 q□ sh□ ng). Its qi is light and nature moderate and not suitable for single medicinal prescription. Thus, for supplementing the spleen and lung, [**Ren**] **Shen** and [**Bai**] **Zhu** must be included as chief medicinals; for supplementing the kidney water, [**Shan**] **Zhu** [**Yu**] and [**Shou**] **Di** [**Huang**] must be included as sovereign medicinals; for astringing turbid vaginal discharge, **Po Gu** [**Zhi**] must be ground together; and for securing emissions and diarrhea, rely on **Tu Si** [**Zi**] for mutual assistance" and "Enters the spleen and lung channels, supplements their insufficiencies, clears their vacuity heat, secures the intestines and stomach, moistens the skin and [body] hair, transforms phlegm-drool, and checks diarrhea and dysentery. Lung is the mother of kidney, thus [**Shan Yao**] also boosts the kidney and strengthens yin and treats vacuity-detriment taxation damage (虛損勞傷 x□ sun láo sh□ ng). The spleen is the son of the heart, thus [**Shan Yao**] can boost heart qi and treat forgetfulness and seminal emission. Crush raw and topically apply on welling-abscesses and sores and [it] disperses swelling and hardness."

In contemporary texts, it is described as having a sweet flavor and balanced nature; entering the spleen, lung, and kidney channels; and having qi-boosting yin-nourishing, spleen-, lung-, and kidney-supplementing, and essence-securing vaginal discharge-checking actions.

Shan Yao contains a broad spectrum of amino acids, proteins, hormones, steroids, vitamins, and trace minerals that can provide exceptional efficacy when administered as processed decocting pieces or simply eaten as medicinal food (藥膳 yào shàn).

Dr. Lee includes **Shan Yao** in a wide range of Yu Sheng formulas for its moderating action (Jian Ling Tang and Yu Sheng Wan), its spleen-, lung- and kidney-supplementing actions (Mai Men Dong Tang and Asthma Formula), and its kidney-supplementing and yin-enriching actions (You Gui Yin and Zuo Gui Yin).

Shan Zha (山楂/Fructus Crataegi/Hawthorn Fruit/aka **Xian Zha)**

In classical literature on pharmacopoeia, it is described as follows: "Sour, sweet, and salty [in flavor] and warm [in nature]," "**Shan Zha** is sour and sweet [in flavor], grinds and disperses meat-type food, treats mounting (疝 shàn) and moves stasis, and disperses bloating and fortifies the stomach," and "Fortifies the spleen and moves qi, dissipates stasis and transforms phlegm, disperses food and grinds accumulations, effuses infantile pox, and relieves infant's-pillow (postpartum abdominal) pain."

In contemporary texts, it is described as having a sour and sweet flavor and a slightly warm nature; entering the spleen, stomach, and liver channels; and having food-dispersing accumulation-transforming, qi-moving stasis-dispersing, and tapeworm-expelling actions.

Shan Zha is an essential medicinal for promoting digestion of greasy, rich and meat-type food accumulation and stagnation; and its **seed (pit)** (核 hé) is also prescribed in combination with **Li Zhi He** and **Ju He** for the treatment of stomach pain and mounting qi (hernia) pain.

Dr. Lee commonly adds the medicinal pair **Shan Zha** and **Cang Zhu** (dries dampness and fortifies the spleen and dispels wind-damp), and sometimes the combination **Shan Zha**, **Cang Zhu**, and **Ji Nei Jin** (disperses food (accumulations) and fortifies the stomach and astringes essence and checks (seminal) emission and enuresis) into formulas containing large doses of medicinals (e.g., heat-clearing toxin-resolving, yin-nourishing blood-supplementing, blood-quickening stasis-transforming, yin-enriching yang-subduing) that may impair digestion and cause sloppy stools in some patients. The medicinal pair **Shan Zha** and **Cang Zhu** is also added into formula variants for the treatment of hyperlipidemia and hypertrigliceridemia. Additionally, Dr. Lee adds **Shan Zha** into formula variants for the treatment of static blood pattern pathoconditions, such as postpartum infant's-pillow pain (postpartum abdominal pain) and coronary artery spasm.

*For more details, refer to **The Digestants** and **The Seeds** profiles.

She Tui (蛇蛻/Periostracum Serpentis/Snake Slough/aka **She Pi)**

In classical literature on pharmacopoeia, it is described as follows: "Miraculous in nature (性靈 xìng líng) repels evil, thus [it] treats ghosts and goblins (鬼魅 gui mèi) and gu toxin (蠱毒 gu dú). Scurrying in nature (竄性 cuàn xìng) excels at dispelling wind, thus [it] treats fright epilepsy and wind malaria, and double tongue (重舌 chóng shé) and throat wind. Toxic in nature kills insects, thus [it] treats scab, lichen, and malign sores, and swollen clove sores and hemorrhoids and fistulas. It is skin so [its] nature excels at sloughing, thus [it] treats skin sores, difficult delivery and eye screen."

In contemporary texts, it is described as having a sweet and salty flavor and balanced nature; entering the liver channel; and having wind-dispelling, swelling-dispersing, worm-killing, fright-stabilizing, and screen-abating actions.

Dr. Lee classifies **She Tui** as an exterior membrane conductor (i.e., eyes, skin) based on its innate substance as slough (shed epithelial tissue) and its inherent capacity to *peel off* the agglutinated protein build-up on the membranous surfaces of the eyes. This is an example of the classical TCM treatment method of resembling forms treat respective body parts and resembling organs treat respective organs (以形治形、以臟治臟 yi xíng zhì xíng, yi zàng zhì zàng).

Dr. Lee typically prescribes the medicinal pair **She Tui** and **Chan Tui** (courses wind and dissipates heat, outthrusts papules and relieves itch, brightens the eyes and abates screens, and checks fright) for the treatment of ophthalmological pathoconditions, such as lens opacities (e.g., cataract) and corneal opacities (e.g., eye screen (目翳 mù yì), scarring), and for dermatological pathoconditions presenting with intense pruritis.

*For more details, refer to **The Eye Brighteners** and **The Itch Relievers** profiles.

Shen Qu (神曲 /Massa Medicata Fermentata/Medicated Leaven)

Shen Qu is a non-standardized proprietary medicinal whose medicinal composition and ingredients vary among different proprietors. Traditionally, some of the most common medicinals include **Qing Hao**, **Cang Er Zi**, **Xing Ren**, **Chi Shao Dou**, and **Bai Zhu**, however, many proprietors have their own secret formulas that they are unwilling to reveal. Variations on the medicinals and ingredients chosen may be determined by cost, availability, and region and climatic differences.

The production of **Shen Qu** entails mixing ground or crushed medicinals together with wheat flour, bran, and water, kneading this "dough," spreading it out on a flat surface or pan, and covering it with a cloth until the fermentation process produces a fine, yellowish-colored mold. Then, it is cut into small pieces and sun dried.

In classical literature on pharmacopoeia, it is described as follows: "Acridity dissipates qi, sweetness regulates the center, and warmth opens the stomach. [**Shen Qu**] transforms grain and water and disperses accumulations and stagnation. Treats phlegm reversal and concretions and binds, diarrhea and distention and fullness, and terminates lactation and aborts the fetus. [It] also treats eye disorders.

In contemporary texts, it is described as having a sweet and acrid flavor and warm nature, entering the spleen and stomach channels, and having food-dispersing stomach-harmonizing actions. Traditionally, **Shen Qu** is added into formulas that contain minerals or shells to promote digestion and absorption of the bioactive constituents.

Dr. Lee includes **Shen Qu** in Ban Xia Tian Ma Bai Zhu San, one of his most commonly prescribed formulas for the treatment of foot Tai Yin spleen channel, spleen and stomach vacuity, phlegm-damp obstruction, and vacuity wind harassing the upper body pattern pathoconditions. Additionally, Dr. Lee may also prescribe **Shen Qu** paired or in combination with other food-dispersing digestion-promoting, spleen-arousing stomach-opening, and spleen-fortifying stomach-harmonizing medicinals, such as **Cang Zhu**, **Shan Zha**, **Gu Ya**, **Mai Ya**, and **Ji Nei Jin**, for accumulation and stagnation of all types of food and drink that causes distention in the stomach duct and abdomen, indigestion (dyspepsia), loss of appetite, and loose stools.

In the past, Dr. Lee had prescribed this medicinal more frequently, but over the years its quality has fluctuated, with obvious variability in the medicinals and ingredients used to produce it. This inconsistency makes it difficult for the practitioner to get a handle on the optimal dosage and potential efficacy in clinical application. That is the main reason Dr. Lee does *not* prescribe this medicinal as much anymore.

The principal bioactive constituents of this medicinal are yeast, enzymes, vitamin B complex, ergosterol, volatile oils, and glycosides. The yeast and enzymes provide probiotic actions, making sure the "good" bacteria outnumber the "bad" bacteria and restoring the "balance" of microorganisms in the stomach and small intestines (gut microbiota). This promotes digestion and nutrient absorption and boosts the immune system. Vitamin B complex also promotes digestion and increases appetite as well.

*For more details, refer to **The Digestants** profile.

Sheng Di Huang (生地黃/Radix Rehmanniae/Rehmannia Root/aka Gan Di Huang)

Clarification is warranted for the confusing parallel nomenclature used to describe the **Rehmannia Root (Di Huang)** throughout history. To clarify this ambiguity, contemporary texts make the clear distinction between **Xian Di Huang** (鮮 xi□n = **fresh**) and **Sheng Di Huang** (生 sh□ng = **raw** = minimally processed), with the term **Sheng Di Huang** now used synonymously in reference to **Gan Di Huang** (乾 g□n = **dried**). It's the same thing! **Gan Di Huang** is the *term* still used at Dr. Lee's clinic for this medicinal; however, since most readers may be more familiar with the term **Sheng Di Huang**, it is referred to as such for the purpose of this text.

In classical literature on pharmacopoeia, it is described as follows: "Sweet and bitter [in flavor] and cold [in nature] and sinks yin and downbears," "Enters the hand and foot Shao Yin and Jue Yin and hand Tai Yang channels," and "Enriches yin, abates yang, and engenders and cools blood. It treats blood vacuity heat effusion, taxation damage cough, wilting and impediment fright palpitations, blood ejection and bloody urine, blood dizziness and flooding, heat and pain on the underside of the foot, and sinew expiration from fractures and falls. It replenishes the bone marrow, generates flesh, disinhibits stool and urine, regulates menstruation, and quiets the fetus. It can also kill worms and treats acute pain in the heart [region] and abdomen."

In contemporary texts, it is described as having a sweet and bitter flavor and cold nature; entering the heart, liver, and lung channels; and having heat-clearing blood-cooling and yin-nourishing liquid-engendering actions.

Based on traditional clinical consensus, **He Shou Wu** is superior for supplementing heart blood and promoting cerebral blood flow and perfusion, whereas **Di Huang** is superior for promoting peripheral blood flow and perfusion.

Xian Di Huang (鮮地黃/Fresh Rehmannia Root)

It has a sweet and bitter flavor and a cold nature; enters the heart, liver and lung channels; and has heat-clearing blood-cooling and yin-nourishing liquid-engendering actions. Due to the cost concerns of shipping and storage, Dr. Lee does *not* keep **Xian Di Huang** in his dispensary and uses **Sheng Di Huang** instead. In cases where the heat-abating action of **Xian Di Huang** is preferred, Dr. Lee will typically prescribe the medicinal pair **Sheng Di Huang** and **Huang Bo** (clears heat and dries dampness, drains fire and resolves toxin, and abates heat and eliminates steaming).

Shu Di Huang (熟地黃/Cooked Rehmannia Root)

It has a sweet flavor and a slightly warm nature; enters the liver and kidney channels; and has blood-supplementing yin-enriching and essence-boosting marrow-replenishing actions. The traditional processing method—steeping **Sheng Di Huang** in yellow wine mixed with **Sha Ren (砂仁)** and steaming and sun-drying repeatedly a total of nine times—is extremely time-consuming, labor-intensive and expensive, and thus seldom implemented anymore. The modern method of processing **Shu Di Huang** results in inferior quality that differs in nature and property compared to its predecessor.

Taking these factors into consideration, in cases where the blood-supplementing yin-enriching and essence-boosting marrow-replenishing actions of **Shu Di Huang** are preferred, Dr. Lee typically pairs **Sheng Di Huang** with medicinals such as **Fu Zi** (frees the twelve channels), **Rou Gui** (enters the liver and kidney blood aspect and supplements life gate ministerial fire), **Ma Huang** (frees the nine orifices), and **Shi Chang Pu** (opens heart hole [passage] and disinhibits the nine orifices).

However, Dr. Lee *does* keep traditionally processed **Shu Di Huang** in his dispensary for inclusion in Du Huo Ji Sheng Tang, which is typically prescribed for impediment pattern (痹症 bì zhèng) pathoconditions such as postpartum blood vacuity engendering wind, pulling of the extremities, hypertonicity of the sinews and vessels, intermittent convulsions, and hemiparesis.

Sheng Gan Cao – refer to **Gan Cao**

Sheng Jiang (生薑/Rhizoma Zingiberis Recens/Fresh Ginger)

In classical literature on pharmacopoeia, it is described as follows: "Moves yang aspect, thus dispels cold and effuses the exterior; diffuses lung qi, thus resolves depression and regulates the center; and opens the appetite, thus eliminates phlegm and allows food to go down. Treats cold damage headache, wind damage nasal congestion, cough and counterflow and retching, chest congestion and phlegm blockage, and cold pain and damp diarrhea. Disperses water qi, moves blood impediment, frees spirit light (神明 shén míng), eliminates foulness, rescues sudden collapse, treats foxy smell (armpit odor), rub on frozen ears (chilblain), kills Ban Xia, Nan Xing, fungus and plants, and wild beast toxins, and repels mist and dew mountain forest miasmic qi (山嵐瘴氣 sh□n lán zhàng qì). Crush to extract the juice and decoct with **Oxhide Glue** (黃明膠/Huang Ming Jiao) and apply on wind-damp impediment pain."

In contemporary texts, it is described as having an acrid flavor and warm nature; entering the lung, spleen, and stomach channels; having sweat-promoting (-effusing) exterior-resolving, center-warming vomit-checking, lung-warming phlegm-transforming, and cough-suppressing actions.

Sheng Jiang is recognized as a sage medicinal for people suffering from retching and vomiting and is traditionally prescribed for the treatment of externally contracted wind-cold, stomach cold vomiting, and cold-phlegm cough.

Dr. Lee includes **Sheng Jiang** in his Yu Sheng versions of Ge Gen Tang, Mai Men Dong Tang, Xiao Chai Hu Tang, Chai Ling Tang, Da Qing Long Tang, and Gui Zhi Jia Long Gu Mu Li Tang. However, he will use **Gan Jiang** in place of **Sheng Jiang** in Yu Sheng versions of Gui Qi Jian Zhong Tang and Xiang Sha Liu Jun Zi Tang. Exceptions to this rule would be Xiang Sha Liu Jun Zi Tang including **Sheng Jiang** for the treatment of morning sickness during the first trimester of pregnancy and **Gan Jiang** replacing **Sheng Jiang** in Ge Gen Tang for the treatment of crick in the neck (落枕 lào zh□n) and painful stiff nape (頭項強痛 tóu xiàng qiáng tòng).

Sheng Long Gu (Crude Dragon Bone) – refer to **Long Gu**

Sheng Mu Li (Crude Oyster Shell) – refer to **Mu Li**

Sheng Shi Gao (Crude Gypsum) – refer to **Shi Gao**

Shi Gao (石膏/Gypsum Fibrosum/Gypsum)

Gypsum is a soft sulfate mineral composed of calcium sulfate dehydrate ($CaSO_4 \cdot 2H_2O$). It is heavy in substance and requires the prescription of relatively large doses in order to achieve therapeutic efficacy.

In classical literature on pharmacopoeia, it is described as follows: "A great cold foot Yang Ming channel medicinal, the color white enters the lung, and also enters the triple burner" and "Cold [in nature] clears heat and downbears fire, acrid [in flavor] promotes sweating and resolves the flesh, and sweet [in flavor] moderates the spleen and boosts qi and engenders liquid and allays thirst. [**Shi Gao**] treats cold damage binding depression (鬱結 yù jié) in the absence of sweating, Yang Ming headache, heat effusion and aversion to cold, late afternoon tidal heat, vigorous heat of the flesh, turbid reddish urine, great thirst with fluid intake, summerheat strike (中暑 zhòng shu) and spontaneous sweating, and parched tongue and toothache. Also, [since] stomach governs the flesh and the lung governs skin and hair, [it] is an essential medicinal for [treating] macular (班 b□n) and papular (疹 zh□n) eruptions. However, when used in small amounts, actions will not become apparent."

In contemporary texts, it is described as having an acrid and sweet flavor and extremely cold nature; entering the liver and stomach channels; and having heat-clearing fire-draining, vexation-eliminating thirst-allaying, astringing, and flesh-engendering actions. **Shi Gao** is recognized as an essential medicinal for clearing and draining *qi* aspect repletion heat of the lung and stomach channels.

Sheng Shi Gao (生石膏/Crude Gypsum) is traditionally prescribed for oral intake and **Duan Shi Gao (煅石膏/Calcined Gypsum)** for topical application. Despite the fact that **Duan Shi Gao** offers superior astringing efficacy for topical application in the treatment of external medicine pathoconditions, it also causes more *intense* skin and tissue irritation (e.g., stinging pain) that may last up to an hour after application. Based on clinical experience, Dr. Lee believes **Sheng Shi Gao** still provides adequate astringing efficacy with *mild*, *if any*, skin irritation, thus he only prescribes the **Sheng (crude)** form for both internal and external administration.

Sheng Shi Gao is by far Dr. Lee's most commonly prescribed medicinal for the treatment of interior repletion heat pattern and exterior damp-heat pattern pathoconditions. Dr. Lee includes this medicinal in the orally administered heat-draining, lung-diffusing panting-calming, and cough-suppressing formulas Ma Xing Shi Gan Tang and Da Qing Long Tang; the external medicine formulas Xian Fang Huo Ming Yin and Seborrheic Dermatitis Formula; and also in the topically applied formulas Body Soothing Powder and Antler Aconite Ginger Gypsum Powder.

Typically, Dr. Lee prescribes a base minimum oral daily dosage of 1 liang up to a maximum of 4 liang, depending on the extent of heat.

Shu Di Huang – refer to **Sheng Di Huang**

Tao Ren (桃仁/Semen Persicae/Peach Kernel)

In classical literature on pharmacopoeia, it is described as follows: "[**Tao Ren**] is a Jue Yin [channel] blood aspect medicinal" and "Bitter [in flavor] discharges blood stagnation; sweet [in flavor] moderates liver qi and engenders new blood and frees the large intestines and blood constipation. Treats heat entering the blood chamber, blood dryness and blood glomus (痞 pi), damage from accumulated blood, blood dysentery (diarrhea) and menstrual block, cough and counterflow ascent, blood heat dryness and itchiness of the skin, and blood amassment heat [effusion] (fever) as if crazed."

In contemporary texts, it is described as having a bitter and sweet flavor, balanced nature, and toxicity; entering the heart, liver, and large intestine channels; and having blood-quickening stasis-dispelling and intestine-moistening stool-freeing actions. **Tao Ren** is a commonly prescribed stasis-dispersing medicinal for the treatment of menstrual block, concretions and conglomerations (癥瘕 zhèng jia), heat disease blood amassment, wind impediment, malaria, knocks and falls, static blood with painful swelling, and blood dryness constipation.

Dr. Lee commonly utilizes the blood-quickening stasis-dispelling action of **Tao Ren** paired or in combination with **Dang Gui**, **Hong**

Hua, **Chi Shao**, **Mu Dan Pi**, and **Da Huang** in numerous formulas—Ru Mo Si Wu Tang, Gui Zhi Fu Ling Wan, Formula Paralysis #1 (Di Long San Variant), Tao Ren Cheng Qi Tang, Di Dang Tang, Sheng Hua Tang, and Po Xiao Dang Bao Tang—for the treatment of all types of internal medicine, gynecological and obstetric, and traumatological pathoconditions. For intestinal dryness constipation, Dr. Lee will also add Tao Ren into formulas either paired or combined with other intestine-moistening stool-freeing medicinals, such as **Huo Ma Ren**, **Bo Zi Ren**, **Xing Ren**, and **Yu Li Ren**.

The bioactive constituent of the **Peach Kernel** that may cause toxicity in high enough doses is amygdalin. Amygdalin is present only in the embryo of the kernel. Thus, to preserve the integrity of the other constituents in this compound for achieving maximum therapeutic efficacy and eliminate the potential for toxicity, Dr. Lee simply crushes the kernels in his processing facility, which breaks open the endosperm and allows the amygdalin inside to undergo thorough thermal degradation upon decoction.

The Digestants (消化藥)

The people of China have traditionally valued foodstuffs for both there nutritional value and medicinal effects in maintaining health and remedying ailments since antiquity. Able to be cultivated in even the least arable of soils, **Scallions**, **Garlic**, and **Fresh Ginger** are still among the most commonly used foodstuffs to this day for opening the stomach, dispersing food stagnation, warming the center and fortifying the spleen, and resolving toxin. They contain ample amounts of bioactive constituents that stimulate the secretion of digestive enzymes to promote digestion and enhance the absorption of nutrients.

Scallions, **Garlic**, and **Fresh Ginger** all have an acrid flavor and warm nature and enter the lung, spleen, and stomach channels. **Scallions** promote sweating and resolve the exterior, free yang and dissipate cold, expel worms, and resolve toxin. **Garlic** warms the center and fortifies the spleen, disperses food and rectifies qi, and resolves toxin and kills worms. **Fresh Ginger** promotes sweating and resolves the exterior, warms the center and checks vomiting, and warms the lung and suppresses cough.

For minor digestive maladies (e.g., poor appetite, indigestion), people can rely on these foodstuffs/medicinals to do the trick, especially when it comes to **Fresh Ginger**. However, once dyshomeostasis goes beyond the medicinal action threshold of these foodstuffs, that's when **The Digestants** can be considered.

The Digestants—Cang Zhu, **Shan Zha**, **Gu Ya**, **Mai Ya**, **Ji Nei Jin**, and **Shen Qu**—are the medicinals that Dr. Lee most commonly prescribes to disperse food and promote digestion, arouse the spleen and open the stomach, and fortify the spleen and harmonize the stomach.

Cang Zhu—An all-purpose aromatic medicinal for all types of indigestion (dyspepsia), food stagnation, and loose stools. Overall, it is among Dr. Lee's most commonly prescribed medicinals in his pharmacopoeia and his first choice for dispelling dampness and fortifying the spleen.

Shan Zha—Specializes in promoting digestion of greasy, rich and meat-type foods. It is commonly paired with **Cang Zhu** in an empowering (相使 xi□ ng shi) relationship for cases involving pronounced food accumulation and stagnation.

Ji Nei Jin—Specializes in promoting digestion of starchy foods (cereal, Dioscorea tubers, and taro) and greasy, rich and meat-type foods. It may be combined in an empowering relationship with **Cang Zhu** and **Shan Zha** for cases involving more pronounced food accumulation and stagnation. Dr. Lee also adds **Ji Nei Jin** into formulas for children with poor appetites and poor digestion, because it directly stimulates the secretion of gastric acid in the stomach and duodenum to promote digestion of proteins and absorption of other nutrients.

Gu Ya—Contains low concentrations of digestive enzymes and specializes in promoting digestion of starchy foods (cereal, Dioscorea tubers, and taro). Dr. Lee commonly prescribes the medicinal pair **Gu Ya** and **Mai Ya** in a mutual need (相須 xi□ ng x□) relationship.

Mai Ya—Contains high concentrations of digestive enzymes and specializes in promoting digestion of starchy foods (cereal, Dioscorea tubers, and taro). Dr. Lee commonly prescribes the medicinal pair **Mai Ya** and **Gu Ya** in a mutual need (相須 xi□ ng x□) relationship. Dr. Lee also adds **Mai Ya** into formulas for elderly patients with poor appetite and aversion to food.

Shen Qu—Contains high concentrations of yeast, enzymes, and vitamin B complex and specializes in promoting the digestion of water and grains. However, it can be prescribed paired or in combination with other medicinals in **The Digestants** category for the accumulation and stagnation of all types of food and drink that causes distention in the stomach duct and abdomen, indigestion (dyspepsia), loss of appetite, and loose stools.

Dr. Lee stocks only the **Sheng** (生 sh□ng = **raw**) form of **The Digestants**, as opposed to **Chao** (炒 chao = **stir-fried**), in his in-house dispensary. Prescribing the **Sheng** (**raw** = minimally processed, but not submitted to heat!) form preserves their full capacity to either *directly* provide, or *indirectly* stimulate the secretion of, digestive enzymes that function to disperse food, promote digestion, and increase the absorption of nutrients. Conversely, submitting these medicinals to heat, as in the **Chao (stir-fried)** form, thermally degrades their bioactive constituents (e.g., volatile oils, digestive enzymes, antioxidants) and diminishes their efficacy.

However, there are some trade-offs involved here because **stir-frying** does enhance other qualities of these medicinals, such as providing superior efficacy at fortifying the spleen and harmonizing the stomach. **Stir-frying** also arouses the brain to *indirectly* promote the secretion of digestive enzymes, but overall provides inferior efficacy at opening the stomach (increases appetite), dispersing food, and promoting digestion.

Dr. Lee believes that the benefits of the **Sheng (raw)** form of **The Digestants** by far outweigh the disadvantages. Thus, unless specified differently, whenever **Cang Zhu**, **Shan Zha**, **Gu Ya**, **Mai Ya**, **Ji Nei Jin**, and **Shen Qu** are used throughout this text, it refers to the **Sheng (raw)** form.

The Eye Brighteners (明目藥)

Dr. Lee commonly adds pairs or combinations of **Qian Li Guang**, **Mi Meng Hua**, **She Tui**, **Chan Tui**, **Ci Ji Li**, and **Zao Jiao Ci** into formula variants for the treatment of ophthalmological disorders.

Qian Li Guang and **Mi Meng Hua** can be classified as eye orifice conductor medicinals, which are prescribed for the treatment of all types of heat (e.g., exterior wind-heat, residual heat, liver channel repletion heat, liver channel vacuity heat, blood stasis heat, blood desiccation with heat, and yin vacuity heat) pattern ophthalmological pathoconditions that present with sore, red, swollen and itchy eyes (e.g., acute and chronic conjunctivitis, uveitis, retinitis, ocular hypertension).

She Tui and **Chan Tui** can be classified as exterior membrane (i.e., eyes, skin) conductor medicinals, which are prescribed specifically for the treatment of lens opacities (e.g., cataract) and corneal opacities (e.g., eye screen (目翳 mù yì), scarring), with their capacity to *peel off* the agglutinated protein build-up on the membranous surfaces of the eyes.

Ci Ji Li and **Zao Jiao Ci** are typically prescribed for the treatment of exterior wind-heat or wind-heat-damp pattern ophthalmological pathoconditions that affect the lacrimal drainage system (e.g., dacryocystitis, dacryoadenitis) and epidemic keratoconjunctivitis ("pinkeye").

The Four Lings (四苓)

This medicinal combination derives from Si Ling Tang (四苓湯)—**Fu Ling**, **Ze Xie**, **Zhu Ling**, and **Bai Zhu**—recorded in the *Teachings of Dan Xi* (丹溪心法 *Dan Xi Xin Fa*). However, Dr. Lee usually substitutes **Cang Zhu** in place of **Bai Zhu** for its spleen-fortifying dampness-drying and antimicrobial actions, which are ideal for Taiwan's humid subtropical climate.

Fu Ling, **Ze Xie**, and **Zhu Ling** all have a similar flavor and nature (sweet, bland, and balanced); enter the kidney and urinary bladder channels; and share the complementary actions of disinhibiting water, percolating dampness, fortifying the spleen, and discharging heat. **Cang Zhu** has an acrid and bitter flavor and warm nature; enters the spleen and stomach channels; and has spleen-fortifying dampness-drying, wind-damp-dispelling sweat-promoting, and antimicrobial actions. The combination of these medicinals fortifies the spleen, disinhibits water, and percolates dampness for the treatment of water-damp collecting internally, inhibited urination, diarrhea, swelling (edema), and bloody urine.

The Four Lings—Fu Ling, **Ze Xie**, **Zhu Ling**, and **Cang Zhu**—form one of the pillars of Dr. Lee's therapeutic approaches administered for a broad scope of pathoconditions involving water amassment or water-rheum collecting internally, which causes obstruction and/or stagnation and leads to the disruption of physiological mechanisms and pathological disorders. The resulting homeostatic imbalance may manifest in pathoconditions such as generalized edema, ascites, pericardial effusion, pleural effusion, and increased intracranial pressure (ICP) (e.g., traumatic injury, hemorrhage, tumor, herniation, heart failure, obstruction of cerebrospinal fluid).

Dr. Lee includes **The Four Lings** in Wu Ling San (Calculi Formula), Wu Ling San (Nephritis Formula), and Chai Ling Tang, and also adds pairs or combinations of these medicinals into formula variants based on presenting signs, symptoms, and pattern identification. For pathoconditions involving diarrhea, ascites, and ICP, Dr. Lee commonly includes **Da Huang** to enhance the draining and precipitating action and adds **Ren Shen** as a counterbalance that aides in the reabsorption of nutrients and electrolytes.

For patients presenting with pronounced water amassment or water-rheum collecting internally (e.g., generalized edema, ascites, pericardial effusion, pleural effusion, increased intracranial pressure (ICP)), Dr. Lee may prescribe large doses (up to 8 qian–1 liang each) of **The Four Lings** (especially **Fu Ling** and **Ze Xie**!) to ensure that an adequate level of water disinhibition is achieved.

The Itch Relievers (止癢藥)

Dr. Lee commonly prescribes pairs or combinations of **Ci Ji Li**, **Zao Jiao Ci**, **Lu Lu Tong**, **She Tui**, and **Chan Tui** for the treatment of all types of skin pathoconditions resulting from inflammatory responses and the build-up of metabolic waste that block pores and disrupt epidermal homeostasis (i.e., epidermopoiesis and its regulation). This may present clinically in manifestations such as pruritis, erythema, macules, papules, scaling, lichenification, pustules, furuncles, abscesses, wheals, and plaques.

Ci Ji Li, **Zao Jiao Ci**, and **Lu Lu Tong** can be classified as pore conductors with their capacity to regulate—*opening* and *closing* (開闔 k□i hé)—the pores and promote dermal circulation. This medicinal combination can be added into formula variants for the treatment of all types of acute (e.g., exterior wind-heat, exterior wind-damp-heat) and chronic (e.g., blood desiccation with exterior wind-heat or exterior wind-heat-damp) dermatological pathoconditions.

She Tui and **Chan Tui** can be classified as exterior membrane (i.e., eyes, skin) conductor medicinals with their capacity to promote epidermal cell proliferation. This medicinal pair can be added into formula variants for the treatment of both acute (e.g., exterior wind-heat, damp-heat) and chronic (e.g., vacuity heat, yang vacuity, blood desiccation) dermatological pathoconditions. However, due to their lightness in substance, high cost, tendency for patient aversion, and the fact that renewal of the dermis will eventually occur naturally—*peeling off* on its own, Dr. Lee rarely prescribes this medicinal pair for skin pathoconditions unless the case is particularly severe and/or recalcitrant (e.g., eczema, atopic dermatitis, psoriasis).

The Seeds (種子)

Dr. Lee commonly prescribes pairs or combinations of **Long Yan He (Longan Seed)**, **Li Zhe He (Litchi Seed)**, **Ju He (Tangerine Seed)**, and **Shan Zha He (Hawthorn Berry Seed)** for pathoconditions of the male genitourinary system (e.g., benign prostatic hyperplasia (BPH), scrotal dermatitis, epididymitis, hydrocele, erectile dysfunction (ED), infertility, prostate cancer).

These medicinals share the common traits of entering the liver channel, having qi-moving bind-dissipating actions, and serving as male genitourinary system conductors for their likeness of the gonads in both external appearance and physiological function. This is an example of the classical TCM treatment method of "resembling forms supplement respective body parts and resembling organs supplement respective organs (以形補形、以臟補臟 yi xíng bu xíng, yi zàng bu zàng)."

Dr. Lee's choice of these particular seeds (pits) is simply based on the fact that these fruits are grown locally, inexpensive and easily accessible. The seeds (pits) of many other fruits contain either identical or similar bioactive constituents and can be readily prescribed in place of those mentioned above for effective results. Prior to decoction, the seeds (pits) must be crushed to facilitate extraction of their bioactive constituents during decoction.

Note: The term seed (種子 zhong zi) and pit (果核 guo hé) are used interchangeably here. Many seed medicinals also have a pit and are thus designated as such in pharmacopoeia nomenclature. For example, **Long Yan He (龍眼核/Longan Seed)** also has a pit (核 hé), but it is commonly translated as a seed, since the seed is indeed enclosed within the pit. To clarify, a *seed* is an ovule containing an embryo, while a *pit* is the part of the fruit that protects the seed until growth time.

The Sweets (甜味藥)

The Sweets—Gan Cao, **Da Zao**, and **Long Yan Rou**—share the common traits of having a sweet flavor and warm nature; entering the heart and spleen channels; and having heart and spleen (center)-supplementing, qi-supplementing, and spirit-quieting actions. **Da Zao** and **Long Yan Rou** share the blood (yin)-nourishing action; and **Gan Cao** and **Da Zao** share the medicinal nature-harmonizing (moderating) action.

The Sweets contain bioactive constituents that promote the production and release of serotonin, which inhibits dopamine production and creates a balanced interplay amidst these pivotal hormones (neurotransmitters) that have a regulatory and moderating affect on mood and behavior.

Dr. Lee includes **The Sweets** in the classical formula Gan Mai Da Zao Tang (already contains **Gan Cao** and **Da Zao**, plus he adds **Long Yan Rou**) for the treatment of disquieted heart spirit (心神不寧 x□n shén bù níng), visceral agitation (臟燥 zàng zào), and essence spirit failing to keep its composure (精神不寧 j□ng shén bù níng). Additionally, Dr. Lee commonly adds combinations of **The Sweets** into other formula variants to supplement the heart and spleen and nourish the blood and quiet the spirit heart (e.g., palpitations, fatigue, anxiety, stress, depression, visceral agitation, menopausal transition, Tourette syndrome) and to harmonize the nature of other medicinals.

The following provides a brief historical background in the evolution of foodstuffs that were commonly used as energy sources (i.e., carbohydrates that include monosaccharides, disaccharides, oligosaccharides, and polysaccharides) in ancient China, including **The Sweets**:

The development of civilization in China during antiquity—starting as far back as the Neolithic period (est. 8,500 BCE) into the Han dynasty (206 BCE–220 CE) and up through the Song dynasty (960–1279 CE)—occurred primarily in the north along the Yellow River basin (semiarid and dry, cool to mid temperate zones), with poor soil and little rainfall, and eventually spread further south to the Yangtze River basin (semihumid, warm temperate zone), with fertile soil and ample rainfall.

By the Han dynasty, the main trade route was to the West, traveling overland in expeditions by camel or horse through present-day Mongolia and Xinjiang into Central Asia and as far as Greece, a time-consuming and laborious process at best that may have taken many years up to a decade roundtrip. Overland transportation routes were even more precarious to the South, remaining undeveloped due to the hilly terrain and humid, wet climate.

Nutritional intake was poor among the general population and undernourishment was widespread. People ate what they hunted, gathered, raised, grew, or could buy. Fresh fruits and vegetables were hard to come by, particularly during the winter months. One of the main sources of carbohydrates was cereal (oligosaccharides and polysaccharides), such as barley, wheat, rice and millet. **Barley Sprouts (Mai Ya)** (oligosaccharides) were also used together with cereal to make **Maltose (Yi Tang)** (disaccharides) as an important energy source. **Jujube (Da Zao)** (monosaccharides and disaccharides) was another, especially since it grew wild and was easily cultivated all year round in the northern temperate climate along the Yellow River basin, and could also be preserved easily and stored for long periods.

Licorice Root (Gan Cao) (oligosaccharides and polysaccharides), grown in the present-day provinces of Gansu and Inner Mongolia and the autonomous region of Xinjiang, was accessible in sufficient supply and a potentially excellent energy source. However, it was predominantly used as an essential medicinal, as opposed to a foodstuff, widely recognized as having the capacity to resolve the toxicity of the hundred medicinals.

Other fruits such as **Wolfberry Fruit (Gou Qi Zi)** (polysaccharide), grown in the present-day autonomous region of Xinjiang, was an excellent energy source that could be preserved easily and stored for long periods, but it was not widely cultivated and the transportation costs made it too expensive for the common folk. Similarly, **Longan** or **Dried Longan Pulp (Long Yan Rou)** (monosaccharides and disaccharides), grown in southern China, was an excellent energy source, but it was limited in supply and availability for the same reasons.

It wasn't until the Song dynasty when domestic maritime shipping routes opened up that the transport of goods from southern China became much more convenient and prevalent. After that, access to "the big four fruit staples of southern China"—litchi, longan, bananas, and pineapples—brought a boom in energy sources to the growing population in the north.

The Three Great Yang-Supplementers (三大補陽)

The medicinal combination **Gan Jiang**, **Fu Zi**, and **Rou Gui** comprises one of the pillars of Dr. Lee's therapeutic approaches. These great spleen and kidney yang-supplementing medicinals are prescribed for the post-acute and chronic stages of pathoconditions that present with yang vacuity and cold stasis pattern. They are also prescribed following surgery, radiotherapy, and the administration of chemotherapeutic agents—*suppress* bone marrow function, thus *inhibiting* hematopoiesis—and corticosteroids—*suppress* the hypothalamic-pituitary-adrenal (HPA) axis, thus *decreasing* corticotropin-releasing hormone (CRH), adrenocorticotropic hormone (ACTH), and endogenous cortisol)—which result in yang vacuity and cold stasis pattern.

Additionally, Dr. Lee may prescribe this medicinal combination when the therapeutic regimen has reached a point where marginal or no significant improvement is being made. In this instance, the treatment method of returning and reinforcing yang is applied to "boost" the metabolism and immune system, giving the body the strength and capacity to bolster right qi and win the struggle between right and evil.

These great yang-supplementing medicinals boost the metabolism and immune system by innervating the central nervous system (CNS), peripheral nervous system (PNS), and autonomic nervous system (ANS), and by engaging a cascade of endocrine and hormonal factors. And when **Ren Shen**, **Huang Qi**, and **Lu Rong** (or **Lu Jiao Shuang**) are prescribed together with **The Three Great Yang-Supplementers** in a formula, this combination promotes the body's capacity for self-repair, regeneration (e.g., nerves, skin, tissue, bone), and hematopoiesis.

An initial dose of 2–3 qian for each medicinal will be prescribed, increasing incrementally up to 5–8 qian each. Once the combined dose reaches 10–12 qian, then 3–5 qian of either one or a combination of **The Three Yellows** (**Huang Qin**, **Huang Bo**, and **Huang Lian**) are added to counteract excessive heat and mitigate the potential adverse effects.

The Three Insects (三蟲)

This term refers to the combination of **Quan Xie**, **Wu Gong**, and **Bai Jiang Can**. These arthropods have evolutionary ancestry dating back nearly 500 million years and are composed of relatively smaller, more basic fundamental amino acid and protein archetypes, offering exceptional efficacy at regulating the transmission of neurotransmitters across chemical synapses.

These three medicinals all enter the liver channel and share the common actions of extinguishing wind and checking tetany, with **Quan Xie** and **Wu Gong** attacking toxins, dissipating binds, and freeing the network vessels and relieving pain, and **Bai Jiang Can** dispelling wind and relieving pain and transforming phlegm and dissipating binds.

Dr. Lee typically adds **The Three Insects** into formula variants for the treatment of neuropathic pain (e.g., trigeminal neuralgia), intractable headache (e.g., migraine, cluster headache), tetany (e.g., periodic painful muscular spasms, tremors, tics, twitches, and hypertonicity), and other neurological disorders (e.g., epileptic seizures, Tourette syndrome).

The Three Yellows (三黃)

This term refers to the combination of **Huang Qin**, **Huang Bo**, and **Huang Lian**. The heat-clearing toxin-resolving (antimicrobial and anti-inflammatory) actions of these medicinals make them among the most important and commonly used medicinals in Dr. Lee's pharmacopoeia, comprising one of the pillars of Dr. Lee's therapeutic approaches. They provide exceptional efficacy for the treatment of all kinds of infections and inflammation (e.g., upper respiratory tract, gastrointestinal, hepatic, renal, autoimmune, musculoskeletal), and are also added into Yu Sheng formula variants to counteract the great heat of **The Three Great Yang-Supplementers—Gan Jiang**, **Fu Zi**, and **Rou Gui**.

Classical literature on pharmacopoeia differentiates the specific actions of these three medicinals as follows: "…**Huang Lian** drains heart fire and middle burner fire, **Huang Qin** drains upper burner fire, [and] **Huang Bo** drains lower burner fire…."

Dr. Lee also acknowledges these distinctions, using **Huang Lian** for the gastrointestinal tract, **Huang Qin** for the upper respiratory tract, and **Huang Bo** for the kidneys and genitourinary tract. However, from his clinical experience, these specific distinctions are *not* vital to achieve efficacy. He often says: "In the treatment of evil qi (i.e., microbial infection) and inflammation, the combination of **The Three Yellows** provides effective broad-spectrum antimicrobial and anti-inflammatory action!"

Tian Ma (天麻/Rhizoma Gastrodiae Elatae/Gastrodia Rhizome)

In classical literature on pharmacopoeia, it is described as follows: "Acrid [in flavor] and warm [in nature]," "Enters the liver channel qi aspect," and "Boosts qi and strengthens yin, frees the blood vessels, strengthens the sinews, and courses phlegm qi. Treats all types of wind dizziness and shaking, dizzy head and eye blackening [spots in visual field], speech not complying (語言不逐 yu yán bù zhú), wind-damp insensitive impediment (頑痹 wán bì) [paralysis of the extremities], and infantile fright epilepsy."

In contemporary texts, it is described as having a sweet flavor and balanced nature; entering the liver channel; and having wind-extinguishing tetany-checking, liver yang uprising-repressing, wind-dispelling, and network vessel-freeing actions.

Tian Ma shares many common properties with **The Three Insects**, thus Dr. Lee typically administers this medicinal either along with them or in combination with **Chuan Xiong**, **Chai Hu**, **Ban Xia**, and **Ge Gen** for the treatment of dizziness, vertigo (e.g., Meniere disease, benign paroxysmal positional vertigo (BPPV), idiopathic), and intractable headache (e.g., migraine, cluster headache). Dr. Lee also prescribes this medicinal for the treatment of neurogenic hypertension caused by brainstem dysfunction.

Depending on the severity of the patient's signs and symptoms, Dr. Lee may prescribe a dose of 3 qian up to 1 liang.

Tian Men Dong (天門冬/Radix Asparagi/Asparagus Root/aka Tian Men)

In classical literature on pharmacopoeia, it is described as follows: "Sweet and bitter [in flavor] and great cold [in nature]" and "[**Tian Men Dong**] enters hand Tai Yin qi aspect, clears metal and downbears fire, boosts the upper source of water, and frees foot Shao Yin kidney below. Enriches the kidney and moistens dryness, allays thirst and disperses phlegm, moisturizes the skin, and disinhibits the urine and stool. Treats lung wilting and lung welling-abscess, spitting up of pus and blood, phlegm cough and hasty panting, dispersion-thirst and dry throat, heat and pain on the underside of the foot, vacuity taxation and steaming bone, and yin vacuity with fire pattern."

In contemporary texts, it is described as having a sweet and bitter flavor and cold nature; entering the lung and kidney channels; and having yin-nourishing dryness-moistening, fire-clearing, and liquid-engendering actions.

Tian Men Dong and **Mai Men Dong** (nourishes yin and moistens the lung, boosts the stomach and engenders liquid, and clears the heart and eliminates vexation) are members of the lily family (Liliaceae) and share similar flavors, natures, actions, and indications. However, **Tian Men Dong** provides *superior* efficacy at nourishing and supplementing the lung and kidney, whereas **Mai Men Dong** provides *superior* efficacy at clearing and moistening lung dryness.

Dr. Lee commonly adds either the medicinal pair **Tian Men Dong** and **Mai Men Dong**, or combinations that include other yin-nourishing dryness-moistening medicinals, such as **Yuan Shen**, **Sha Shen**, and **Bai He** (also a member of the Liliaceae family!), for the treatment of yin vacuity dryness pattern pathoconditions (e.g., yin vacuity cough, pulmonary tuberculosis, Sjogren's syndrome, caustic mucous membrane damage following radiotherapy).

Tian Xiong – refer to **Fu Zi**

Tu Si Zi (菟絲子/Semen Cuscutae Chinensis/Cuscuta)

This medicinal is processed in-house in Dr. Lee's own medicinal processing and decoction facility. **Tu Si Zi** is **plain stir-fried** (清炒 q□ ng chao = **Qing Chao**) over a low flame until faint crackling sounds can be heard and an aromatic scent arises. At this time, these seeds will be dark yellow to light brown in color. The purpose for processing in this way is to crack open the seed coat, thus allowing the constituents to be easily extracted upon decoction. Thus, unless specified differently, whenever **Tu Si Zi** is used throughout this text, it refers to **Qing Chao Tu Si Zi**.

In classical literature on pharmacopoeia, it is described as follows: "Sweet and acrid [in flavor] and harmonious and balanced [in nature] and condenses qi of right yang (凝正陽之氣 níng zhèng yáng zh□ qì)," "Enters the three yin [channels] of the foot," and "Strengthens yin and boosts essence, warms without drying, and does not reinforce ministerial fire. Treats the five taxations and seven damages, seminal cold and dribbling, and bitterness of mouth with dryness and thirst. Dispels wind and brightens the eyes, supplements defense qi, aides the sinews and vessels, boosts qi and bodily strength, and fattens and fortifies the body."

In contemporary texts, it is described as having a sweet flavor and a warm nature; entering the liver, kidney, and spleen channels; and having kidney-supplementing essence-securing, liver-nourishing eye-brightening, diarrhea-checking, and fetus-quieting actions.

Dr. Lee includes the medicinal pair **Tu Si Zi** and **Sha Yuan Ji Li** (supplements the kidney and secures essence and nourishes the liver and brightens the eyes) in Atopic Dermatitis Formula and Blood Desiccation Formula. Additionally, he commonly adds the pair into formula variants for their balanced and moderate liver and kidney yin-nourishing actions. Together, these medicinals offer superior capacity for retaining moisture (cellular hydration) and maintaining cell metabolic activity.

Wu Gong (蜈蚣/Scolopendra Subspinipes/Centipede)

In classical literature on pharmacopoeia, it is described as follows: "Mobile and able to dissipate, [it] treats umbilical wind clenched jaw, fright epilepsy and scrofula, snake concretions and nail sores, and kills worms and aborts the fetus."

In contemporary texts, it is described as having an acrid flavor, a warm, mobile and penetrating nature able to reach the interior and exterior, and toxicity; entering the liver channel; and having wind-extinguishing tetany-checking, toxin-attacking bind-dissipating, and network vessel-freeing pain-relieving actions.

Traditionally, **Wu Gong** is commonly paired with **Quan Xie** (i.e., Zhi Jing San) for the treatment of pathoconditions presenting with spasm and convulsion, such as acute and chronic fright wind, tetanus, wind striking the channels and network vessels, and deviated eyes and mouth; and **Quan Xie** and **Bai Jiang Can** (i.e., She Feng San) for the treatment of tetanus, spasm, and convulsion with arched-back rigidity

Since **Wu Gong** is such an expensive medicinal, Dr. Lee typically only prescribes it in cases where the neuropathic pain is "unbearable." He has found that the much more economical **Qi Cao (White Grub)** can be prescribed as a substitute with very good efficacy for most neuropathies that present with spasms, tremors, hypertonicity, tics, twitches, seizures, and pain, with the exception of certain types of tumors (e.g., sarcomas) and phantom pain.

*For more details, refer to **The Three Insects** profile.

Xi Lu Rong – refer to **Lu Rong**

Xian Di Huang – refer to **Sheng Di Huang**

Xian Zha – refer to **Shan Zha**

Xie – refer to **Quan Xie**

Xing Ren (杏仁/ Semen Armeniacae/Apricot Kernel)

In classical literature on pharmacopoeia, it is described as follows: "Acrid, bitter and sweet [in flavor], warm [in nature], and disinhibits (moistens the intestines)" "[**Xing Ren**] drains the lung and resolves flesh, eliminates wind and dissipates cold, downbears qi and moves phlegm, moistens dryness and disperses accumulations, and frees the large intestine and qi constipation (氣秘 qì mì). Treats seasonal headache, upper burner wind dryness, cough and counterflow qi ascent, and vexation heat and hasty panting. Contains mild toxicity, [thus] can kill worms and treat sores, and control rabid dog bite and tin poisoning."

In contemporary texts, it is described as having a bitter flavor, slightly warm nature, and toxicity; entering the lung and large intestine channels; and having cough-suppressing panting-calming and intestine-moistening stool-freeing actions. Traditionally, it is a commonly prescribed medicinal for the treatment of both wind-heat and wind-cold cough and panting and dryness-heat cough, and also intestinal dryness with constipation.

The bioactive constituent of the **Apricot Kernel** that may cause toxicity in high enough doses is amygdalin. Amygdalin is present only in the embryo of the kernel. Thus, to preserve the integrity of the other constituents in this compound for achieving maximum therapeutic efficacy and eliminate the potential for toxicity, Dr. Lee simply crushes the kernels in his processing facility, which breaks open the endosperm and allows the amygdalin inside to undergo thorough thermal degradation upon decoction.

Xing Ren is one of Dr. Lee's commonly prescribed medicinals and is included in numerous formulas—Ma Huang Tang, Ma Xing Gan Shi Tang, Ma Xing Yi Gan Tang, Da Qing Long Tang, Mai Men Dong Tang, She Gan Ma Huang Tang, Asthma Formula, Atopic Dermatitis Formula, Seborrheic Dermatitis Formula, and Tearing on Exposure to Wind Formula—for the treatment of both respiratory tract and dermatological pathoconditions.

Xiong Huang (雄黃/Realgar)

In classical literature on pharmacopoeia, it is described as follows: "Acrid [in flavor] and warm [in nature] with toxicity and obtains qi of right yang," "Enters the liver channel qi aspect," and "Tracks (down) the liver (搜肝 s□u g□n) and strengthens the spleen, dissipates great wind of the hundred joints (百節大風 bai jié dà f□ng), kills hundred toxin, and repels ghosts and goblins. Treats fright epilepsy and phlegm-drool, headache and dizziness, summerheat malaria and afflux dysentery (澼痢 pì lì), and diarrhea and accumulations and gatherings. [It] can also transform blood into water, dry dampness and kill worms, and treat taxation gan (劳疳 láo g□n), sores and boils, and snake bite."

In contemporary texts, it is described as having an acrid flavor, warm nature, and toxicity; entering the heart, liver and stomach channels; and having toxin-resolving worm-killing, dampness-drying, and wind-dispelling actions.

This medicinal contains the toxic constituent arsenic sulfide (As2S2). To get rid of the impurities, eliminate the potential for harmful side effects, and ensure safety, a rigorous and time-consuming traditional water grind (elutriation) processing method must be performed (calcination is *strictly* prohibited!). This processed pulverized powder form of **Xiong Huang** is then used for clinical application

Administered orally, this medicinal can only be prescribed in minuscule doses and added within a well-balanced formula composition due to the potential risk of adverse effects if taken in excessive dosages (e.g., suppression of hematopoiesis). **Xiong Huang** powder is included in the Yu Sheng formula compositions of Bao An Wan Ling Dan, Vaginal Suppository, Antimicrobial Wash, Body Soothing Powder, and Yu Sheng Medicated Thread. Dr. Lee also uses this medicinal as an external application for the treatment of herpes zoster skin rash.

Xiong Huang is experimentally and clinically proven to contain potent and effective toxin-resolving, worm-killing (i.e., antimicrobial), and anticancer (i.e., suppresses cell differentiation, induces apoptosis, and inhibits tumor growth and angiogenesis) actions.

Xu Duan (續斷/Radix Dipsaci/Teasal Root)

In classical literature on pharmacopoeia, it is described as follows: "An essential medicinal for supplementing and joining the blood vessels" and "Bitterness and warmth supplement the kidney and acridity and warmth supplement the liver. [**Xu Duan**] perfuses blood vessels and rectifies sinew and bone, thus supplements insufficiency during injury, relaxes the uterus, reduces urination, and breaks static blood. [It] treats lumbar pain and fetal spotting, flooding and vaginal discharge and seminal emission, intestinal wind and blood dysentery, and welling-abscesses, hemorrhoids, and toxin swelling. [It] treats incised wounds, breaks, and knocks and falls, relieves pain and engenders flesh, and is considered a first-class medicinal for women's medicine and external medicine."

In contemporary texts, it is described as having a bitter, sweet, and acrid flavor and slightly warm nature; entering the liver and kidney channels; and having liver- and kidney-supplementing, sinew- and bone-strengthening, blood-stanching, and fetus-quieting actions for the treatment of injuries and mending breakages.

Dr. Lee commonly includes **Xu Duan** paired or in combination with other medicinals containing similar properties in his formulas as follows: **Xu Duan** and **Du Zhong** (supplements the liver and kidney, strengthens sinew and bone, and quiets the fetus)—serve as lumbus (spine) and lower limb conductors—in Dang Gui San; **Xu Duan** and **Gu Sui Bu** (quickens the blood and transforms stasis, breaks blood, and treats injury and mends breakages) in the medicinal paste Diao Fen Gao (Suspension Powder); and **Xu Duan**, **Gu Sui Bu**, and **Niu Xi** (quickens the blood and frees the channels, supplements the liver and kidney, strengthens sinew and bone, disinhibits water and frees strangury, and conducts fire (blood) downward)—serve as lumbus (spine) and lower limb and hard tissue conductors—in Tong Jing Fang.

Additionally, Dr. Lee commonly adds the medicinal pair **Xu Duan** and **Gu Sui Bu**—serve as hard tissue conductors—into formula variants for the treatment of skeletal bone, marrow, and dental pathoconditions (e.g., fractures, osteoporosis, periodontitis).

Yi Tang (飴糖/Maltosum/Maltose/aka **Mai Ya Tang)**

In classical literature on pharmacopoeia, it is described as follows: "[**Yi Tang**] treats fulminant damage of the center burner and construction qi, dizziness, dispersion-thirst (消渴 xi□ o k□), center dispersion, and fearful throbbing and vexation and derangement." "Supplements spleen essence, transforms stomach qi, engenders liquid, nourishes blood, relaxes tension, and relieves abdominal pain."

In contemporary texts, it is described as having a sweet flavor and warm nature; entering the spleen, stomach, and lung channels; having spleen-supplementing qi-boosting, tension-relaxing pain-relieving, and lung-moistening cough-suppressing actions.

The main bioactive constituents of this medicinal (and foodstuff!) include maltose, glucose, dextrin, vitamin B, and iron.

*For more details, refer to **The Sweets** profile.

Yi Yi Ren (薏苡仁/Semen Coicis/Coix Seed)

In classical literature on pharmacopoeia, it is described as follows: "[**Yi Yi Ren**] belongs to earth and [thus] is a Yang Ming medicinal" and "Sweet [in flavor] boosts the stomach, earth overcomes water, and bland percolates dampness. Drains water by boosting earth, and thus fortifies the spleen [for the] treatment of swelling (edema) and damp impediment, leg qi and mounting qi, and diarrhea and dysentery and heat strangury. Boosts earth by engendering metal, thus supplements the lung and clears heat [for the] treatment of lung wilting and lung abscess, and coughing and spitting of pus and blood. Supports earth by repressing wood, thus treats wind-heat and tension of the sinews and hypertonicity."

In contemporary texts, it is described as having a sweet and bland flavor and slightly cold nature; entering the spleen, stomach, and lung channels; and having water-disinhibiting dampness-percolating, spleen-fortifying, impediment-eliminating, heat-clearing pus-expelling, and lung-supplementing actions. Traditionally, it is both eaten as a foodstuff (e.g., mixed with rice, grains, and lentils) and taken as a medicinal to resolve damp-heat of the skin and joints and lung and intestinal welling-abscesses.

Dr. Lee includes **Yi Yi Ren** in Ma Xing Yi Gan Tang and Seborrheic Dermatitis Formula for the treatment of dermatological pathoconditions and Si Shen Tang for the treatment of spleen and stomach vacuity pathoconditions.

Yi Yi Ren is an adaptogen that regulates the mucous membranes, improves the capacity of the epithelial cells to produce secretions, enhances the capacity of the immune system to fight off microbial infections (e.g., bacteria, fungus, virus), and normalizes both overactive ("hyper") and underactive ("hypo") autoimmune response. Thus, Dr. Lee commonly advises patients to eat **Yi Yi Ren** on their own as a medicinal food for all types of *chronic* pathoconditions involving the mucous membranes throughout the entire body. This includes the skin (e.g., tinea), lungs (e.g., lung welling-abscess), intestines (e.g., intestinal welling-abscess), genitourinary tract, endometrium, placenta (e.g., retention of dead fetus), and eyes (e.g., chronic conjunctivitis, chalazion), as well as for autoimmune disorders (e.g., rheumatoid arthritis (RA)) and cancer.

Yin Xing Ye (銀杏葉/Folium Ginkgo/Ginkgo Leaf/aka **Bai Guo Ye)**

This medicinal is the leaf of *Ginkgo biloba* L. and its seed is **Bai Guo** (constrains the lung and stabilizes panting, checks discharge, and reduces urine).

In classical literature on pharmacopoeia, it is described as follows: "Grind into powder, knead into dough, make into cake, roast and eat cooked, [it] checks diarrhea and dysentery."

In contemporary texts, it is described as having a bitter, sweet and astringent flavor, balanced nature, and mild toxicity; entering the heart, lung, and spleen channels; and having blood-quickening heart-nourishing and lung-constraining intestine-astringing actions.

Traditionally, it is prescribed for the treatment of chest impediment heart pain, panting with phlegm cough, diarrhea and dysentery, and white vaginal discharge. Experimental animal studies have shown that the flavonols (i.e., quercetin, kaempferol, and isorhamnetin) and biflavonols in **Yin Xing Ye** have the capacity to dilate coronary blood vessels, increase coronary blood flow, lower serum cholesterol, and inhibit platelet aggregation. Dr. Lee explains that "one of its main physiological mechanisms involves increasing exchanges across blood vessel membranes."

This is a commonly prescribed medicinal in Dr. Lee's pharmacopoeia and is prescribed for the treatment of conditions such as coronary artery disease (CAD), angina pectoris, hyperlipidemia, atherosclerosis, hypertension, cerebral vasospasm, and aneurysms. It is also an essential medicinal in (Yu Sheng) Bu Yang Huan Wu Tang, which Dr. Lee commonly prescribes for a broad array of blood stasis and qi stagnation pattern pathoconditions, such as sequelae of cerebrovascular accident (CVA), Parkinson's disease (PD), Alzheimer's disease (AD), and other cerebrovascular, cardiovascular and neurodegenerative pathoconditions.

Yu Gui – refer to **Rou Gui**

Zao Jiao Ci (皂角刺/Spina Gleditsiae/Chinese Honeylocust Spine)

In classical literature on pharmacopoeia, it is described as follows: "Acrid [in flavor] and warm [in nature]. **[Zao Jiao Ci]** tracks (down) wind and kills worms, just like **Zao Jia (皂荚)** [**Zao Jiao**], but it is sharp [and] can reach the affected site [to] break and disperse welling- and flat-abscesses for the treatment of welling-abscess toxin, begrudging milk [excess of breast milk] (妒乳 dù ru), pestilential wind [leprosy] (癘風 lì f□ng) and malign sores, and retention of the placenta. [It is] contraindicated for welling- and flat-abscesses that have already ruptured [and] for pregnant women" and "[**Zao**] **Jiao Ci** opens the orifices for all welling- and flat-abscesses that have not yet ruptured; and for those that have already ruptured, [it] can conduct medicinals to the sore, thus is an essential medicinal for all types of malign sores and lichen and pestilential wind [leprosy]."

In contemporary texts, it is described as having an acrid flavor and warm nature; entering the liver and stomach channels; and having blood-quickening swelling-dispersing and pus-expelling milk-freeing actions.

Traditionally, **Zao Jiao Ci** is prescribed for the early stage of swelling and toxin of welling-abscesses and sores, pus formation that fails to rupture, and breast milk stoppage. It can also be applied topically for the treatment of sores and lichen. The medicinal combination **Zao Jiao Ci**, **Ci Ji Li**, and **Chan Tui** can be prescribed to promote the dispersion and rupture of welling-abscesses and sores and relieve itching.

Dr. Lee commonly adds the medicinal pair **Zao Jiao Ci** and **Ci Ji Li** (calms and courses the liver and dispels wind and brightens the eyes) into formula variants for the treatment of exterior wind-heat or wind-heat-damp pattern ophthalmological pathoconditions affecting the lacrimal drainage system (e.g., dacryocystitis, dacryoadenitis), epidemic keratoconjunctivitis ("pinkeye"), and damp-heat pattern dermatological pathoconditions (e.g., lipomas, flat warts).

Dr. Lee classifies **Zao Jiao Ci**, **Ci Ji Li**, and **Lu Lu Tong** (expels wind and frees the network vessels and disinhibits water and eliminates dampness) as pore conductors with their capacity to regulate—*opening* and *closing* (開闔 k□i hé)—the pores and promote dermal circulation. Thus, he adds this medicinal combination into formula variants for the treatment of exterior wind-heat (or wind-heat-damp) and blood desiccation with exterior wind-heat (or with exterior wind-heat-damp) pattern skin pathoconditions that present with pruritic papules and maculopapular and vesicular eruptions (e.g., dyshidrotic eczema (pompholyx), palmoplantar pustulosis (PPP), wind papules (urticaria), acute stage atopic dermatitis).

Dr. Lee explains that blood-quickening stasis-transforming medicinals (e.g., **Dang Gui**, **Chuan Xiong**, **Ru Xiang**, **Mo Yao**) promote an increase of angiogenic proteins, the precursors necessary for angiogenesis, while the medicinal pair **Zao Jiao Ci** and **Ci Ji Li** has the capacity to open up pathways in the granulation tissue and collagen deposition formed during the wound healing process. The prescription of these mutually complementary medicinals reestablishes patent vasculature and perfusion at the site of the fibrous tissue (i.e., scar) formation, restores the natural skin coloration, and shrinks the size of the scar, thus improving the cosmetic appearance of both hypertrophic and keloid scars.

*For more details, refer to **The Eye Brighteners** and **The Itch Relievers** profiles.

Ze Xie (澤瀉/Rhizoma Alismatis Orientalitis/Alisma)

In classical literature on pharmacopoeia, it is described as follows: "Enters the urinary bladder [channel], disinhibits urine, drains fire evil in the kidney channel, and specializes in disinhibiting dampness and moving water."

In contemporary texts, it is described as having a sweet and bland flavor and cold nature; entering the kidney and urinary bladder channels; and having water-disinhibiting dampness-percolating and heat-discharging actions. It is experimentally proven to increase urine output and the excretion of urea and chloride, lower blood pressure, and lower blood sugar levels.

As a general rule, for patients presenting with pronounced water amassment or water-rheum collecting internally (e.g., generalized edema, ascites, pericardial effusion, pleural effusion, increased intracranial pressure (ICP)), Dr. Lee will prescribe the medicinal pair **Fu Ling** and **Ze Xie** in equivalently large doses (≥ 8 qian) for their mutually accentuating water-disinhibiting actions.

*For more details, refer to **The Four Lings** profile.

Zhi Gan Cao – refer to **Gan Cao**

Zhi Zi (栀子/Fructus Gardeniae/Gardenia Fruit/aka **Shan Zhi Zi)**

Dr. Lee stocks only **raw** (生 sh□ng = **Sheng**) in his in-house dispensary. Thus, unless specified differently, whenever **Zhi Zi** is used throughout this text, it refers to **Sheng Zhi Zi**.

In classical literature on pharmacopoeia, it is described as follows: "Bitter [in flavor] and cold [in nature]…," "Used **raw** [it] drains fire, **stir-fried until black** (炒黑 chao h□i = **Chao Hei**) [it] stanches bleeding, **stir-fried with ginger juice** (姜汁炒 ji□ng zh□ chao = **Jiang Zhi Chao**) [it] treats vexation and vomiting, [and] for interior heat use the seed and for exterior heat use the skin," "Red [in] color enters the heart," "Drains evil heat in the heart and lung and bends [conducts] it downwards [to be] excreted via the urine, thus resolving depressed fire in the triple burner, calming heat reversal and heart pain, and extinguishing vomiting of blood, blood strangury, and blood dysentery. Treats heart vexation and anguish and sleeplessness (insomnia), five yellows, five stranguries, blood collapse and desiccation of fluid, dry mouth and red eyes, purple patches and white lai (癞 lài), and sores."

In contemporary texts, it is described as having a bitter flavor and cold nature; entering the heart, liver, lung, stomach, and triple burner channels; having fire-draining vexation-eliminating, heat-clearing dampness-disinhibiting, blood-cooling toxin-resolving, and swelling-dispersing pain-relieving actions. Traditionally, **Zhi Zi** is prescribed for heat pattern diseases that present with vexation and oppression (e.g., Huang Lian Jie Du Tang, Zhi Zi Shi Tang) and damp-heat jaundice (e.g., Yin Chen Hao Tang).

Dr. Lee includes **Zhi Zi** in Huang Lian Jie Du Tang for the treatment of triple burner heat toxin pattern pathoconditions, Long Dan Xie Gan Tang for the treatment of liver and gallbladder repletion fire and lower burner damp-heat pattern pathoconditions, and Liang Ge San for the treatment of accumulated heat in the upper and middle burner pattern pathoconditions. Dr. Lee also commonly prescribes the medicinal pair **Zhi Zi** and **Mu Dan Pi** for the treatment of acute inflammation of vasculature (e.g., vasculitis, arteritis) that affects the endothelial cells located on the intima.

It is important to note that long-term administration (≥ 3 months) of **Zhi Zi** may cause transient blue-gray or bronze skin dyspigmentation in some patients. Studies have suggested that a metabolite (i.e., genipin) of geniposide, the main bioactive constituent in this medicinal, is the causative factor involved in the discoloration. For this reason, Dr. Lee only administers **Zhi Zi** for short-term regimens (≤ 3 months). In cases where long-term administration is necessary, he will prescribe other heat-clearing toxin-resolving (e.g., **The Three Yellows**), yin-enriching fire-draining (e.g., **Qing Hao**, **Zhi Mu**), and blood-cooling (e.g., **Di Gu Pi**, **Mu Dan Pi**) medicinals, instead.

Zhu Ling (豬苓/Sclerotium Polyporus Umbellati/Polyporus)

In classical literature on pharmacopoeia, it is described as follows: "Bitter [in flavor] drains stagnation, bland [in flavor] disinhibits the orifices, and sweet [in flavor] assists yang. Enters the urinary bladder [and] kidney channels, upbears thus can downbear, opens the interstices and promotes sweating, disinhibits urine and moves water, and has similar actions as **Fu Ling** except that it does not supplement…."

In contemporary texts, it is described as having a sweet and bland flavor and a balanced nature; entering the kidney and urinary bladder channels; and having water-disinhibiting dampness-percolating actions. **Zhu Ling** has a *superior* water-disinhibiting action compared to **Fu Ling**, but an *inferior* supplementing action. The physiological mechanism of its urine-disinhibiting (diuretic) action primarily involves inhibiting the absorption of water and electrolytes (specifically potassium (K+), sodium (Na+), and chlorine (Cl-)) in the renal tubules of the nephron.

*For more details, refer to **The Four Lings** profile.

Zhu Ru (竹茹/Caulis Bambusae in Taenia/Bamboo Shavings)

In classical literature on pharmacopoeia, it is described as follows: "Sweet [in flavor] and slightly cold [in nature]" and "Opens depression in stomach-earth, clears dryness in lung-metal, [and] cools the blood and eliminates heat. Treats upper burner vexation heat, warm qi cold and heat, dysphagia-occlusion and retching and hiccup, blood ejection and spontaneous external bleeding, lung wilting and fright epilepsy, [and] flooding stirring fetus." "Clears house of the stomach heat, [and] is an essential medicinal for vacuity vexation and vexation thirst and stomach vacuity retching counterflow."

In contemporary texts, it is described as having a sweet flavor and slightly cold nature; entering the lung and stomach channels; and having heat-clearing phlegm-transforming and vexation-eliminating vomit-checking actions. **Zhu Ru** is recognized as being particularly effective for treating pathoconditions involving phlegm-heat that results in cough, vexation and sleeplessness (insomnia), and both stomach repletion heat and stomach vacuity heat retching and vomiting.

Traditionally, this medicinal is paired with **Chen Pi** (rectifies qi and fortifies the spleen and dries dampness and transforms phlegm) and

Zhi Shi (breaks qi and eliminates impediment and transforms phlegm and disperses accumulations).

Dr. Lee also utilizes the medicinal combination **Zhu Ru**, **Chen Pi**, and **Zhi Shi** in Wen Dan Tang, a commonly prescribed formula for all types of Shao Yang depressed heat with phlegm and damp-heat pattern pathoconditions from the common cold and otitis to vexation and sleeplessness, infertility, and myasthenia gravis.

Zhu Sha (硃砂/Cinnabaris/Cinnabar/aka **Dan Sha)**

This medicinal is an inorganic mercury ore which contains mercuric sulfide (HgS), but is often found mixed with impurities such as realgar, apatite, and bitumen. To get rid of the impurities, eliminate the potential for harmful side effects, and ensure safety, a rigorous and time-consuming traditional water grind (elutriation) processing method must be performed (calcination is *strictly* prohibited!).

In classical literature on pharmacopoeia, it is described as follows: "[**Zhu Sha**'s] form is yang and property is yin, [its] flavor is sweet and [nature] is cool, [and its] color is red and belongs to fire," "Drains evil heat in the heart channel, settles the heart and clears the liver, brightens the eyes and promotes sweating, stabilizes fright and dispels wind, repels evil and resolves toxin, and suppresses cough and quiets the fetus," and "**Dan Sha (丹砂)** combined with **Yuan Zhi** and **Long Gu** nourishes heart qi; combined with **Dang Gui** and **Dan Shen** nourishes heart blood; combined with **Gou Ji** and **Di Huang** nourishes the kidney; combined with **Hou Po** and **Chuan Jiao** nourishes the spleen; and combined with **Nan Xing** and **Chuan Wu** dispels wind. [It] can brighten the eyes, quiet the fetus, resolve toxin, and promote sweating; [its] actions depend on the assistant and courier and thus [it] has no limitations."

In contemporary texts, it is described as having a sweet flavor, cold nature, and toxicity; entering the heart channel; and having heart-settling spirit-quieting and heat-clearing toxin-resolving actions.

Traditionally, **Zhu Sha** is prescribed in combination with **Di Huang** and **Bo Zi Ren** for heart and yin vacuity pattern pathoconditions (e.g., disquieted heart spirit, palpitations, insomnia); paired with **Ci Shi** for ascendant hyperactivity of liver yang pattern pathoconditions (e.g., fright wind, epilepsy); and in combination with **Xiong Huang**, **Da Ji**, and **Shan Ci Gu** as a topical application (e.g., Zi Jin Ding) for the treatment of swelling and toxin of sores.

For the treatment of profuse menstruation (e.g., menorrhagia, hypermenorrhea), Dr. Lee will typically prescribe **Zhu Sha** in combination with **Sheng Mu Li**, **Chuan Qi**, and **Dai Zhe Shi**. However, since this medicinal is becoming more difficult to obtain and increasingly expensive, for the treatment of pathoconditions involving hyperactivity of ascendant liver yang pattern, Dr. Lee will typically prescribe **Dai Zhe Shi** instead (e.g., Jian Ling Tang). And for the treatment of welling-abscesses, flat-abscesses, and clove sores, Dr. Lee also utilizes **Zhu Sha** in the topically applied medicinal paste Zi Jin Ding.

DR. LEE'S FORMULAS

This section introduces the formulas Dr. Lee commonly prescribes and includes details about the dose and action of each medicinal, the composite action of each formula, and the types of pathoconditions for which each formula is typically administered. Many of these formulas are variants on Han dynasty classical formulas from the *Treatise on Cold Damage and Miscellaneous Diseases* (傷寒雜病論 *Shang Han Za Bing Lun*), some are variants on more contemporary classic formulas from the Tang, Song, Ming, and Qing dynasties, and others are original formulas designed by Dr. Lee. Additionally, other formulas that Dr. Lee mentions as alternatively effective therapeutic options in the text are also listed for reference, but with only the compositions provided.

Throughout the text, the name "(Yu Sheng)" may be included in front of a formula's name to distinguish that it is a Dr. Lee variant on an existing formula or his own unique composition. Even when not included, it is still implied that all of the formulas Dr. Lee prescribes are indeed (Yu Sheng) formulas. The term Yu Sheng simply refers to Yu Sheng Chinese Medicine Clinic of which Dr. Lee is the founder, director, and chief physician.

The following formulas are set compositions designed to treat the extensive scope of pathoconditions that Dr. Lee commonly incurs in his clinical practice. The medicinals comprising the formulas are either purchased already processed or processed in-house, and then pre-weighed and pre-packaged into semiporous decocting packets (not yet sealed) for convenient storage and administration. Upon prescription, Dr. Lee will subsequently make modifications to these formulas by adding medicinals based on each individual patient's signs, symptoms, and pattern identification. The packets are then sealed and ready for administration and decoction. This is not an exhaustive listing: when special cases present, Dr. Lee will compose formulas specifically designed for a particular case.

As time evolves, social and environmental factors impact the manifestation of maladies in the human body, mind, and spirit. Dr. Lee continues to search for the best approaches to provide the most effective treatment in our modern world.

*__Disclaimer__: The formula compositions and medicinal doses provided in Dr. Lee's commonly prescribed formulas listed below and throughout this entire three-volume series are *for reference purposes only* and are *not* intended for indiscriminate administration by other individuals or parties. Prescription of these formulas should only be administered by a licensed traditional Chinese medicine (TCM) physician or practitioner who has carefully evaluated the patient's history, signs, and symptoms, and conducted pattern identification as the basis for determining treatment. Licensed TCM practitioners must be aware that these formula compositions and medicinal doses are *for reference purposes only* and solely intended for administration by Dr. Lee in his own clinical practice.

An Zhong San (安中散/Center-Quieting Powder)
Gui Zhi, Yan Hu Suo, Mu Li, Xiao Hui Xiang, Sha Ren, Gan Cao, Liang Jiang

Antimicrobial Wash (洗劑/Xi Ji)

Liu Huang, Xiong Huang, Da Huang	5 qian each
She Chuang Zi, Long Dan Cao	1 liang each

This formula composition is identical to **Vaginal Suppository (Sai Ji)** except for the addition of Long Dan Cao. The core toxin-resolving, worm-killing, and itch-relieving medicinals—She Chuang Zi, Xiong Huang, Liu Huang, and Da Huang—are the same. The combination of these medicinals clears heat and resolves toxin, kills worms and relieves itch, dispels wind and eliminates dampness, and closes sores and engenders flesh.

Antimicrobial Wash is an immersion and wash therapy that can be prescribed for all types of microbial infections of the skin and mucous membranes. However, Dr. Lee most commonly prescribes this formula for microbial infections of the vulva and vaginal opening, including bacterial vaginosis (i.e., *Gardnerella vaginalis*), yeast (candidiasis), parasites (trichomoniasis), and sexually transmitted diseases (STDs) (e.g., genital herpes, gonorrhea, Chlamydia) that present with itching, irritation, and watery or viscous vaginal discharge.

Antler Aconite Ginger Gypsum Powder (鹿附乾石粉/Lu Fu Gan Shi Fen)

Lu Jiao Shuang	100 g
Fu Zi	16 g
Gan Jiang	16 g
Sheng Shi Gao	16 g

This is a specially designed topical medicinal powder for the treatment of yang vacuity pattern ulcerations. These chronic, noninfectious and nonhealing ulcers are typically caused by peripheral vascular disease (e.g., stasis ulcers resulting from venous insufficiency) and present as an open sore (ulcer) with *no* putrid odor. If *clear* exudate presents (indicating *mild* inflammatory response), then add Huang Bo (16 g); and if *purulent* exudate presents (indicating more *pronounced* inflammatory response), then add Da Huang (16 g) instead.

These medicinals are all ground into a fine powder and thoroughly blended together to form a homogenous mixture. The powder is applied inside the open sore (ulcerated lesion), covered in gauze, and fit with a tubular elastic net, which must be kept dry at all times. It should be left in place until the wound bed fills with new connective tissue and contraction of the wound margins occurs. At that time, in order to prevent hyperplastic growth of new connective tissue, any remaining powder or debris should be debrided; and in its place, Da Huang (powder) should be topically applied on the wound up until the collagen fibers regorganize, the new tissue remodels and matures (extracellular matrix remodeling), and scarring occurs.

Lu Jiao Shuang, the sovereign medicinal, is composed primarily of calcium phosphate and calcium carbonate, along with an array of fundamental amino acids. It has kidney-warming yang-assisting, astringing, and blood-stanching actions, which function to activate fibroblast growth factors that promote fibroblast and keratinocyte (granulation tissue) influx and re-epithelialization (proliferative phase of wound healing). This process fills the wound with connective tissue and lays the lattice for new blood vessels (angiogenesis) to develop, stimulates stem cell activation and promotes extracellular matrix remodeling (maturation phase of wound healing).

Fu Zi, Gan Jiang, and Sheng Shi Gao serve as the minister and assistant medicinals. Fu Zi returns yang and stems counterflow, reinforces yang and supplements fire, and dissipates cold and relieves pain; and Gan Jiang warms the center, expels cold, and returns yang and frees the vessels. Together, Fu Zi and Gan Jiang boost the metabolism and promote tissue perfusion, which enhances Lu Jiao Shuang's capacity to initiate and accelerate the proliferative and maturation phase of wound healing. Sheng Shi Gao (Gypsum/CaSO4·2H2O/aqueous calcium sulfate) clears heat and drains fire and astringes and engenders flesh. Calcium sulfate assists in the process of fibroblast and keratinocyte (granulation tissue) formation during the proliferative phase and extracellular matrix remodeling during the maturation phase of wound healing.

Huang Bo and Da Huang also serve as assistant medicinals. Huang Bo clears heat and dries dampness, drains fire in the lower burner and resolves toxin, and abates heat and eliminates steam; and Da Huang clears heat and drains fire, resolves toxin and erodes pus, and quickens the blood and dispels stasis. The antimicrobial and anti-inflammatory actions of these medicinals destroy bacteria and ensure that infection does *not* interfere with the growth of new tissue.

Asthma Formula (氣喘方/Qi Chuan Fang)

Ma Huang	1.5 qian
Dan Shen, Cang Zhu, Fu Ling, Gan Cao	3 qian each
Mu Xiang, Sha Ren, Wu Wei Zi	3 qian each
Chen Pi, Ban Xia, Xing Ren, Bai Guo	4 qian each
Shan Yao, Rou Gui	5 qian each

This original Yu Sheng formula contains the qi-boosting spleen-fortifying and qi-moving phlegm-transforming actions of **Xiang Sha Liu Jun Zi Tang** adding Ma Huang, Wu Wei Zi, Xing Ren, Bai Guo, Shan Yao, and Rou Gui.

Ma Huang promotes sweating and resolves the exterior; Wu Wei Zi constrains the lung and stabilizes panting; Xing Ren suppresses cough and calms panting; Bai Guo constrains the lung and dispels phlegm;

Shan Yao supplements the spleen, lung, and kidneys and nourishes yin; and Rou Gui supplements fire and assists yang for the treatment of vacuity asthma debilitation of the life gate fire. Dr. Lee will also add Ren Shen (powder), which enters the lung and spleen channels, greatly supplements original qi, and supplements the spleen and boosts the lung. As its name indicates, this formula is designed for the treatment of asthma, and specifically for the *spleen yang vacuity* pattern type that presents with panting (asthma) and shortness of breath (dyspnea).

Spleen yang vacuity pattern presents in the early stages of this pathocondition, when it can be more readily managed and often even cured. If this pathocondition progresses to the more severe, chronic stage of *kidney yang vacuity* pattern, Dr. Lee typically prescribes **You Gui Yin** variant. For acute flare-ups, heat-clearing toxin-resolving, lung-depurating phlegm-transforming, and cough-suppressing panting-calming medicinals will be added to the formula; or the original formula will be substituted with a heat-clearing, cough-suppressing, and panting-calming formula variant (e.g., **Ma Xing Gan Shi Tang**, **Da Qing Long Tang**) until the flare-up subsides.

Atopic Dermatitis Formula (異位性皮膚炎方/Yi Wei Xing Pi Fu Yan Fang)

Ma Huang	1.5 qian
Dan Shen, Cang Zhu, Fu Ling, Gan Cao	3 qian each
Chen Pi, Ban Xia, Mu Xiang, Sha Ren	3 qian each
Xing Ren, Bai Guo, Wu Wei Zi, Shan Yao	3 qian each
Dang Gui, He Shou Wu, Tu Si Zi, Sha Yuan Zi	5 qian each

This is an Yu Sheng original compound formula derived from **Asthma Formula** (subtracting Rou Gui) and **Blood Desiccation Formula** (subtracting Ci Ji Li). **Asthma Formula** supplements the spleen, lung, and kidneys, nourishes yin, resolves the exterior, opens the pores, and dispels phlegm; and **Blood Desiccation Formula** nourishes blood, enriches yin, and dispels wind. As its name indicates, Dr. Lee administers **Atopic Dermatitis Formula** for the treatment of atopic dermatitis, and specifically, the *spleen yang vacuity* pattern type.

Depending on the patient's presenting signs, symptoms and pattern, the following medicinals are commonly added: for severe pruritis—Sheng Shi Gao, Lu Lu Tong, and Hua Shi; for flare-ups with excessive suppuration—Bai Xian Pi, Huang Qin, and Yi Yi Ren; and for chronic persistent cases with erythematous lesions (in body creases or generalized), cracking, suppuration, pruritis, and agitation—the doses of the **Blood Desiccation Formula** medicinals will be increased, with small amounts of The Three Great Yang-Supplementers (Gan Jiang, Fu Zi, and Rou Gui) added to supplement kidney and spleen vacuity and return and reinforce yang.

Ba Xian Chang Shou Wan (八仙長壽丸/Eight Immortals Longevity Pill)

Sheng Di Huang, Shan Zhu Yu, Huai Shan, Fu Ling, Mu Dan Pi, Ze Xie, Mai Men Dong, Wu Wei Zi

Ba Zheng San (八正散/Eight Corrections Powder)

Mu Tong, Qu Mai, Che Qian Zi, Bian Xu, Hua Shi, Gan Cao, Da Huang, Zhi Zi, Deng Xin Cao

Bai He Gu Jin Tang (百合固金湯/Lily Bulb Metal-Securing Decoction)

Bai He, Sheng Di Huang, Shu Di Huang, Yuan Shen	3 qian each
Jie Geng, Gan Cao, Mai Men Dong	3 qian each
Dang Gui, Chi Shao, Cang Zhu	3 qian each

Bai Hu Tang (白虎湯/White Tiger Decoction)

Zhi Mu, Shi Gao, Gan Cao, Jing Mi

Ban Xia Hou Po Tang (半夏厚朴湯)

Ban Xia, Hou Po, Fu Ling, Sheng Jiang, Gan Su Ye

Ban Xia Tian Ma Bai Zhu San (半夏天麻白朮散)

Dang Gui	2 qian
Ban Xia, Bai Zhu, Fu Ling, Cang Zhu	3 qian each
Ze Xie, Chen Pi, Shen Qu	3 qian each
Mai Ya, Gan Jiang, Huang Bo	3 qian each
Fu Zi, Tian Ma	5 qian each
Huang Qi	1 liang

The Yu Sheng version is similar to the original formula—**Ban Xia Tian Ma Bai Zhu Tang (半夏天麻白朮湯)**—except for the addition of Dang Gui and Fu Zi, and the fact that Ren Shen (powder) is either taken separately or added into the formula after decoction.

Dang Gui supplements and quickens the blood and Fu Zi returns yang and stems counterflow, supplements fire and reinforces yang, and dissipates cold and relieves pain. These additions complement this foot Tai Yin spleen channel formula's overall spleen- and stomach-supplementing, phlegm-damp transforming, and wind-stabilizing actions. The classical TCM pathomechanisms of this formula are explained as follows: "Phlegm reversal [refers to] phlegm-damp reverse flow ascending. Phlegm counterflow leads to upper body repletion, causing headache, dizzy head, and black [spots] in front of the eyes [visual field]."

Ban Xia Tian Ma Bai Zhu San is among Dr. Lee's most commonly prescribed formulas, administered for a wide range of pathoconditions including Meniere disease, benign paroxysmal positional vertigo (BPPV), psychosomatic symptoms (e.g., abdominal distention, malaise, and fatigue), migraine and cluster headaches, traumatic brain injury resulting in increased intracranial pressure, and benign brain tumors. It is also one of the commonly prescribed formulas in Dr. Lee's cancer treatment protocol, specifically administered for malignant brain tumors.

Bao An Wan Ling Dan (保安萬靈丹/Safeguard Unlimited Efficacy Elixir)

Tian Ma, Chuan Xiong, Chuan Wu, Wu Cao	1 liang each
Fang Feng, Jing Jie, Ma Huang, Xi Xin	1 liang each
Qiang Huo, He Shou Wu, Dang Gui	1 liang each
Shi Hu, Quan Xie, Gan Cao	1 liang each
Cang Zhu	8 liang
Xiong Huang	6 qian

Dr. Lee uses the *Orthodox Manual of External Medicine* (外科正宗 *Wai Ke Zheng Zong*) version of this formula and commonly abbreviates the name, calling it simply **Wan Ling Dan**. This is a pill specially prepared for Dr. Lee by an outsourced medicinal processing facility.

It is composed of medicinals that dispel wind, eliminate dampness, dissipate cold, extinguish wind, quicken and supplement the blood, check tetany, free the network vessels, open the orifices, resolve toxin, dissipate binds, and relieve pain. Xiong Huang is among the principal medicinals in this composition with its antimicrobial and anticancer actions (e.g., suppresses cell differentiation, induces apoptosis, and inhibits tumor growth and angiogenesis).

As its name implies, **Safeguard Unlimited Efficacy Elixir** has been traditionally administered for the treatment of a broad spectrum of pathoconditions including welling- and flat-abscesses, deep pus sores, clove toxin, mouth-level nape flat abscess, jowl effusion, damp phlegm streaming sore, bone flat-abscesses, crane's-knee wind, wind-cold-damp impediment, paralysis, tetanus, and migraine headaches.

Dr. Lee prescribes **Wan Ling Dan** for various types of acute, chronic, and intractable pathoconditions including innominate toxin-swelling, benign tumors, and paralysis resulting from parasitic infection. It also constitutes one of the pillars of Dr. Lee's cancer treatment protocol, prescribed as a part of the regimen for all types of solid tumors (e.g., carcinomas, sarcomas, lymphomas) and hematological cancers (i.e., leukemia and myeloma). Combined with other formulas, it has the capacity to induce partial or complete remission and lower the chances of recurrence and metastasis.

Blood Desiccation Formula (血枯方/Xue Ku Fang)

Cang Zhu, Ci Ji Li	4 qian each
Dang Gui, He Shou Wu, Tu Si Zi, Sha Yuan Zi	8 qian each

The term blood desiccation first appears in *The Yellow Emperor's Inner Canon* (黃帝内經 *Huang Di Nei Jing*) and refers to this pathocondition as blood vacuity following hemorrhage. Indeed, Dr. Lee's adaptation of this term covers a much broader scope of applications.

This Yu Sheng original formula contains the same core medicinals—Dang Gui, He Shou Wu, and Ci Ji Li.—as **Dang Gui Yin Zi** and thus shares similar actions and clinical applications. However, **Blood Desiccation Formula** replaces Shao Yao, Chuan Xiong, and Sheng Di Huang with large doses of Dang Gui and He Shou Wu; subtracts Fang Feng, Jing Jie, and Huang Qi; and adds Sha Yuan Zi, Tu Si Zi, and Cang Zhu.

Sha Yuan Zi and Tu Si Zi both supplement the kidney, secure essence, and nourish the liver; and Cang Zhu dispels wind-damp and dries dampness and fortifies the spleen to counteract the potential for digestion impairment and loose stools resulting from the blood-nourishing yin-enriching medicinals. These additions complement this formula's overall actions of nourishing the blood, moistening dryness, dispelling wind, and relieving itch for the treatment of yin vacuity, blood vacuity, and blood desiccation pattern.

For the treatment of skin pathoconditions, the relatively hardier Ma Huang is added to resolve the exterior instead of Fang Feng and Jing Jie (their volatile oils readily degrade upon decoction and thus require large doses to achieve efficacy); and if itch presents, Ci Ji Li, Zao Jiao Ci, and Lu Lu Tong are added.

Dr. Lee typically prescribes **Blood Desiccation Formula** for pathoconditions that can be identified as blood vacuity with wind-dryness pattern, presenting with dry, itchy skin, and possibly mild redness (e.g., pruritis, erythema, urticaria, eczema, atopic dermatitis); liver blood vacuity pattern, presenting with darkened skin and compromised hematopoiesis (e.g., late stage hepatic cirrhosis); and vacuity of the thoroughfare and controlling vessel pattern, presenting with endometrial hypoperfusion (e.g., causing infertility or miscarriage).

Bo Zi Ren Wan (柏子仁丸)
Bo Zi Ren, Ren Shen, Bai Zhu, Ban Xia, Wu Wei Zi, Mu Li, Ma Huang Gen, Mai Fu

Body Soothing Ointment – refer to **Body Soothing Powder**

Body Soothing Powder (爽身粉/Shuang Shen Fen)

Bing Pian	. 2 qian
Da Huang, Sheng Mu Li, Sheng Long Gu each	. 1 liang
Lu Gan Shi, Hua Shi, Sheng Shi Gao each	. 1 liang
Xiong Huang	. 5 qian

This is a hybrid formula that contains a compilation of the most commonly prescribed topically applied essential medicinals in the Chinese medicine pharmacopoeia for exterior *damp-heat* pattern skin pathoconditions that present with *intense itch* and/or *excessive perspiration*. As its name indicates—**Shuang Shen (爽身)** means to "soothe the body"—this formula functions to soothe the skin, relieve itch, absorb sweat, calm agitation and vexation, and has antimicrobial and anti-inflammatory actions.

Bing Pian (Borneol) opens the orifices and arouses the spirit and clears heat and relieves pain; Da Huang (Rhubarb Root) clears heat and drains fire, resolves toxin and erodes pus, and quickens the blood and dispels stasis; Sheng Mu Li (Oyster Shell) calms the liver and subdues yang, softens hardness and dissipates binds, and astringes and secures; Sheng Long Gu (Dragon Bone) subdues yang and quiets the spirit and astringes and secures; Lu Gan Shi (Calamine) resolves toxin, clears the eyes and abates screens and absorbs dampness, engenders flesh, and closes sores; Hua Shi (Talc) disinhibits water and frees strangury, clears and resolves summerheat-heat, and dispels dampness and closes sores; Sheng Shi Gao (Gypsum) clears heat and drains fire and astringes and engenders flesh; and Xiong Huang (Realgar) resolves toxin and kills worms (antimicrobial), dries dampness and dispels phlegm, and dispels wind.

These medicinals are all ground into a fine powder and thoroughly blended to form a homogenous mixture. Together, they combine to provide effective toxin- and itch-resolving with clearing coolness, wind-dissipating dampness-dispelling, sore-closing flesh-engendering, heat-clearing worm-killing, and sweat-checking actions.

Dr. Lee prescribes **Body Soothing Powder** as a part of the therapeutic regimen for both acute and chronic exterior *damp-heat* pattern skin pathoconditions (e.g., all types of dermatitis, eczema, urticaria, tinea, miliaria, psoriasis, and hyperhidrosis) that present with *intense itch* to the extent of agitation and vexation and/or *excessive perspiration*.

For *dry lesions*, Dr. Lee will prescribe this formula in powder form, which can be dabbed on with a cosmetic sponge. For *oozing and crusting lesions*, Dr. Lee will prescribe **Body Soothing Ointment (爽身**

膏)—simply **Body Soothing Powder** mixed in petroleum jelly—an ointment that can be rubbed on.

Bu Yang Huan Wu Tang (補陽還五湯/Yang-Supplementing Five-Returning Decoction)

Dang Gui, Chuan Xiong, Chi Shao	4 qian each
Dan Shen, Yin Xing Ye	4 qian each
Huang Qi	2 liang

The Yu Sheng version is based on the original formula, but only contains 2 liang of Huang Qi as opposed to 4 liang; excludes Di Long, Tao Ren, and Hong Hua; and adds Yin Xing Ye and Dan Shen.

Though not listed above, Ren Shen *is* included in this composition just as in the original formula, except in pulverized powder form, and is often paired with Chuan Qi (aka Ren Shen/Chuan Qi Powder). This medicinal pair serves to complement the qi-supplementing action of Huang Qi and the blood-quickening action of Dan Shen.

Dr. Lee has chosen a relatively smaller dose of Huang Qi for this composition, because starting out with an excessive dose may result in the rupture of compromised blood vessels or a sudden increase in intracranial pressure in patients with arteriosclerosis, atherosclerosis, hematoma, or adhesions in the subarachnoid space of the meninges.

Yin Xing Ye is an essential medicinal in this formula. Dr. Lee utilizes its capacity of increasing exchanges across blood vessel membranes (e.g., promotes lymphatic circulation) and phlegm-transforming actions to reduce blood viscosity and eliminate plaque for patients with cerebrovascular and neurodegenerative pathoconditions, such as cerebrovascular accident (CVA) (stroke) sequelae, transient ischemic attack (TIA) sequelae, Parkinson's disease (PD), and Alzheimer's disease (AD).

Tao Ren, Hong Hua, and Di Long are excluded, because unlike stroke patients in the 18th and 19th centuries when this formula was designed, modern biomedicine has already intervened during the acute stage to accelerate reperfusion with drugs and surgical decompression. This intervention obviates the need for these potent blood-quickening stasis-dispelling and network vessel-freeing medicinals.

Nowadays, the primary role of TCM is to treat the neurological sequelae and prevent subsequent attacks. This requires the administration of dual blood- and qi-supplementing, blood-quickening, and phlegm-transforming medicinals to reduce blood viscosity, maintain plaque-free vasculature, and prevent the development of emboli or thrombi. Prescribed for the treatment of neurodegenerative diseases (e.g., AD, PD, Huntington's disease), **Bu Yang Huan Wu Tang** slows down the rate of degeneration, enhances quality of life, and extends life expectancy.

Bu Zhong Yi Qi Tang (補中益氣湯/Center-Supplementing Qi-Boosting Decoction)

Huang Qi	1 liang
Dang Gui	2 qian
Dan Shen, Cang Zhu, Chen Pi	3 qian each
Gan Cao, Sheng Ma, Chai Hu	3 qian each

The Yu Sheng version is similar to the original formula except that Dan Shen replaces Ren Shen for its blood-quickening stasis-dispelling action, and Cang Zhu replaces Bai Zhu for its spleen-fortifying dampness-drying action, which aids digestion and is more suitable for Taiwan's humid subtropical climate. However, depending on the presenting signs, symptoms, and pattern, Dr. Lee may also add Ren Shen (powder) or Ren Shen/Chuan Qi Powder.

Dr. Lee prescribes this qi-boosting, yang-upbearing fall-raising, and spleen-supplementing stomach-regulating formula for pathoconditions such as anal prolapse, uterine prolapse, gastroptosis, nephroptosis, inguinal hernia, anal fissures, hemorrhoids, myasthenia gravis (qi-vacuity type), leukorrhea (qi-vacuity type), and proteinuria (intrinsic renal disease) in pediatric patients. Additionally, this formula's exceptional efficacy at promoting tissue repair and mucous membrane healing makes **Bu Zhong Yi Qi Tang** an essential formula for patients with post-surgical wounds and cancer patients who have undergone (or are currently receiving) radiotherapy and/or chemotherapy.

Chai Hu Gui Zhi Tang (柴胡桂枝湯)

Chai Hu, Gui Zhi, Ren Shen, Gan Cao, Ban Xia, Huang Qin, Shao Yao, Da Zao, Sheng Jiang

Chai Hu Jia Long Gu Mu Li Tang (柴胡加龍骨牡蠣湯)
Chai Hu, Long Gu, Huang Qin, Sheng Jiang, Qian Dan, Ren Shen, Gui Zhi, Fu Ling, Ban Xia, Da Huang, Mu Li, Da Zao

Chai Ling Tang (柴苓湯)

Huang Qin, Fu Ling, Zhu Ling, Ze Xie	3 qian each
Cang Zhu, Yan Hu Suo, Mu Xiang, Gui Zhi	3 qian each
Dan Shen, Ban Xia, Gan Cao, Sheng Jiang	5 qian each
Da Zao	3 pieces
Chai Hu	6 qian

The Yu Sheng version is similar to the original formula except for the addition of Yan Hu Suo, Mu Xiang, and Dan Shen; Cang Zhu replaces Bai Zhu; Ren Shen pulverized powder is used instead of decocting pieces; and unlike other Yu Sheng formulas, Gui Zhi *is* included (instead of Rou Gui) for its yang-assisting qi-transforming actions. Yan Hu Suo and Mu Xiang relax smooth muscle and thus relieve pain.

Chai Ling Tang is a compound formula that includes elements of **Xiao Chai Hu Tang (小柴胡湯)** and **Wu Ling San (Calculi Formula) (五苓散) (結石方)**. It. functions to eliminate heat, disinhibit water, and transform phlegm for the treatment of water amassment collecting above and below the diaphragm, amassed phlegm and collecting rheum (蓄痰停飲 xù tán tíng yin), cold damage with residual Shao Yang heat, chest and rib-side distention and impediment, difficult urination, and vomiting and diarrhea upon drinking water.

Dr. Lee typically prescribes **Chai Ling Tang** for the treatment of ascites, portal hypertension, pleural effusion, pleuritis, pericardial effusion, cerebral edema, and increased intracranial pressure that manifest in pathoconditions such as in chronic liver disease (e.g., hepatitis, cirrhosis, fulminant hepatitis, hepatorenal syndrome (HRS), hepatocellular carcinoma), encephalitis, trauma, and side effects of radiotherapy.

Chai Ling Tang is also one of the commonly prescribed formulas in Dr. Lee's cancer treatment protocol, specifically administered for Shao

Yang depressed heat pattern cancers, which manifest in the membranous tissues of organs such as the liver, kidney, and lung.

Chai Ping Tang (柴平湯)

Chai Hu, Ren Shen, Ban Xia, Huang Qin, Gan Cao, Chen Pi, Hou Po, Cang Zhu, Sheng Jiang, Da Zao

Chong He Tang (沖和湯/Harmonious Flow Decoction)

Ren Shen, Chen Pi, Huang Qi, Bai Zhu, Dang Gui, Bai Zhi, Fu Ling, Chuan Xiong, Zao Jiao Ci, Ru Xiang, Mo Yao, Jin Yin Hua, Gan Cao

Chou Feng Tang (抽風湯/Tugging Wind Formula)

Fang Feng, Yuan Ming Fen, Chai Hu, Da Huang, Huang Qin, Che Qian Zi, Jie Geng, Xi Xin

Da Chai Hu Tang (大柴胡湯/Major Bupleurum Decoction)

Chai Hu, Huang Qin, Ban Xia, Zhi Shi, Da Huang, Shao Yao, Sheng Jiang, Da Zao

Da Huang Zhe Chong Wan (大黃哲蟲丸)

Da Huang, Huang Qin, Gan Cao, Tao Ren, Xing Ren, Bai Shao, Shou Di Huang, Gan Qi, Meng Chong, Shui Zhi, Qi Cao, Tu Bie Chong, Feng Mi (Honey)

Da Qing Long Tang (大青龍湯/Major Green-Blue Dragon)

Ma Huang	2 qian
Xing Ren, Cang Zhu	4 qian each
Rou Gui, Sheng Jiang, Gan Cao	3 qian each
Sheng Shi Gao	1 liang
Da Zao	5 pieces

The Yu Sheng version is virtually identical to the original formula, which is a derivative of **Ma Huang Tang** that includes large doses of Ma Huang and Gan Cao and adds Sheng Shi Gao, Sheng Jiang, and Da Zao. However, as is the case in many of Dr. Lee's formulas, Rou Gui replaces Gui Zhi, and Cang Zhu is added due to considerations for Taiwan's humid subtropical climate.

Its name, **Major Green-Blue Dragon**, refers to the notion that after taking this formula, sweat flows and evil abates as if a dragon rose up to the skies and brought rain pouring down, thus resulting in the immediate elimination of depressed heat.

This formula is traditionally prescribed for the treatment of external contraction wind-cold exterior repletion with interior heat pattern that presents in pathoconditions such as the common cold, influenza, bronchitis, measles papules, wind papules, urticaria, and itchy skin.

Similarly, Dr. Lee prescribes **Da Qing Long Tang** for the treatment of Tai Yang cold damage with vexation and agitation from interior heat; however, for external medicine (i.e., dermatology) manifestations, he may consider prescribing formula variants, such as **Yue Bi Tang**, **Gui Zhi Ma Huang Ge Ban Tang**, or **Ma Xing Gan Shi Tang**, instead.

Da Zao Wan (大造丸/Great Creation Pill)
Zi He Che, Gui Ban, Huang Bo, Du Zhong, Niu Xi, Tian Men Dong, Mai Men Dong, Ren Shen, Di Huang

Dang Gui Bu Xue Tang (當歸補血湯)
Huang Qi, Dang Gui

Dang Gui Liu Huang Tang (當歸六黃湯)
Dang Gui, Sheng Di Huang, Shu Di Huang, Huang Qin, Huang Lian, Huang Bo, Huang Qi

Dang Gui Long Hui Wan (當歸龍薈丸)
Dang Gui, Long Dan Cao, Zhi Zi, Huang Qin, Huang Lian, Huang Bo, Da Huang, Lu Hui, Chi Fu Ling, Mu Xiang, She Xiang

Dang Gui San (當歸散)

Dang Gui, Chuan Xiong, Sheng Bai Shao	3 qian each
Sheng Di Huang, Chao Bai Zhu, Xu Duan	3 qian each
Du Zhong, Gan Cao	3 qian each
Shan Yao, Ai Ye	5 qian each
Huang Qin	2 qian

The Yu Sheng version is composed of the same essential medicinals as the original formula— Dang Gui, Chuan Xiong, Sheng Bai Shao, Chao Bai Zhu, and Huang Qin—and Shan Yao, Ai Ye, Sheng Di Huang, Xu

Duan, Du Zhong, and Gan Cao have been added. These additions complement and enhance the original formula's blood-nourishing stasis-transforming and blood-cooling fetus-quieting actions.

Sheng Di Huang clears heat and cools the blood and nourishes yin and engenders liquid; the medicinal pair Du Zhong and Xu Duan conduct medicinals downward to the lumbus (spine) and lower limbs, supplement the liver and kidney, strengthen sinew and bone, and quiet the fetus; Ai Ye warms the channels and stanches bleeding, dissipates cold and regulates menstruation, and quiets the fetus; Shan Yao boosts qi and nourishes yin, supplements the spleen, lung, and kidney, and secures essence and checks vaginal discharge; and Gan Cao boosts qi and supplements the center, clears heat and resolves toxin, relaxes tension and relieves pain, and harmonizes the nature of medicinals

Dang Gui San promotes a healthy pregnancy and treats all types of prenatal and postpartum pathoconditions. It is traditionally prescribed for women with a history of habitual abortion and/or premature labor, stirring fetus, scant blood with heat, heat vexation and thirst, hysteria, and aching lumbus and abdominal pain.

Dang Gui San is Dr. Lee's first-line formula for a broad spectrum of obstetric pathoconditions, including the prevention of spontaneous abortions due to poor implantation of the blastocyst embryo during the first two weeks of pregnancy, absence of cervical mucus, ovulation disorders (e.g., anovulation, oligoovulation), thin endometrial lining, morning sickness, preeclampsia, gestational diabetes, postpartum depression ("baby blues"), perineal pain, uterine infection, and mastitis.

Dang Gui Shao Yao San (當歸芍藥散)
Dang Gui, Shao Yao, Chuan Xiong, Fu Ling, Ze Xie, Bai Zhu

Dang Gui Si Ni Tang (當歸四逆湯)
Dang Gui, Gui Zhi, Bai Shao, Xi Xin, Gan Cao, Tong Cao, Da Zao,

Dang Gui Si Ni Jia Wu Zhu Yu Sheng Jiang Tang (當歸四逆加吳茱萸生薑湯)
Dang Gui, Gui Zhi, Bai Shao, Xi Xin, Gan Cao, Tong Cao, Da Zao, Wu Zhu Yu, Sheng Jiang

Dang Gui Yin Zi (當歸飲子)
Dang Gui, Bai Shao, Chuan Xiong, Sheng Di Huang, Bai Ji Li, Fang Feng, Jing Jie, He Shou Wu, Huang Qi, Gan Cao, Sheng Jiang

Di Dang Tang (抵擋湯/Dead-On Decoction)

Tao Ren	1 g
Meng Chong	2 g
Shui Zhi	2 g
Da Huang	3 g

Note: This formula is administered as a pulverized medicinal powder.

Di Gu Pi Yin (地骨皮飲)

Dang Gui, Chuan Xiong, Chi Shao	3 qian each
Sheng Di Huang, Gan Cao, Huang Qin	3 qian each
Cang Zhu	4 qian
Di Gu Pi, Mu Dan Pi	5 qian each

The Yu Sheng version is based on the *On Blood Pathoconditions* (血症論 *Xie Zheng Lun*) formula. It is composed of **Si Wu Tang**—Dang Gui, Chuan Xiong, Chi Shao, Sheng Di Huang—adding Di Gu Pi, Mu Dan Pi, Huang Qin, and Cang Zhu.

Si Wu Tang supplements and quickens the blood; Di Gu Pi nourishes yin and cools the blood, downbears latent heat in the lung, and supplements right qi; Mu Dan Pi drains latent heat in the blood and harmonizes, cools, and engenders blood; Huang Qin clears heat and dries dampness and drains fire and resolves toxin; and Cang Zhu fortifies the spleen and dries dampness to counteract the digestion impairment and loose stools some patients experience when administered blood-nourishing yin-enriching medicinals.

The blood-nourishing yin-enriching and heat-clearing blood-cooling actions of this formula are traditionally prescribed for the treatment of fire effulgence due to yin-vacuity, steaming bone taxation heat, heat entering the blood chamber, antepartum heat, and alternating tidal heat.

Similarly, Dr. Lee typically prescribes **Di Gu Pi Yin** for yin-vacuity blood heat with stasis heat (or Shao Yang depressed heat) pattern and steaming bone taxation heat (fever) pattern that manifest in pathoconditions such as autoimmune diseases, leukemia, lymphoma, idiopathic thrombocytopenic purpura (ITP), menopausal transition symptoms, sweating of the five hearts, dengue fever, tuberculosis, and vasculitis.

Di Huang Yin Zi (地黄飲子)

Sheng Di Huang, Ba Ji Tian, Shan Zhu Yu, Shi Hu, Rou Cong Rong, Wu Wei Zi, Rou Gui, Fu Ling, Mai Men Dong, Fu Zi, Shi Chang Pu, Yuan Zhi, Sheng Jiang, Da Zao, Bo He

Di Long San (地龍散)

Rou Gui, Di Long, Huang Bo, Gan Cao, Qiang Huo, Su Mu, Ma Huang, Tao Ren, Dang Gui, Du Huo

Di Tan Tang (滌痰湯/Phlegm-Flushing Decoction)

Ban Xia, Tian Nan Xing, Ju Hong, Zhi Shi, Fu Ling, Ren Shen, Shi Chang Pu, Zhu Ru, Gan Cao, Sheng Jiang, Da Zao

Diao Fen Gao (吊粉膏/Suspension Powder Paste)

Da Huang, Huang Bo	1 part
Ru Xiang, Mo Yao	1 part
Xu Duan, Gu Sui Bu	1 part
Chuan Wu, Cao Wu	1 part
Rice Wine	

It comprises equal parts heat-dispersing inflammation-resolving (Da Huang and Huang Bo), blood-quickening stasis-transforming and swelling-dispersing flesh-engendering (Ru Xiang and Mo Yao), sinew- and bone-strengthening and injury-treating breakage-mending (Xu Duan and Gu Sui Bu), and anesthetic and pain-relieving (Chuan Wu and Cao Wu) medicinals.

These medicinals are pulverized into medicinal powder and then mixed with rice wine (27% alcohol) to form a medicinal paste (藥膏 yào g□ o) that is applied topically as a compress in the acute stage of inflammation. This is the stage presenting with heat, pain, redness (or purplish), and swelling in traumatic injuries (e.g., sprains, subluxation, fractures).

To apply, first determine the size of the compress needed based on the site of injury and then prepare the materials (i.e., thick paper, burlap cloth, gauze, bandage, and elastic net dressing). Then, place the fine burlap cloth on the thick paper, spread **Suspension Powder Paste** on the fine burlap cloth and cover it with gauze. Apply to the site of injury and sufficiently wrap with bandage and secure it with tubular elastic net dressing (should be wrapped just tight enough to secure the cloth in place without adversely affecting circulation!).

For best efficacy, it is recommended that the medicinal paste be left on for 6 to 8 hours. However, it should be removed ahead of the recommended time in the rare case of allergic reaction (e.g., patient feels itchiness, tingling, stinging, and discomfort).

Ding Xiang San (丁香散)

Ding Xiang, Shi Di, Gan Cao, Liang Jiang

Du Huo Ji Sheng Tang (獨活寄生湯)

Shu Di Huang	8 qian
Ren Shen, Gan Jiang, Fu Zi, Qin Jiao, Xu Duan	5 qian each
Gu Sui Bu, Gui Ban, Bie Jia, Du Zhong	5 qian each
Niu Xi, Chen Pi, Du Huo, Wu Jia Pi	5 qian each
Fu Ling, Chao Shao Yao, Chao Bai Zhu	4 qian each
Dang Gui, Chuan Xiong, Rou Gui, Huang Qin	3 qian each
Fang Feng, Xi Xin, Gan Cao	3 qian each
Dang Shen, Huang Qi, Sang Ji Sheng	1 liang each

Er Chen Tang (二陳湯/Two Matured Ingredients Decoction)

Huang Qin	3 qian
Chen Pi, Ban Xia, Fu Ling, Gan Cao	4 qian each

The Yu Sheng version is similar to the original except for the subtraction of Sheng Jiang and Wu Mei and the addition of Huang Qin. Huang Qin's heat-clearing dampness-drying actions are acclimated for Taiwan's humid subtropical climate and complement this formula's overall dampness-drying phlegm-harmonizing and qi-normalizing center-harmonizing actions.

Dr. Lee commonly prescribes derivatives of **Er Chen Tang—Wen Dan Tang** and **Ban Xia Tian Ma Bai Zhu San**—for a broad scope of pathoconditions, ranging from external contraction (common cold), psychosomatic symptoms (e.g., abdominal distention, malaise, and fatigue) to infertility, glaucoma and brain tumors.

Er Miao San (二妙散/Mysterious Two Powder)

Huang Bo, Cang Zhu, Sheng Jiang Zhi (Raw Ginger Juice)

Fang Feng Tong Sheng San (防風通聖散/Saposhnikovia Sage-Inspired Powder)

Fang Feng, Jing Jie, Lian Qiao, Ma Huang, Bo He, Chuan Xiong, Dang Gui, Bai Shao, Bai Zhu, Shan Zhi Zi, Da Huang, Mang Xiao, Huang Qin, Shi Gao, Jie Geng, Gan Cao, Shi Gao, Sheng Jiang, Cong Bai

Feng Shi Fang (風濕方/Rheumatism Formula)

Ma Huang	1.5 qian
Rou Gui, Chi Shao, Gan Cao, Gan Jiang	3 qian each
Fu Zi, Huang Qin, Huang Bo, Fu Ling	3 qian each
Zhu Ling, Ze Xie, Cang Zhu, Sheng Shi Gao	3 qian each
Jin Yin Hua, Wu Wei Zi, Yin Yang Huo	3 qian each
Da Zao	5 pieces

This Yu Sheng original formula was designed by Dr. Lee early on in his clinical practice. It was specifically prescribed for patients with rheumatic disorders (e.g., osteoarthritis (OA), rheumatoid arthritis (RA)) who were either currently *being* administered or recently *had been* administered immunosuppressants (e.g., corticosteroids).

In years past, Western medical doctors in Taiwan indiscriminately prescribed systemic corticosteroids for the treatment of all types of inflammatory pain (including rheumatic pain!), without any consideration given to the deleterious side effects. This practice has been largely superseded by a more responsible approach that has in part been driven by the advent of new drugs and drug combinations.

Attuned to the pulse of our ever-evolving modern environment, nowadays, Dr. Lee typically prescribes **(Yu Sheng) Hyperactive Immune Formula**—clears heat and dries dampness, drains fire and resolves toxin (anti-inflammatory), cools the blood and eliminates steaming, and enriches yin and clears vacuity heat)—for these types of pathoconditions instead.

Fu Ling Ze Xie Tang (茯苓澤瀉湯)
Fu Ling, Ze Xie, Gan Cao, Gui Zhi, Bai Zhu, Sheng Jiang

Fu Yuan Huo Xue Tang (復原活血湯/Origin-Restorative Blood-Quickening Decoction)
Da Huang, Chai Hu, Dang Gui, Tao Ren, Hong Hua, Chuan Shan Jia, Gua Lou Gen, Gan Cao

Gan Jiang Ren Shen Ban Xia Wan (乾薑人參半下丸)
Gan Jiang, Ren Shen, Ban Xia, Sheng Jiang

Gan Lu Yin (甘露飲/Sweet Dew Beverage)
Sheng Di Huang, Shu Di Huang, Tian Men Dong, Mai Men Dong, Shi Hu, Yin Chen, Huang Qin, Zhi Ke, Pi Pa Ye, Gan Cao

Gan Mai Da Zao Tang (甘麥大棗湯)
Gan Cao, Xiao Mai, Da Zao

Gan Mai Da Zao Tang Combining Ban Xia Hou Po Tang (甘麥大棗湯合併半夏厚朴湯)

Ban Xia, Hou Po, Zi Su Zi, Fu Ling	4 qian each
Gan Cao	5 qian
Da Zao	10 pieces
Fu Xiao Mai	1 liang

This is a compound formula (複方 fù f□ng) that comprises the combination of the two minor formulas (小方 xiao f□ng) **Gan Mai Da Zao Tang** and **Ban Xia Hou Po Tang**. The composition of **Gan Mai Da Zao Tang Combining Ban Xia Hou Po Tang** is virtually identical to those two minor formulas except for the subtraction of Sheng Jiang.

Gan Mai Da Zao Tang has center-harmonizing spirit-quieting and tension-relaxing agitation-calming actions, and is traditionally prescribed for the treatment of visceral agitation. **Ban Xia Hou Po Tang** has qi-moving counterflow-downbearing and stagnation-dissipating phlegm-transforming actions, and is traditionally prescribed for the treatment of seven-affect binding depression (七情鬱結 q□ qíng yù jié) (e.g., anxiety, depression, hypomania), insomnia, palpitations, gastrointestinal neurosis, vocal cord nodules and polyps, plum-pit qi, and symptoms of menopausal transition.

Considering that the actions and indications of these two minor formulas are complementary, Dr. Lee has combined them to form **Gan Mai Da Zao Tang Combining Ban Xia Hou Po Tang**, which he prescribes for the treatment of a broad spectrum of mood, psychosomatic, and neuropsychiatric disorders (e.g., mild cases of Tourette syndrome), including those mentioned above.

For patients presenting with phlegm reversal and ascending counterflow symptoms (e.g., abdominal distention, headache, malaise, fatigue), Dr. Lee may prescribe this compound formula combined with **Ban Xia Tian Ma Bai Zhu San**. And for relatively mild pathoconditions, he may simply prescribe one of these minor formulas on its own.

Ge Gen Qin Lian Tang (葛根芩連湯/aka **Ge Gen Huang Qin Huang Lian Tang)**

Ge Gen, Huang Qin, Huang Lian, Gan Cao

Ge Gen Tang (葛根湯)

Ma Huang	1.5 liang
Huang Qin, Cang Zhu	3 qian each
Ge Gen, Chi Shao, Gan Cao, Rou Gui, Sheng Jiang	5 qian each
Da Zao	5 pieces

The Yu Sheng version is similar to the original formula, which is a derivative of **Gui Zhi Tang**. However, just as in many of Dr. Lee's other formulas, Rou Gui replaces Gui Zhi and Chi Shao replaces Bai Shao, and Cang Zhu and Huang Qin are added due to considerations for Taiwan's humid subtropical climate. This formula promotes sweating and resolves the exterior and upbears liquid and courses the channels.

Dr. Lee commonly prescribes variants of this formula for external contraction with Yang Ming headache and body ache, heat effusion (fever) without sweating, aversion to cold, stretched stiffness of the nape and back (項背強几几 xiàng bèi qiáng sh□ sh□), crick in the neck, and sinusitis. This formula is also prescribed for patients with acute stage facial palsy (caused by trauma or tumor), Bell's palsy (caused by a virus), or trigeminal neuralgia, who have *not* been prescribed corticosteroids.

The inclusion of Huang Qin and Cang Zhu in the Yu Sheng version of this formula also makes it easily modified into **Ge Gen Huang Qin Huang Lian Tang** (by adding Huang Lian) for the treatment of heat evil entering the interior causing diarrhea or dysentery (gastroenteritis) and exterior evil that has not yet resolved.

Ge Xia Zhu Yu Tang (膈下逐瘀湯/Infradiaphragmatic Stasis-Expelling Decoction)
Wu Ling Zhi, Dang Gui, Chuan Xiong, Tao Ren, Mu Dan Pi, Chi Shao, Wu Yao, Yan Hu Suo, Gan Cao, Xiang Fu, Hong Hua, Zhi Ke

Gua Lou Niu Bang Zi Tang (栝蔞牛蒡子湯)
Gua Luo Ren, Niu Bang Zi, Hua Fen, Huang Qin, Sheng Zhi Zi, Lian Qiao

Gui Lu Er Xian Jiao (龜鹿二仙膠/Tortoise Shell and Deerhorn Two Immortals Glue)
Lu Jiao, Gui Ban, Ren Shen, Gou Qi Zi

Gui Ma Ge Ban Tang – refer to **Gui Zhi Ma Huang Ge Ban Tang**

Gui Pi Tang (歸脾湯/Spleen-Returning Decoction)
Ren Shen, Huang Qi, Bai Zhu, Fu Ling, Dang Gui, Suan Zao Ren, Gui Yuan Rou, Yuan Zhi, Mu Xiang, Gan Cao, Sheng Jiang, Da Zao

Gui Qi Jian Zhong Tang (歸耆建中湯/Chinese Angelica and Astragalus Center-Fortifying Decoction)

Dang Gui	2 qian
Gan Jiang, Huang Qin, Cang Zhu	3 qian each
Rou Gui, Chi Shao, Gan Cao, Fu Zi	5 qian each
Da Zao	5 pieces
Huang Qi	1 liang

This formula is derived from **Xiao Jian Zhong Tang** adding Dang Gui and Huang Qi. The Yu Sheng version of this formula is similar to the original version, but includes large doses of Huang Qi; Chi Shao replaces Bai Shao, Gan Jiang replaces Sheng Jiang, and a large dose of Rou Gui (superior quality and efficacy!) replaces Gui Pi. Plus, Cang Zhu, Huang Qin, Da Zao, and a large dose of Fu Zi are added.

Huang Qin's heat-clearing dampness-drying and fire-draining toxin-resolving actions counteract the great heat of The Three Great Yang-Supplementers—Gan Jiang, Rou Gui, and Fu Zi. Huang Qi functions as a conductor for the *upper* limbs and Rou Gui functions as a conductor for the *four* extremities (limbs).

The additions to the Yu Sheng version of this formula enhance its qi-supplementing center-fortifying, tension-relaxing interior-harmonizing, and blood supplementing actions, while also equipping it with the capacity to treat vacuity cold pathoconditions specifically for, but *not* limited to, the *upper* body.

Dr. Lee commonly prescribes this formula for cold impediment of the Tai Yang small intestine channel, neuropathy, frozen shoulder, and Raynaud disease (and phenomenon); and for skin pathoconditions (e.g., non-erupting papules (acne), menopausal pruritis).

Gui Zhi Fu Ling Wan (桂枝茯苓丸)

Rou Gui, Fu Ling	4 qian each
Mu Dan Pi, Chi Shao, Tao Ren	4 qian each
Gan Cao, Cang Zhu	3 qian each

Gui Zhi Jia Hou Po Xing Ren Tang (桂枝加厚朴杏仁湯)

Gui Zhi, Bai Shao, Gan Cao, Sheng Jiang, Da Zao, Hou Po, Xing Ren

Gui Zhi Jia Long Gu Mu Li Tang (桂枝加龍骨牡蠣湯)

Cang Zhu	4 qian
Rou Gui, Chi Shao, Gan Cao, Sheng Jiang	5 qian each
Sheng Long Gu, Sheng Mu Li, Shan Yao, Dang Shen	5 qian each
Da Zao	5 pieces

The Yu Sheng version contains all of the essential medicinals of the original formula with the exception of Rou Gui replacing Gui Zhi and the addition of Dang Shen, Shan Yao, and Cang Zhu. The qi-boosting spleen-fortifying and essence-securing dampness-drying actions of these additional medicinals complement this formula's overall action of neutrally supplementing yin and yang, subduing and settling, and securing essence and containing urine.

This formula is traditionally prescribed for pathoconditions such as vacuity taxation with dual yin and yang vacuity, dreaming with seminal emission, hypertonicity of the lesser abdomen, lower burner vacuity cold, stirring palpitations below the umbilicus resulting from urinary incontinence, and hysteria.

In addition to these pathoconditions, Dr. Lee also prescribes **Gui Zhi Jia Long Gu Mu Li Tang** for the treatment of juvenile acne, stress-related hair loss (e.g., alopecia areata, hair shedding (telogen effluvium), hair pulling disorder (trichotillomania)), and children with hyperactivity or impulsivity (e.g., attention deficit hyperactivity disorder (ADHD)). Early on in Dr. Lee's clinical practice, he would prescribe this formula for obstetrics pathoconditions, but in recent years he typically prescribes **Dang Gui San** variants instead.

Gui Zhi Ma Huang Ge Ban Tang (桂枝麻黃各半湯)
Gui Zhi, Ma Huang, Shao Yao, Sheng Jiang, Xing Ren, Gan Cao, Da Zao

Gui Zhi Ren Shen Tang (桂枝人參湯)
Gui Zhi, Gan Cao, Bai Zhu, Ren Shen, Gan Jiang

Gui Zhi Tang – refer to **Yang Dan Tang**

He Che Da Zao Wan (河車大造丸/Placenta Great Creation Pill)
Ren Shen, Huang Qi, Bai Zhu, Dang Gui, Suan Zao Ren, Yuan Zhi, Bai Shao, Shan Yao, Fu Ling, Gou Qi Zi, Shou Di, Zi He Che, Lu Jiao, Gui Ban

Hei Xi Dan (黑錫丹)
Hei Xi, Liu Huang, Chen Xiang, Fu Zi, Hu Lu Ba, Yang Qi Shi, Xiao Hui Xiang, Bu Gu Zhi, Rou Dou Kou, Chuan Lian Zi, Mu Xiang, Rou Gui

Huan Hun Tang (還魂湯)

Ma Huang, Xing Ren, Gan Cao

Huan Shao Dan (還少丹/Rejuvenation Elixir)
Shu Di Huang, Shan Yao, Niu Xi, Gou Qi, Shan Zhu Rou, Fu Ling, Du Zhong, Yuan Zhi, Wu Wei Zi, Chu Shi, Xiao Hui Xiang, Ba Ji Tian, Rou Cong Rong, Shi Chang Pu

Huang Lian Jie Du Tang (黃連解毒湯/Coptis Toxin-Resolving Decoction)

Huang Lian, Huang Qin, Huang Bo, Zhi Zi	3 qian each
Cang Zhu	4 qian
Gan Cao	5 qian

The Yu Sheng version is virtually the same as the original formula except for the addition of Cang Zhu and Gan Cao. The essential medicinals of this formula are The Three Yellows—Huang Qin, Huang Bo, and Huang Lian—which Dr. Lee commonly utilizes for their heat-clearing dampness drying and fire-draining toxin-resolving (antimicrobial and anti-inflammatory) actions.

Cang Zhu fortifies the spleen, dries dampness, and dispels wind-damp; and Gan Cao boosts qi and supplements the center, clears heat and resolves toxin, dispels phlegm and suppresses cough, relaxes tension and relieves pain, and harmonizes the nature of medicinals. Together, the medicinal pair Cang Zhu and Gan Cao promotes digestion and protects the stomach from the bitter flavor and cold nature of the essential medicinals.

Plus, Huang Bo clears heat and dries dampness, drains lower burner fire, resolves toxin, and serves as a foot Tai Yang channel conductor. Together, the medicinal pair Cang Zhu and Huang Bo clears heat and dries dampness, disperses swelling and relieves pain, and eliminates dampness for the treatment of damp-heat pouring downward pattern (e.g., strangury-turbidity, dribbling urinary block, vaginal discharge, damp-heat diarrhea) and wilting pattern (e.g., myasthenia gravis) pathoconditions.

Huang Lian Jie Du Tang is a commonly administered formula for triple burner heat toxin pattern. Huang Lian drains heart fire and middle burner fire; Huang Qin drains upper burner fire; Huang Bo drains lower burner fire; and Zhi Zi frees and drains heat in all three burners, abducting heat downward where the heat evil is excreted in the urine. The combination of these medicinals contains potent heat-clearing toxin-resolving actions that provide exceptional broad-spectrum antimicrobial and anti-inflammatory efficacy for the treatment of all types of infections and inflammation throughout the entire body (e.g., upper respiratory, gastrointestinal, hepatic, renal, genitourinary, musculoskeletal, autoimmune disorders).

It is important to note here that long-term administration (≥ 3 months) of Zhi Zi may cause transient blue-gray or bronze skin pigmentation in some patients. In cases where long-term administration is necessary, Dr. Lee will either subtract Zhi Zi or prescribe another formula, such as **Hyperactive Immune Formula** (clears heat and dries dampness, drains fire and resolves toxin (anti-inflammatory), cools the blood and eliminates steaming, and enriches yin and clears vacuity heat), instead.

Huang Long Tang (黃龍湯/Yellow Dragon Decoction)
Da Huang, Mang Xiao, Zhi Shi, Hou Po, Gan Cao, Ren Shen, Dang Gui, Sheng Jiang, Da Zao, Jie Geng

Huang Qin Tang (黃芩湯)
Huang Qin, Bai Shao, Gan Cao, Da Zao

Hui Yang Sheng Xian Tang (回陽升陷湯/Yang-Returning Fall-Upbearing Decoction)
Huang Qi, Gan Jiang, Dang Gui, Gui Zhi, Gan Cao

Huo Luo Dan (活絡丹/Network-Quickening Elixir)

Dang Gui, Ru Xiang, Mo Yao	5 jin each
Dan Shen, Di Long, Chuan Wu	5 jin each
Wu Cao, Tian Nan Xing, Ma Huang	5 jin each

The Yu Sheng version is similar to the original formula, which is also known as **Xiao Huo Luo Dan (小活絡丹/Minor Network-Quickening Elixir)**, except for the addition of Dang Gui, Dan Shen, and Ma Huang.

Dang Gui supplements and quickens the blood; Dan Shen quickens the blood and dispels stasis; and Ma Huang "opens up" and transports medicinals across all membranes. These additions complement and enhance this formula's overall wind-dispelling dampness-dispersing, blood-quickening stasis-dispelling, and network vessel-freeing pain-relieving actions.

This formula is traditionally prescribed for the treatment of wind-cold-damp evil invading the channels and network vessels, contraction and pain of the sinews and vessels, inhibited bending and stretching of the joints, and wandering aches and pain; insensitivity of the limbs following stroke and phlegm-damp dead blood in the channels and network vessels; and knocks and falls (traumatic injury) and stasis obstruction in the channels and network vessels causing pain.

Dr. Lee utilizes **Huo Luo Dan**'s blood-quickening stasis-dispelling and channel- and network vessel-freeing actions to achieve exceptional efficacy in relieving pain, particularly for wind-damp impediment and traumatic injuries involving the lumbus and lower limbs. This pill is produced and processed in-house, using a strictly controlled fermentation method and oven-roast process that safely ensures elimination of the potential for toxicity.

Hyperactive Immune Formula (免疫過抗方/Mian Yi Guo Kang Fang)

Huang Lian, Huang Qin, Huang Bo, Cang Zhu	5 qian each
Qing Hao, Zhi Mu, Di Gu Pi	5 qian each

This formula was designed relatively later in Dr. Lee's clinical practice, primarily for the treatment of connective tissue diseases, degenerative disorders, and systemic inflammation in patients who have *not* been administered immunosuppressants (e.g., systemic corticosteroids, high dose methotrexate (MTX)), those who *have* been administered immunosuppressants for ≤ 1 week, or those who *have* previously been administered immunosuppressants, but sufficient *time has elapsed* for its suppressive effects to wear off.

It is composed of the essential medicinals from **(Yu Sheng) Huang Lian Jie Du Tang**—The Three Yellows (Huang Lian, Huang Qin, and Huang Bo) and Cang Zhu—along with the addition of Qing Hao, Zhi Mu, and Di Gu Pi. These medicinals combine to form a potent combination of heat-clearing dampness drying, fire-draining toxin-resolving (anti-inflammatory), blood-cooling steam-eliminating, and yin-enriching vacuity heat-clearing actions for the treatment of effulgent yin vacuity fire, yin vacuity internal heat, and yin vacuity taxation heat with blood heat pattern pathoconditions.

As mentioned in the **Feng Shi Fang (Rheumatism Formula)** profile, the evolving practices of Western medicine in Taiwan have been trending away from the indiscriminate administration of systemic corticosteroids. In response, Dr. Lee now commonly prescribes **Hyperactive Immune Formula** for treating patients with a broad scope of autoimmune and degenerative pathoconditions that present with both acute and chronic inflammation, including osteoarthritis (OA), rheumatoid arthritis (RA), ankylosing spondylitis (AS), systemic lupus erythematosus (SLE), polymyositis, dermatomyositis, scleroderma, multiple sclerosis (MS), Behcet disease (BD), Sjogren's syndrome (SS), immune thrombocytopenic purpura (ITP), inflammatory bowel disease (IBS), and vasculitis.

In addition to applying eight-principle and six-channel pattern identification, lab tests that include inflammatory indices (e.g., erythrocyte sedimentation rate (ESR), antinuclear antibody (ANA), rheumatoid factor (RF)) are invaluable diagnostic tools for determining the severity of inflammation and gauging clinical efficacy.

Hyperactive Immune Formula provides reliable and lasting effectiveness in resolving inflammation and relieving symptoms (i.e., treat the tip). Once the inflammation is under control, the patient can proceed on to other nourishing and supplementing TCM formulas in the process of bringing the pathocondition into complete remission (i.e., treat the root).

Jia Wei Er Miao San (加味二妙散/Supplemented Mysterious Two Powder)
Cang Zhu, Huang Bo, Gui Ban, Bi Xie, Zhi Mu

Jia Wei Xiao Chai Hu Tang (加味小柴胡湯/Supplemented Minor Bupleurum Decoction)
Chai Hu, Huang Qin, Zhi Mu, Dang Shen, Bie Jia, Ban Xia, Chang Shan, Cao Guo, Gan Cao, Jiu Qu, Sheng Jiang, Da Zao

Jia Wei Xiao Yao San (加味逍遙散/Supplemented Free Wanderer Powder)

Dang Gui, Fu Ling, Zhi Zi, Bo He, Shao Yao, Chai Hu, Gan Cao, Bai Zhu, Mu Dan Pi, Wei Jiang

Jian Ling Tang (健瓴湯/Sweeping Down Decoction)

Ci Shi	3 qian
Bo Zi Ren	4 qian
Niu Xi, Chi Shao, Sheng Long Gu	5 qian each
Sheng Mu Li, Sheng Di Huang, Shan Yao	5 qian each
Dai Zhe Shi	8 qian

The Yu Sheng version is virtually the same as the original formula except for Chi Shao replacing Bai Shao and the addition of Ci Shi. As in many Yu Sheng formulas, Chi Shao is selected for its superior blood-quickening stasis-dispelling actions.

The essential medicinals of this spirit-quieting by heavy settling formula are Dai Zhe Shi—enters the blood aspect of the liver and heart channels, eliminates heat, calms the liver and subdues yang, and downbears counterflow by heavy settling; Ci Shi—enters the liver and kidney channels, governs the lung and kidney, settles fright and quiets the spirit, and calms the liver and subdues yang; Sheng Long Gu—enters the heart, liver, and kidney channels, subdues yang, and quiets the spirit; and Sheng Mu Li—calms the liver and subdues yang, softens hardness and dissipates binds, and astringes and secures.

Dr. Lee typically reserves **Jian Ling Tang** for only the most severe cases of ascendant hyperactivity of yang pattern or yin vacuity with hyperactivity of yang pattern that manifest in pathoconditions such as hyperglycemia (diabetes), hypertension, hyperthyroidism, recalcitrant insomnia, schizophrenia, and Tourette syndrome. This includes cases in which Western medicine drug therapy has been administered without efficacy, or with initial efficacy, but is no longer able to effectively control the pathocondition.

Jin Suo Gu Jing Wan (金鎖固精丸/Golden Lock Essence-Securing Pill)

Sha Yuan Zi, Qian Shi, Lian Xu, Long Gu, Mu Li, Lian Zi Fen

Jing Fang Bai Du San (荊防敗毒散/Schizonepeta and Saposhnikovia Toxin-Vanquishing Powder)
Jing Jie, Fang Feng, Chai Hu, Fu Ling, Jie Geng, Chuan Xiong, Qiang Huo, Du Huo, Zhi Ke, Gan Cao, Sheng Jiang

Ju He Wan (橘核丸)
Ju He, Hai Zao, Kun Bu, Hai Dai, Chuan Lian Zi, Tao Ren, Ho Po, Yu Zhi Zi, Zhi Shi, Yan Hu Suo, Gui Xin, Mu Xiang

Ju Pi Zhu Ru Tang (橘皮竹茹湯)
Ju Pi, Zhu Ru, Da Zao, Dang Shen, Gan Cao, Sheng Jiang

Li Zhong Tang (理中湯/Center-Rectifying Decoction/aka **Ren Shen Tang)**
Bai Zhu, Ren Shen, Gan Jiang, Gan Cao

Liang Ge San (涼膈散/Diaphragm-Cooling Powder)

Lian Qiao, Huang Qin, Bo He Ye	3 qian each
Zhu Ye, Shan Zhi Zi, Gan Cao	3 qian each
Da Huang, Mang Xiao	1 qian each
Cang Zhu	4 qian

Ling Gui Zao Gan Tang (苓桂棗甘湯)
Fu Ling, Gui Zhi, Da Zao, and Gan Cao

Ling Gui Zhu Gan Tang (苓桂朮甘湯)
Fu Ling, Gui Zhi, Bai Zhu, Gan Cao

Liu Jun Zi Tang (六君子湯/Six Gentlemen Decoction)
Ren Shen, Gan Cao, Fu Ling, Bai Zhu, Chen Pi, Ban Xia, Sheng Jiang, Da Zao

Liu Wei Di Huang Wan (六味地黃丸/Six-Ingredient Rehmannia Decoction)
Shu Di Huang, Shan Zhu Yu, Shan Yao, Ze Xie, Fu Ling, Mu Dan Pi

Liu Yi San (六一散/Six-To-One Powder)
Hua Shi, Gan Cao

Liu Yu Tang (六鬱湯/Six Depressions Decoction)

Xiang Fu, Cang Zhu, Shen Qu, Shan Zhi Ren, Lian Qiao, Chen Pi, Chuan Xiong, Bei Mu, Zhi Ke, Bai Fu Ling, Su Geng, Gan Cao

Long Dan Xie Gan Tang (龍膽瀉肝湯/Gentian Liver-Draining Decoction)

Long Dan Cao, Huang Qin, Zhi Zi, Dang Gui	3 qian each
Sheng Di Huang, Mu Tong, Chai Hu, Che Qian Zi	3 qian each
Cang Zhu, Ze Xie	4 qian each
Sheng Gan Cao	5 qian

The Yu Sheng version is identical to the original except for the addition of Cang Zhu, with its wind-damp dispelling actions further complementing this formula's potent overall liver and gallbladder repletion fire-draining and lower burner damp-heat-clearing actions.

Traditionally, this formula is prescribed for *liver and gallbladder repletion fire flaming upward* pattern pathoconditions presenting with rib-side pain (e.g., herpes zoster) and headache (e.g., acute hepatitis, acute cholecystitis), red eyes (e.g., acute conjunctivitis, keratitis) and bitter taste in mouth, and deafness and swelling of the ear (e.g., otitis media, sinusitis); and *liver channel damp-heat pouring downward* pattern pathoconditions presenting with urinary dribbling and strangury-turbidity (e.g., urinary tract infection, enlarged prostate), pudendal itch, genital swelling (e.g., acute epididymitis), and vaginal discharge (e.g., vaginitis).

In addition to these pathoconditions, Dr. Lee also administers **Long Dan Xie Gan Tang** for pain wind (痛風 tòng f□ng) (gout and pseudogout) and patients infected with the human immunodeficiency virus (HIV+) in order to lower viral load and increase CD4 cell counts.

Lu Fu Gan Shi Fen – refer to **Antler Aconite Ginger Gypsum Powder**

Ma Huang Fu Zi Xi Xin Tang (麻黃附子細辛湯)
Ma Huang, Fu Zi, Xi Xin

Ma Huang Jia Zhu Tang (麻黃加朮湯)
Ma Huang, Gui Zhi, Gan Cao, Xing Ren, Bai Zhu

Ma Huang Lian Yao Chi Xiao Dou Tang (麻黃連軺赤芍豆湯)
Ma Huang, Lian Yao (aka Lian Qiao Gen), Xing Ren, Chi Xiao Dou, Da Zao, Zi Bai Pi, Sheng Jiang, Gan Cao

Ma Huang Tang (麻黃湯)
Ma Huang, Gui Zhi, Gan Cao, Xing Ren

Ma Xing Gan Shi Tang (麻杏甘石湯)

Ma Huang	1.5 qian
Cang Zhu	3 qian
Xing Ren	4 qian
Gan Cao	5 qian
Shi Gao	1 liang

The Yu Sheng version is identical to the original formula except for the addition of Cang Zhu, which is included for its wind-damp dispelling dampness-drying actions.

This formula's heat-draining, lung-diffusing panting-calming, and cough-suppressing actions are traditionally administered for the treatment of externally contracted wind-cold and exuberant lung heat, failure to resolve generalized heat (fever), and panting counterflow and rapid breathing.

Dr. Lee typically prescribes **Ma Xing Gan Shi Tang** for the treatment of the common cold (exterior wind-heat external contraction), acute bronchitis, and pneumonia. Additionally, Dr. Lee may also add Yi Yi Ren to form a **Ma Xing Yi Gan Tang** variant for the treatment of wind-damp exterior pattern external medicine (dermatological) pathoconditions (e.g., eczema, urticaria, seborrheic dermatitis).

Ma Xing Yi Gan Tang (麻杏薏甘湯/aka **Ma Huang Xing Ren Yi Yi Ren Gan Cao Tang)**
Ma Huang, Gan Cao, Yi Yi Ren, Xing Ren

Mai Men Dong Tang (麥門冬湯)

Ma Huang	1.5 qian
Xing Ren, Cang Zhu	4 qian each
Mai Men Dong, Xuan Shen, Ban Xia	5 qian each

Gan Cao, Shan Yao, Sheng Jiang	5 qian each
Da Zao	5 pieces

The Yu Sheng version contains the entire composition of the original formula—Mai Men Dong, Ban Xia, Ren Shen (pulverized powder instead of decocting pieces), Gan Cao, and Da Zao—except for the subtraction of Jing Mi. Plus, Dr. Lee has added Ma Huang, Xing Ren, Cang Zhu, Xuan Shen, Shan Yao, and Sheng Jiang. Just as in **Jia Wei Mai Men Dong Tang**, Shan Yao replaces Jing Mi. These additions complement the overall yin-enriching, lung- and stomach-nourishing, and counterflow-downbearing qi-precipitating actions of this classic formula.

Xuan Shen (clears heat and cools the blood and nourishes yin and resolves toxin) and Shan Yao (boosts qi and nourishes yin, supplements the spleen, lung, and kidneys, and secures essence) complement the actions of Mai Men Dong (nourishes yin, engenders liquid, and moistens the lung) and Ren Shen (supplements the spleen, boosts the lung, and engenders liquid). Ma Huang promotes sweating and resolves the exterior, diffuses the lung and calms panting, disinhibits water and disperses swelling, frees the nasal orifice, and relieves itch; Xing Ren suppresses cough, calms panting, and dispels phlegm; and Cang Zhu dries dampness, fortifies the spleen, and dispels wind-damp.

Traditionally, **Mai Men Dong Tang** is prescribed for the treatment of lung yin vacuity, lung wilting, upflaming vacuity fire, and qi counterflow panting and coughing. These types of pathoconditions typically result from microbial infections (i.e., bacteria, virus, fungi) that damage the mucous membranes of the respiratory tract (e.g., larynx, trachea, bronchi) and inhibit the secretion of epithelial lining fluid (ELF). In health, this fluid maintains epithelial moisture, traps particulate material and pathogens moving through the airway, and transports mucous (e.g., metabolic waste, pus, phlegm-rheum) upwards through the trachea towards the mouth, where it is either coughed out or swallowed.

Dr. Lee classifies these types of pathoconditions as yin vacuity cough (陰虛發咳 y□n x□ f□ ké) (aka dryness cough) in the lung and kidney channels. **Mai Men Dong Tang** functions to promote healing of these mucous membranes and serves to restore normal regulation of fluid secretion in the respiratory tract. He will also prescribe this formula for caustic damage of the mucous membranes (e.g., mouth, throat) and skin (e.g., redness, blistering and peeling) caused by the side effects of radiotherapy in cancer (e.g., head and neck) patients.

Additionally, Dr. Lee utilizes the medicinal pair Ma Huang and Xing Ren—exterior-resolving skin conductor—along with this formula's overall yin-enriching and lung- and stomach-nourishing actions for the treatment of yin vacuity pattern dermatological pathoconditions (e.g., palmer hyperhidrosis, recalcitrant contact dermatitis).

Medicated Thread – refer to **Yu Sheng Medicated Thread**

Paralysis Formula Series (截癱方系)

These three formulas were specially designed early on in Dr. Lee's clinical practice for the treatment of paresis and paralysis (correlating with wilting pattern (**痿證** w□i zhèng) in TCM classical pathologic terminology) that results from traumatic injury (including iatrogenic), microbial infection, and degenerative diseases of autoimmune and hereditary etiology.

Each formula in this series has a specific function throughout the various stages of the pathocondition. Since the determination of treatment is based on signs, symptoms, and pattern identification, in addition to the selections in this **Paralysis Formula** series, Dr. Lee may also prescribe other formulas for the treatment of paresis, paralysis, and neuropathies. For instance, in cases involving paralysis induced by viral infection, if the patient has *not* yet been administered corticosteroids and it is still in the acute stage (approximately < 3 to 4 days), Dr. Lee will approach this as an external contraction exterior wind-heat pattern, prescribing a formula such as **Ge Gen Tang** variant, with its cool acrid exterior-resolving actions combined with other orifice-freeing medicinals (e.g., Di Long).

The typical protocol is as follows:

Paralysis Formula #1 (Di Long San Variant) (截癱一號方 (地龍散加方))—acute stage (approximately ≤ 1 week following the onset of symptoms, *unless* corticosteroids have already been administered)—presenting with static blood and metabolic waste (e.g., hyaline degeneration, inflammatory factors) that congests the vasculature, channels, and network vessels, which can be identified as collection of static blood pattern; **Paralysis Formula #2 (Shi Quan Da Bu Tang Variant) (截癱二號方 (十全大補湯加方))**—post-acute and chronic stage (approximately ≥ 1 week)—presenting with enduring symptoms that can be identified as dual qi and blood vacuity pattern, and specifically, for cases involving cervical and thoracic spine injuries; and **Paralysis Formula #3 (You Gui Yin Variant) (截癱三號方 (右歸飲加方))**—post-acute and chronic stage (approximately ≥ 1 week)—presenting with enduring symptoms that can be identified as kidney yang vacuity pattern, and specifically, for cases involving lumbar spine injuries.

Formula Paralysis #1 (Di Long San Variant)
(截癱一號方 (地龍散加方))

Ma Huang, Hong Hua	1.5 qian each
Tao Ren, Gan Cao, Gan Jiang, Rou Gui	3 qian each
Di Long, Dang Gui, Huang Bo	3 qian each
Du Zhong	4 qian
Wei Ling Xian, Niu Xi, Fu Zi	5 qian each

The Yu Sheng version is composed of the original formula's essential medicinals—Di Long, Tao Ren, Rou Gui, Huang Bo, Gan Cao, Ma Huang, and Dang Gui—along with the addition of Hong Hua, Niu Xi, Wei Ling Xian, Gan Jiang, Fu Zi, and Du Zhong.

Hong Hua, Niu Xi, and Wei Ling Xian enhance the formula's blood-quickening stasis-dispelling, blood-supplementing blood-breaking, and channel-freeing actions. Wei Ling Xian is a Tai Yang urinary bladder channel medicinal that perfuses the twelve channels and network vessels; and Du Zhong and Niu Xi supplement the liver and kidney, strengthen sinew and bone, and serve as lumbus (spine) and lower limb conductors.

The medicinal combination Gan Jiang, Fu Zi, and Rou Gui—The Three Great Yang-Supplementers—form one of the pillars of Dr. Lee's therapeutic approaches, boosting the metabolism by innervating the central nervous system (CNS) and peripheral nervous system (PNS), repairing damaged cells, rejuvenating weakened cells, and promoting tissue regeneration.

Ma Huang "opens up" and transports other medicinals across all membranes of the body down to the cellular level, thus making it an effective "systemic" conductor, and its action of opening the nine orifices innervates the nervous system (i.e., CNS, PNS, ANS). Di Long is a Tai Yang urinary bladder channel medicinal that extinguishes wind, clears heat and disinhibits urine, and frees the channels and quickens the network vessels. Together, the medicinal pair Ma Huang and Di Long serves as a nervous system conductor.

Huang Bo clears heat and resolves toxin, abates heat and dries dampness, drains fire and eliminates steam in the lower burner, and counteracts the heat of The Three Great Yang-Supplementers. And Gan Cao supplements the center, relieves pain, and harmonizes the nature of medicinals.

The original formula is traditionally prescribed for the treatment of knocks and falls, pain in the cervical, thoracic, and lumbar spine, pain in the arms, accumulations and gatherings in the abdomen, and blood stasis and static blood pain.

As mentioned in the **Paralysis Formula Series** introduction, Dr. Lee typically administers **Formula Paralysis #1** during the acute stage (approximately ≤ 1 week following the onset of symptoms, *unless* corticosteroids have already been administered) that presents with static blood and metabolic waste (e.g., hyaline degeneration, inflammatory factors) congesting the vasculature, channels, and network vessels, which can be identified as collection of static blood pattern.

Paralysis Formula #2 (Shi Quan Da Bu Tang Variant)
(截癱二號方 (十全大補湯加方)

Da Huang	5 fen
Ma Huang	1.5 qian
Dan Shen, Chao Bai Zhu, Fu Ling, Gan Cao	3 qian each
Dang Gui, Chuan Xiong, Chi Shao	3 qian each
Sheng Di Huang, Huang Qi, Rou Gui	3 qian each
Di Long, Niu Xi, Huang Qin, Gan Jiang	3 qian each
Fu Zi	5 qian

This formula is composed of **(Yu Sheng) Shi Quan Da Bu Tang** with Chao Bai Zhu replacing Cang Zhu for its emphasis on supplementing qi and fortifying the spleen, along with the addition of Da Huang, Ma Huang, Di Long, and Niu Xi.

Da Huang drains and precipitates, attacks accumulations, clears heat and drains fire, quickens the blood and dispels stasis, and resolves toxin to effectively lower intracranial pressure, relieve tension in the diaphragm, and promote lysis of hyaline degeneration and the removal of metabolic waste that obstructs the flow of neurotransmitters across the synaptic cleft.

Ma Huang "opens up" and transports other medicinals across all membranes of the body down to the cellular level, thus making it an effective "systemic" conductor, and its action of opening the nine orifices innervates the nervous system (i.e., CNS, PNS, and ANS). Di Long is a Tai Yang urinary bladder channel medicinal that extinguishes wind, clears heat and disinhibits urine, and frees the channels and quickens the network vessels. Together, the medicinal pair Ma Huang and Di Long serves as a nervous system conductor. Niu Xi quickens the blood and frees the channels, supplements the liver and kidney, strengthens sinew and bone, and conducts fire (blood) downward.

The addition of the draining and precipitating, water-disinhibiting, accumulation-dispersing, blood-quickening stasis-transforming, wind-extinguishing, and channel-freeing network vessel-quickening medicinals complements and enhances the blood-quickening blood-supplementing, qi-boosting spleen-fortifying, and kidney yang-supplementing actions of **Shi Quan Da Bu Tang**.

As mentioned in the **Paralysis Formula Series** introduction, Dr. Lee typically administers **Paralysis Formula #2** during the post-acute and chronic stage (approximately ≥ 1 week) that presents with enduring symptoms, which can be identified as dual qi and blood vacuity pattern, and specifically, for cases involving cervical and thoracic spine injuries.

Paralysis Formula #3 (You Gui Yin Variant)
(截癱三號方 (右歸飲加方))

Da Huang	5 fen
Ma Huang	1.5 qian

Fu Ling, Dang Gui	2 qian each
Gou Qi Zi, Niu Xi, Du Zhong, Huang Bo	3 qian each
Di Long, Gan Jiang, Rou Gui	3 qian each
Sheng Di Huang, Shan Zhu Yu, Shan Yao, Tu Si Zi	4 qian each
Fu Zi	5 qian

This formula is derived from **(Yu Sheng) You Gui Yin** subtracting Cang Zhu and adding Di Long, Da Huang, and Ma Huang, just as in the **Paralysis #2 Formula (Shi Quan Da Bu Tang Variant)** above.

Ma Huang "opens up" and transports other medicinals across all membranes of the body down to the cellular level, thus making it an effective "systemic" conductor, and its action of opening the nine orifices innervates the nervous system (i.e., CNS, PNS, and ANS). Di Long is a Tai Yang urinary bladder channel medicinal that extinguishes wind, clears heat and disinhibits urine, and frees the channels and quickens the network vessels. Together, the medicinal pair Ma Huang and Di Long serves as a nervous system conductor.

Da Huang drains and precipitates, attacks accumulations, clears heat and drains fire, quickens the blood and dispels stasis, and resolves toxin to effectively lower intracranial pressure, relieve tension in the diaphragm, and promote lysis of hyaline degeneration and the removal of metabolic waste that obstructs the flow of neurotransmitters across the synaptic cleft.

The addition of the draining and precipitating, water-disinhibiting, accumulation-dispersing, blood-quickening stasis-transforming, wind-extinguishing, and channel-freeing network vessel-quickening medicinals complements and enhances the overall kidney yang-warming and -supplementing, blood-quickening stasis-dissipating, sinew- and bone-strengthening, and dampness-eliminating pain-relieving actions of this formula.

As mentioned in the **Paralysis Formula Series** introduction, Dr. Lee typically administers **Paralysis Formula #3** during the post-acute and chronic stage (approximately $\geq$ 1 week) that presents with enduring symptoms, which can be identified as kidney yang vacuity pattern, and specifically, for cases involving lumbar spine injuries.

Ping Wei San (平胃散/Stomach-Calming Powder)
Chen Pi, Hou Po, Cang Zhu, Gan Cao, Sheng Jiang, Da Zao

Po Xiao Dang Bao Tang (朴硝盪胞湯/Po Xiao Uterus-Flushing Decoction)

Da Huang, Mang Xiao	1 qian each
Rou Gui, Fu Ling, Mu Dan Pi, Chi Shao	3 qian each
Tao Ren, Dang Shen, Gan Cao	3 qian each
Niu Xi, Dang Gui, Hou Po, Xi Xin	3 qian each
Jie Geng, Huang Qin, Qing Pi, Shui Zhi	3 qian each
Cang Zhu	4 qian
Gan Jiang, Fu Zi	5 qian each
Meng Chong	20 pieces

The Yu Sheng version is virtually the same as the original formula with the exception of Dang Shen replacing Ren Shen and the addition of Huang Qin, Cang Zhu, and Gan Jiang.

Meng Chong, Shui Zhi, Hou Po, Da Huang, Mang Xiao, and Niu Xi—drain and precipitate, dispel stasis and break accumulations, transform phlegm and disperse accumulations, move qi (and blood) downwards and free the channels—are among the essential medicinals that combine to provide an effective formula for treating female infertility. Po Xiao is a lesser refined grade of mirabilite and generally not used for medicinal purposes anymore, instead being replaced by the more refined form called Mang Xiao.

As its name indicates—**Dang Bao (盪胞)** literally means to "flush the uterus." This formula functions to "flush away" the residual metabolic waste (e.g., pus, cellular matter, blood clots) that may stagnate on the uterine lining and fallopian tube junctions (i.e., uterotubal junction) as a result of inflammation, adhesions, polyps, endometrial hyperplasia, endometriosis, and leiomyomas. This formula also elicits uterine contractions, which sends a definitive feedback signal to the hypothalamus and pituitary gland, so that the body clearly recognizes it should recalibrate normal hormone regulation (autoregulation) and continue the regeneration process once again (i.e., a pathophysiological phenomenon occurring in some women whom have already given birth or have had a spontaneous abortion, either knowingly or unknowingly).

Dr. Lee administers **Po Xiao Dang Bao Tang** specifically as a first-line treatment for female infertility—defined as *absence* of a live birth despite ≥ 1 year of efforts with a male partner (primary infertility), during which they have *not* used contraceptives; or in women who *have* consummated a live birth previously, but are subsequently *unable* to despite ≥ 1 year of efforts (secondary infertility), during which they have *not* used contraceptives.

The therapeutic regimen involves administration of this formula for 1 week, starting a few days before menstruation, with the couple subsequently proceeding in an attempt at natural insemination over a 6-month period. In approximately 70% of these cases, this approach will lead to pregnancy within that 6-month period. If this treatment does *not* result in pregnancy, then Dr. Lee will advise the couple to undergo further evaluation (e.g., ultrasound to determine the thickness of the endometrial lining, scrotal ultrasound) and testing (e.g., postcoital test (PCT), semen analysis to determine the presence of anti-sperm antibodies) prior to conducting further pattern identification and proceeding with other therapeutic approaches.

Qi Bao Mei Ran Dan (七寶美髯丸/Seven-Jewel Beard-Blackening Elixir)
He Shou Wu, Fu Ling, Niu Xi, Dang Gui, Gou Qi Zi, Tu Si Zi, Po Gu Zhi

Qi Chuan Fang – refer to **Asthma Formula**

Qi Fu Tang (耆附湯)
Huang Qi, Fu Zi, Sheng Jiang

Qi Qi Tang (七氣湯/Major Seven Qi Decoction)
Ren Shen, Guan Gui, Gan Cao, Ban Xia, Sheng Jiang

Qian Jin Nei Tuo San (千金內托散/Thousand Gold Pieces Internal Expulsion Powder)
Ren Shen, Dang Gui, Huang Qi, Chuan Xiong, Fang Feng, Jie Geng, Hou Po, Gui Zhi, Bai Zhi, Gan Cao

Qian Zheng San (牽正散/Pull Aright Powder)
Bai Fu Zi, Bai Jiang Can, Quan Xie

Qin Jiao Bie Jia San (秦艽鱉甲散)
Di Gu Pi, Chai Hu, Qin Jiao, Zhi Mu, Dang Gui, Bie Jia, Qing Hao, Wu Mei

Qin Lian Si Wu Tang (芩連四物湯/Scutellaria and Coptis Four Agents Decoction)
Dang Gui, Chuan Xiong, Chi Shao, Gan Di Huang, Huang Qin, Huang Lian

Qing Shang Fang Feng Tang (清上防風湯/Upper-Body-Clearing Saposhnikovia Decoction)
Fang Feng, Lian Qiao, Bai Zhi, Jie Geng, Huang Qin, Chuan Xiong, Huang Lian, Jing Jie, Shan Zhi Zi, Zhi Ke, Bo He, Gan Cao

Qing Wei San (清胃散/Stomach-Clearing Powder)

Huang Lian, Sheng Ma, Dang Gui	3 qian each
Sheng Di Huang, Mu Dan Pi	3 qian each

Qing Xin Lian Zi Yin (清心蓮子飲/Heat-Clearing Lotus Seed Beverage)
Huang Qin, Mai Men Dong, Di Gu Pi, Che Qian Zi, Chai Hu, Gan Cao, Lian Zi, Fu Ling, Huang Qi, Dang Shen

Qing Yan Li Ge San (清咽利膈散/Throat-Clearing Diaphragm-Disinhibiting Decoction)
Jin Yin Hua, Fang Feng, Jing Jie, Bo He, Jie Geng, Huang Qin, Huang Lian, Shan Zhi Zi, Lian Qiao, Xuan Shen, Da Huang, Mang Xiao, Niu Bang Zi, Gan Cao

Qing Zao Jiu Fei Tang (清燥救肺湯/Dryness-Clearing Lung-Rescuing Decoction)
Sang Ye, Shi Gao, Gan Cao, Ren Shen, Hua Ma Ren, E Jiao, Mai Men Dong, Xing Ren, Pi Pa Ye

Ren Shen Bai Du San (人參敗毒散/Ginseng Toxin-Vanquishing Powder)
Ren Shen, Qiang Huo, Du Huo, Chai Hu, Qian Hu, Chuan Xiong, Zhi Ke, Jie Geng, Fu Ling, Gan Cao, Sheng Jiang, Bo He

Ren Shen Yang Rong Tang (人參養榮湯/Ginseng Construction-Nourishing Decoction)

Ren Shen, Bai Zhu, Huang Qi, Gan Cao, Chen Pi, Rou Gui, Dang Gui, Shu Di Huang, Wu Wei Zi, Fu Ling, Yuan Zhi, Bai Shao, Da Zao, Sheng Jiang

Ru Mo Si Wu Tang (乳沒四物湯/Frankincense and Myrrh Four Agents Decoction)

Dang Gui, Chuan Xiong, Chi Shao	3 qian each
Sheng Di Huang, Ru Xiang, Mo Yao	3 qian each
Cang Zhu, Gan Cao, Tao Ren	3 qian each
Hong Hua	1.5 qian

This Yu Sheng formula is a variant of **Tao Hong Si Wu Tang**, with Sheng Di Huang replacing Shu Di Huang, Chi Shao replacing Bai Shao, and the addition of Cang Zhu and Gan Cao.

Sheng Di Huang supplements yin and cools the blood; Chi Shao cools the blood and expels stasis; Tao Ren quickens the blood and dispels stasis; and Hong Hua quickens the blood, dispels stasis, and frees the channels (menstruation). The addition of the medicinal pair Ru Xiang (quickens the blood and moves qi, disperses swelling and engenders flesh, and relieves pain) and Mo Yao (dissipates the blood and transforms stasis, disperses swelling and engenders flesh, and relieves pain) complements **Tao Hong Si Wu Tang**'s blood-nourishing blood-quickening, network vessel-freeing channel (menstruation)-regulating, and stasis-dispelling pain-relieving actions

Ru Mo Si Wu Tang is a commonly prescribed formula for gynecological pathoconditions presenting with blood stasis and concretions, conglomerations, accumulations, and gatherings (e.g., uterine fibroids (leiomyomas), endometrial hyperplasia, ovarian cysts, menstrual irregularities).

Dr. Lee prescribes **Ru Mo Si Wu Tang** for a broad spectrum of pathoconditions involving blockage of the flow of blood both inside the vessels (e.g., thrombus, embolus) and outside in the interstitium (e.g., hemorrhage), where it is capable of promoting absorption of blood and stanching bleeding. And it is also one of the main formulas prescribed in Dr. Lee's cancer treatment protocol, specifically administered for malignant (or benign) tumors of the smooth muscle (soft tissue) (e.g., carcinomas, fibromas, leiomyosarcomas, hamartomas) involving the breast, urinary bladder, uterus, gastrointestinal tract, and respiratory tract.

Sai Ji – refer to **Vaginal Suppository**

San Ao Tang (三拗湯/Rough and Ready Three Decoction)
Ma Huang, Xing Ren, Gan Cao, Sheng Jiang

San Bi Tang (三痹湯/Three Impediment Decoction)
Ren Shen, Huang Qi, Fu Ling, Gan Cao, Dang Gui, Chuan Xiong, Bai Shao, Sheng Di Huang, Du Zhong, Niu Xi, Xu Duan, Gui Xin, Xi Xin, Qin Jiao, Du Huo, Fang Feng

San Ceng Hui Xiang Wan (三層茴香丸/Three-Option Anise Pill)
Ba Jiao Hui Xiang, Chuan Lian Zi, Mu Xiang, Fu Ling, Bei Sha Shen, Bi Ba, Bin Lang, Fu Zi

San Miao Wan (三妙丸/Mysterious Three Pill)
Huang Bo, Cang Zhu, Niu Xi

San Zhong Kui Jian Tang (散腫潰堅湯/Swelling-Dispersing Hardness-Breaking Decoction)
Huang Qin, Zhi Mu, Huang Bo, Long Dan Cao, Tian Hua Fen, Jie Geng, Kun Bu, Chai Hu, Sheng Ma, Lian Qiao, Gan Cao, San Leng, E Zhu, Ge Gen, Dang Gui, Shao Yao, Huang Lian

Seborrheic Dermatitis Formula (脂漏方/Zhi Lou Fang)

Ma Huang	1.5 qian
Huang Qin	3 qian
Xing Ren, Cang Zhu	4 qian
Gan Cao, Jin Yin Hua	5 qian each
Lu Lu Tong	10 pieces
Shi Gao, Yi Yi Ren	1 liang each

This Yu Sheng original formula is composed of **(Yu Sheng) Ma Xing Yi Gan Tang** adding Huang Qin, Jin Yin Hua, and Lu Lu Tong.

Huang Qin clears heat and resolves toxin, dries dampness, and drains fire; Jin Yin Hua clears heat and resolves toxin, courses wind and dissipates heat, disperses welling-abscesses and swelling, and is an essential medicinal for the treatment of all types of yang pattern swollen welling-abscesses and clove sores (carbuncles, furuncles, boils); and Lu Lu Tong dispels wind, eliminates dampness, and resolves toxin for the treatment of wind-damp streaming sores, welling-abscesses, scab, and lichen.

As the name indicates, **Seborrheic Dermatitis Formula** is designed for the treatment of seborrheic dermatitis, and specifically for the acute and post-acute stages that can be identified as *exterior wind-heat* or *exterior wind-heat-damp* pattern. Seborrheic dermatitis correlates with the classical TCM pathologic terms wandering wind of the face (面游風 miàn yóu f□ ng) and white scaling wind (白屑風 bái xiè f□ ng).

Shao Fu Zhu Yu Tang (少腹逐瘀湯/Lesser Abdomen Stasis-Dispelling Decoction)

Xiao Hui Xiang, Gan Jiang, Yan Hu Suo, Mo Yao, Dang Gui, Chuan Xiong, Rou Gui, Chi Shao, Pu Huang, Wu Ling Zhi

She Gan Ma Huang Tang (射干麻黃湯/Belamcanda and Ephedra Decoction)

Ma Huang	2 qian
She Gan, Zi Wan, Kuan Dong Hua	3 qian each
Wu Wei Zi, Xi Xin, Sheng Jiang, Gan Cao	3 qian each
Ban Xia, Xing Ren, Chen Pi, Fu Ling	4 qian each
Hong Zao	3 pieces

Shen Fu Tang (參附湯)

Fu Zi, Gan Cao, Gan Jiang, Ren Shen

Shen Ling Bai Zhu San (參苓白朮散)

Bian Dou, Ren Shen, Bai Zhu, Fu Ling, Gan Cao, Shan Yao, Lian Zi, Yi Yi Ren, Jie Geng, Sha Ren, Da Zao

Shen Qi Wan (腎氣丸/Kidney Qi Pill)

Sheng Di Huang, Shan Zhu Yu	4 qian each
Shan Yao, Cang Zhu, Du Zhong	4 qian each
Fu Ling, Ze Xie, Mu Dan Pi, Huang Bo	2 qian each

Niu Xi, Fu Zi, Rou Gui	5 qian each
Gan Cao, Gan Jiang	3 qian each

Sheng Hua Tang (生化湯/Engendering Transformation Decoction)

Dang Gui, Chi Shao	4 qian each
Chuan Xiong, Yan Hu Suo, Tao Ren	3 qian each
Gan Jiang, Fu Zi, Huang Qin,	3 qian each
Du Zhong, Chao Bai Zhu	3 qian each
Xu Duan, Mu Xiang	5 qian each
Dang Shen	1 liang
Hong Hua	1.5 qian

Sheng Yang Yi Wei Tang (升陽益胃湯/Yang-Upbearing Stomach-Boosting Decoction)

Huang Qi, Ban Xia, Ren Shen, Gan Cao, Du Huo, Fang Feng, Bai Shao, Qiang Huo, Ju Pi, Fu Ling, Chai Hu, Ze Xie, Bai Zhu, Huang Lian, Sheng Jiang, Da Zao

Sheng Yu Tang (聖愈湯/Sagacious Cure Decoction)

Dang Gui, Chuan Xiong, Chi Shao	3 qian each
Sheng Di Huang, Cang Zhu	3 qian each
Dan Shen	5 qian
Huang Qi	1.5 liang

The Yu Sheng version is similar to the original formula except that Sheng Di Huang replaces Shu Di Huang, Dan Shen replaces Ren Shen, and Chi Shao and Cang Zhu are added. These additions complement and enhance this formula's overall blood-nourishing menstruation (blood)-regulating, blood-cooling stasis-dispelling, and yin-nourishing qi-supplementing actions. And depending on the presenting signs, symptoms, and pattern, Dr. Lee may also add Ren Shen (powder) or Ren Shen/Chuan Qi Powder.

Due to the time-consuming and costly method of traditional processing, the Shu Di Huang on the market today is either very expensive or uses modern processing methods that result in inferior quality. Thus, Dr. Lee typically substitutes Shu Di Huang with Sheng Di Huang, which has yin-enriching, blood-nourishing, and blood-cooling actions. Chi Shao cools the blood and expels stasis; Dan

Shen quickens the blood and dispels stasis and regulates menses and relieves pain; and Cang Zhu fortifies the spleen and dries dampness, thus counteracting the potential for digestion impairment and loose stools induced by the blood-nourishing yin-enriching medicinals.

Dr. Lee utilizes **Sheng Yu Tang**'s stasis-dispelling blood-cooling actions for the treatment of vascular wall pathologies, such as chemotherapy-induced nephrotoxicity (e.g., interstitial nephritis), chemotherapy-induced hepatotoxicity (e.g., hepatitis), aneurysm, and retinopathy (e.g., diabetic). For the treatment of chemotherapy side effects manifesting as vascular wall pathoconditions, Dr. Lee will typically prescribe **Xiao Chai Hu Tang** combined with **Sheng Yu Tang**. **Sheng Yu Tang** is an excellent formula for providing *stable* and *lasting* effects in the promotion of blood perfusion, but it neither *controls* blood as effectively as **Blood Desiccation Formula**, nor does it *promote* blood perfusion as rapidly as **Bu Yang Huan Wu Tang**.

Shi Quan Da Bu Tang (十全大補湯/Perfect Major Supplementation Decoction)

Huang Qin	2 qian
Dan Shen, Cang Zhu, Fu Ling, Gan Cao	3 qian each
Dang Gui, Chuan Xiong, Chi Shao	3 qian each
Sheng Di Huang, Gan Jiang, Fu Zi	3 qian each
Rou Gui	5 qian
Huang Qi	1 liang

This formula is virtually identical to the original formula. It combines the blood-quickening blood-supplementing actions of **(Yu Sheng) Si Wu Tang**—Dang Gui, Chuan Xiong, Chi Shao, and Sheng Di Huang—and the qi-boosting spleen-fortifying actions of **(Yu Sheng) Si Jun Zi Tang**—Dan Shen, Cang Zhu, Fu Ling, and Gan Cao—adding Gan Jiang, Fu Zi, Huang Qin, and a large dose of Huang Qi. Huang Qin is added to counteract the heat of The Three Great Yang-Supplementers.

(Yu Sheng) Shi Quan Da Bu Tang provides enhanced blood-quickening blood-supplementing, qi-boosting spleen-fortifying, and kidney yang-supplementing actions applicable for the treatment of a broad range of dual qi and blood vacuity with yang vacuity pattern pathoconditions. Among its many therapeutic applications, Dr. Lee commonly prescribes this formula for pediatric patients with delayed growth (height and/or weight), cerebral palsy (congenital or acquired), and congenital developmental delay (e.g., physical, cognitive, emotional, speech and language).

Shi Xiao San (失笑散/Sudden Smile Powder)
Wu Ling Zhi, Pu Huang, Cu (Vinegar)

Shi Zao Tang (十棗湯/Ten Jujubes Decoction)
Yan Hua, Gan Sui, Da Ji, Da Zao

Shuang Shen Fen – refer to **Body Soothing Powder**

Shun Qi Huo Xue Tang (順氣活血湯/Qi-Normalizing Blood-Quickening Decoction)
Su Geng, Hou Po, Zhi Ke, Sha Ren, Dang Gui, Hong Hua, Mu Xiang, Chi Shao, Tao Ren, Su Mu, Xiang Fu, Mi Jiu (Rice Wine)

Si Jun Zi Tang (四君子湯/Four Gentlemen Decoction)
Ren Shen, Gan Cao, Fu Ling, Bai Zhu

Si Ling Tang (四苓湯/Poria Four Decoction)
Fu Ling, Bai Zhu, Zhu Ling, Ze Xie, Deng Xin Cao

Si Miao Wan (四妙丸/Mysterious Four Pill)
Huang Bo, Cang Zhu, Niu Xi, Yi Yi Ren

Si Ni San (四逆散/Counterflow Cold Powder)
Chai Hu, Zhi Shi, Bai Shao, Gan Cao

Si Ni Tang (四逆湯/Counterflow Cold Decoction)
Gan Cao, Gan Jiang, Fu Zi

Si Qi Tang (四七湯/Four-Seven Decoction)
Ban Xia, Hou Po, Fu Ling, Zi Su

Si Shen Tang (四神湯/Four Spirits Decoction)

Fu Ling, Qian Shi, Bai Guo, Lian Zi	3 qian each
Shan Yao	5 qian
Yi Yi Ren	1 liang

Shan Zha 2 qian

This formula was first mentioned in the *Dictionary of Frequently-Used Taiwan Minnan* (臺灣閩南語常用詞辭典 *Taiwan Minnan Yu Chang Yong Ci Ci Dian*) during the Japanese occupation of Taiwan (1895–1945 CE). **Si Shen Tang** is composed of Shan Yao, Qian Shi, Lian Zi, and Fu Ling, and if eaten as a medicinal food, it is usually boiled together with either pork stomach or pork intestines (function as spleen and stomach channel conductors) into a stew. In Taiwan, it is also known as **Si Chen Tang (四臣湯/Four Ministers Decoction)**, and you can find this medicinal stew in night markets and restaurants. To make it even tastier and healthier, Yi Yi Ren and a bit of rice wine are also commonly added.

The Yu Sheng version is the same as the original except for the addition of Bai Guo, Yi Yi Ren, and Shan Zha. Bai Guo constrains the lung and stabilizes panting, checks discharge, reduces urine, boosts the kidney and enriches yin, and descends damp turbidity and phlegm-drool; Yi Yi Ren disinhibits water and percolates dampness, fortifies the spleen, eliminates impediment, clears heat and expels pus, and supplements the lung; and Shan Zha disperses food and promotes digestion, fortifies the spleen and opens the stomach, and expels tapeworm. These additions complement and enhance this formula's overall spleen-fortifying dampness-disinhibiting, kidney-boosting essence-securing, discharge- and diarrhea-checking, heart-nourishing spirit-quieting, lung-supplementing, and immune system-boosting actions.

Dr. Lee prescribes this formula for patients with spleen, stomach, and lung vacuity pattern type body constitutions (e.g., thin in stature, have poor appetites, inadequate nutritional state) and pathoconditions. This includes children and adolescents with developmental delays, female patients with chronic leucorrhea or interstitial cystitis, and specifically, for patients of all ages with low total protein (T-Pro) and albumin levels (e.g., cirrhosis, nephritic syndrome, cancer, autoimmune diseases).

Typically, Dr. Lee prescribes **Si Shen Tang** combined with other formulas or adds combinations of its composition into another formula. Or, he may simply advise patients to eat these ingredients as medicinal foods on their own, along with a well-rounded diet that includes plenty of fruit and vegetables, dairy products, fresh eggs, meat (especially brain and liver!), seafood, nuts, grains, and legumes.

Si Shen Wan (四神丸/Four Spirits Pill)
Bu Gu Zhi, Wu Zhu Yu, Rou Dou Kou, Wu Wei Zi, Sheng Jiang, Da Zao

Si Wu Tang (四物湯/Four Agents Decoction)
Dang Gui, Chuan Xiong, Bai Shao, Shu Di Huang

Tao Hong Si Wu Tang (桃紅四物湯/Peach Kernel and Carthamus Four Agents Decoction)
Dang Gui, Chuan Xiong, Bai Shao, Shu Di Huang, Tao Ren, Hong Hua

Tao Ren Cheng Qi Tang (桃仁承氣湯/Peach Kernel Qi-Coordinating Decoction)
Tao Ren, Da Huang, Gui Zhi, Gan Cao, Mang Xiao

Tearing on Exposure to Wind Formula (迎風落淚方/Ying Feng Luo Lei Fang)

Ma Huang	1.5 qian
Dan Shen, Cang Zhu, Fu Ling, Gan Cao	3 qian each
Chen Pi, Ban Xia, Mu Xiang	3 qian each
Sha Ren, Xi Xin, Wu Wei Zi	3 qian each
Bai Guo	4 qian
Rou Gui	5 qian

This original Yu Sheng formula contains the qi-boosting spleen-fortifying and qi-moving phlegm-transforming actions of **Xiang Sha Liu Jun Zi Tang**, and its composition is similar to **Asthma Formula** except for the subtractions of Shan Yao and Xing Ren and the addition of Xi Xin.

Xi Xin dispels wind and dissipates cold, frees the orifices and relieves pain, and warms the lung and transforms rheum; Ma Huang promotes sweating, resolves the exterior, and frees the nasal orifices; Wu Wei Zi constrains the lung and stabilizes panting; Bai Guo constrains the lung and dispels phlegm; and Rou Gui warms the kidney and supplements the spleen, resolves the exterior, and frees the channels. These medicinals complement the qi-boosting spleen-fortifying and qi-moving phlegm-transforming actions of **Xiang Sha Liu Jun Zi Tang**.

As its name indicates, **Tearing on Exposure to Wind Formula** is specifically designed for the treatment of tearing on exposure to wind (迎風落淚 yíng f□ ng luò lèi), a classical TCM pathologic term that correlates with post-acute and chronic allergic rhinitis and other related pathoconditions of the sinuses. The underlying pathomechanism of tearing on exposure to wind is *spleen yang vacuity with exterior* pattern, which inhibits the spleen's capacity to absorb and diffuse nutrients throughout the entire body and results in a compromised immune system and inability to govern flesh (and sinew).

Dr. Lee explains that persistent and prolonged sneezing, nasal discharge, and post-nasal drip further irritates the lacrimal drainage system apparatus, resulting in laxity of the lacrimal ducts upstream and/or clogged lacrimal puncta downstream that leads to excessive tearing (epiphora).

Ti Gang San (提肛散/Rectum-Lifting Powder)
Chuan Xiong, Dang Gui, Bai Zhu, Ren Shen, Huang Qi, Chen Pi, Gan Cao, Sheng Ma, Chai Hu, Huang Qin, Huang Lian, Bai Zhi

Tian Tai Wu Yao San (天台烏藥散)
Tian Tai Wu Yao, Mu Xiang, Hui Xiang, Liang Jiang, Qing Pi, Bin Lang, Chuan Lian Zi, Ba Dou

Tian Wang Bu Xin Dan (天王補心丹/Celestial Emperor Heart-Supplementing Elixir)
Tian Men Dong, Ren Shen, Fu Ling, Xuan Shen, Dan Shen, Yuan Zhi, Jie Geng, Dang Gui, Wu Wei Zi, Mai Men Dong, Bo Zi Ren, Suan Zao Ren, Sheng Di Huang

Tinea/Pompholyx Immersion (香港腳/汗皰疹泡藥)
Xiong Huang, Da Huang, Ru Xiang, Hua Shi, Gan Shi, Qing Fen

Tong Guan Wan (通關丸/Gate-Freeing Pill)

Huang Bo, Zhi Mu, and Rou Gui

Tong Jing Fang (通經方/Channel-Freeing Formula)

Cang Zhu	4 qian
Gan Cao	5 qian
Niu Xi, Xu Duan, Gu Sui Bu, Qian Cao	8 qian each

The Yu Sheng version is designed with similar therapeutic actions as its namesake **Tong Jing Wan (Channel-Freeing Pill)**, but Dr. Lee has overhauled the composition by choosing other medicinals with similar and complementary actions. The addition of liver- and kidney-supplementing and sinew- and bone-strengthening medicinals complement the original formula's blood-breaking, channel-freeing, and pain-relieving actions.

Niu Xi quickens the blood and frees the channels, supplements the liver and kidney, strengthens sinew and bone, disinhibits water and frees strangury, and conducts fire (blood) downward; Xu Duan supplements the liver and kidney, strengthens sinew and bone, and stanches bleeding and quiets the fetus; and Gu Sui Bu quickens the blood and transforms stasis, breaks blood, treats injury and mends breakages, and relieves pain. Together, the medicinal combination Gu Sui Bu, Xu Duan and Niu Xi serves as lumbus (spine) and lower limb and hard tissue conductor.

Qian Cao cools the blood, transforms stasis, stanches bleeding, and frees the channels (menstruation); Cang Zhu has the action of drying dampness and fortifying the spleen to counteract the potential of digestion impairment and loose stools resulting from the blood-nourishing yin-enriching medicinals; and Gan Cao boosts qi and supplements the center, relaxes tension and relieves pain, and harmonizes the nature of medicinals.

Dr. Lee typically prescribes **Tong Jing Fang** for the treatment of pathoconditions involving bone (e.g., fractures, osteoporosis), marrow, striated muscle (e.g., traumatic injuries), and the female reproductive system, as well as adjuvant therapy for the side efforts of chemotherapy in bone and gynecologic cancer patients. It is also a commonly prescribed formula in Dr. Lee's cancer treatment protocol, specifically administered for malignant (or benign) tumors of the striated muscle and marrow (e.g., rhabdomyosarcoma, osteosarcoma), with its capacity to inhibit tumor-cell mediated angiogenesis and neovascularization and the proliferation of cancer stem cells.

Tong Jing Wan (通經丸/Channel-Freeing Pill)

San Leng, E Zhu, Dang Gui, Chuan Xiong, Chi Shao, Chuan Shan Jia, Yan Hua, Liu Ji Nu

Tuo Li Xiao Du San (托裏消毒飲/Internal Expulsion Toxin-Dispersing Beverage)

Huang Qi, Chuan Xiong, Dang Gui, Shao Yao, Ren Shen, Bai Zhu, Fu Ling, Jiao Zao Ci, Jie Geng, Bai Zhi, Hou Po, Jin Yin Hua

Vaginal Suppository (塞劑/Sai Ji)

She Chuang Zi	1 g
Xiong Huang, Liu Huang, Da Huang	0.3 g each

This formula composition is identical to **Antimicrobial Wash (Xi Ji)** except for the subtraction of Long Dan Cao. The core toxin-resolving, worm-killing, and itch-relieving medicinals—She Chuang Zi, Xiong Huang, Liu Huang, and Da Huang—are the same. The combination of these medicinals clears heat and resolves toxin, kills worms and relieves itch, and dispels wind and eliminates dampness.

Vaginal Suppository is prescribed for various types of vaginal infections, including bacterial vaginosis (i.e., *Gardnerella vaginalis*), yeast (candidiasis), parasites (trichomoniasis), and sexually transmitted diseases (STDs) (e.g., genital herpes, gonorrhea, Chlamydia) that present with itching, irritation, and watery or viscous vaginal discharge.

This formula is typically prescribed as part of a therapeutic regimen that includes decocted formulas taken orally such as **Long Dan Xie Gan Tang**, **Jin Suo Gu Jing Wan**, or **Bu Zhong Yi Qi Tang**.

Wan Ling Dan – refer to **Bao An Wan Ling Dan**

Wen Dan Tang (溫膽湯/Gallbladder Warming Decoction)

Huang Qin, Zhi Shi	3 qian each
Chen Pi, Ban Xia, Fu Ling, Gan Cao	4 qian each

Zhu Ru	3 pieces
Da Zao	4 pieces

The Yu Sheng version is virtually identical to the original formula except for the addition of Huang Qin and the subtraction of Sheng Jiang.

Huang Qin's heat-clearing dampness-drying and fire-draining toxin-resolving actions enhance this formula's capacity to clear repletion (and residual) heat and transform phlegm-heat and complement its overall qi-moving phlegm-transforming and gallbladder- and stomach-harmonizing actions.

Traditionally, this formula is prescribed for disharmony of the gallbladder and stomach pattern and phlegm turbidity harassing the inner body pattern pathoconditions that present with vacuity vexation and insomnia, oppression in the chest with phlegm, nausea and vomiting, hiccup, fright palpitations, bitter taste in the mouth, slimy tongue fur, and stringlike and slippery pulse.

Dr. Lee prescribes **Wen Dan Tang** for a broad scope of Shao Yang depressed heat with phlegm and damp-heat pattern pathoconditions from external contraction (e.g., the common cold), rhinitis, and otitis to insomnia, glaucoma, infertility (both male and female), and myasthenia gravis (damp-heat pattern type).

Wen Qing Yin (溫清飲/Warm Clearing Beverage)
Dang Gui, Chuan Xiong, Bai Shao, Shu Di Huang, Huang Qin, Huang Bo, Zhi Zi, Huang Lian

Wu Lin San (五淋散/Five Stranguries Powder)
Chi Fu Ling, Dang Gui, Chi Shao Yao, Zhi Zi, Gan Cao, Deng Xin Cao

Wu Ling San (五苓散/Five Poria Powder)
Zhu Ling, Ze Xie, Bai Zhu, Fu Ling, Gui Zhi

Wu Ling San (Calculi Formula) (五苓散 (結石方)/Five Poria Powder (Calculi Formula))

Rou Gui	2 qian
Yan Hu Suo, Mu Xiang, Huang Bo, Gan Cao	3 qian each
Cang Zhu, Zhu Ling, Fu Ling	5 qian each
Dang Gui	8 qian
Ze Xie	1 liang

This Yu Sheng version contains the essential components of the original **Wu Ling San**—Fu Ling, Ze Xie, Bai Zhu, Gui Zhi, and Zhu Ling—except for Rou Gui replacing Gui Zhi and Cang Zhu replacing Bai Zhu. Plus, Dang Gui, Yan Hu Suo, Mu Xiang, Huang Bo, and Gan Cao have been added. These additions complement the original formula's overall yang-warming qi-transforming actions and enhance its water-disinhibiting dampness-percolating actions, while also providing potent qi-moving blood-quickening, heat-draining, and pain-relieving actions.

Wu Ling San (Calculi Formula) includes large doses of Ze Xie for its water-inhibiting dampness-percolating and heat-draining actions, and large doses of Dang Gui for its blood-supplementing and -quickening actions. Together, this medicinal pair promotes smooth muscle contractions of the bile ducts, kidneys, and urinary tract, thus resulting in the dislodgement and evacuation of calculi.

Mu Xiang moves qi and relieves pain; and Yan Hu Suo quickens the blood, moves qi, and relieves pain. Together, the medicinal pair Mu Xiang and Yan Hu Suo serves as a muscle relaxant and analgesic, promoting the evacuation of calculi and relieving pain. Cang Zhu dries dampness and fortifies the spleen; and Huang Bo drains lower burner fire, dries dampness, resolves toxin, and disinhibits the gallbladder to treat inflammation. Together, the medicinal pair Cang Zhu and Huang Bo enhances the dampness-percolating and pain-relieving actions of this formula and provides damp-heat-eliminating actions.

As its name implies, Dr. Lee has specifically designed **Wu Ling San (Calculi Formula)** for the treatment of calculi in the kidneys (nephrolithiasis) and other sites along the urogenital tract (e.g., urethra, bladder), bile ducts (gallstones, aka choledocholithiasis), and the pancreatic duct (pancreatolithiasis).

Wu Ling San (Nephritis Formula) (五苓散 (腎炎方)/Five Poria Powder (Nephritis Formula))

Dang Gui	2 qian
Gan Jiang, Fu Zi, Huang Bo	3 qian each
Zhu Ling, Fu Ling, Cang Zhu, Ze Xie, Rou Gui	5 qian each
Huang Qi	1 liang

This Yu Sheng version contains the essential components of the original **Wu Ling San**—Fu Ling, Ze Xie, Bai Zhu, Gui Zhi, and Zhu Ling—except for Rou Gui replacing Gui Zhi and Cang Zhu replacing Bai Zhu. Plus, Dang Gui, Huang Qi, Gan Jiang, Fu Zi, and Huang Bo have been added. These additions greatly enhance the original formula's yang-warming qi-transforming actions and complement the overall water-disinhibiting dampness-percolating actions.

Huang Qi supplements qi, disinhibits water and disperses swelling, increases myocardial contractility, promotes passage across membranes, and functions as a broad-spectrum antimicrobial, which complements Dang Gui's actions of supplementing and quickening the blood, as these medicinals combine to improve renal blood flow and filtration through the glomeruli.

Gan Jiang warms the center, returns yang, and frees the vessels; Fu Zi reinforces yang, supplements the kidney and life-gate fire, frees the twelve channels, and strengthens cardiac contractility; and Rou Gui reinforces yang, greatly supplements life gate fire, conducts medicinals throughout the entire body, and promotes blood circulation. Together, they form the medicinal combination The Three Great Yang-Supplementers, which "boosts" the metabolism and immune system, increases stroke volume, and reduces heart rate.

Cang Zhu dries dampness, fortifies the spleen, and dispels wind-damp; and Huang Bo clears heat and dries dampness, drains lower burner fire, resolves toxin, serves as a foot Tai Yang channel conductor, and counteracts the heat of The Three Great Yang-Supplementers. Together, the medicinal pair Cang Zhu and Huang Bo clears heat and dries dampness, disperses swelling and relieves pain, and eliminates dampness and checks vaginal discharge for the treatment of damp-heat pouring downward pattern and wilting pattern pathoconditions.

Wu Ling San is traditionally administered for the treatment of exterior evil in the outer body and water-damp collecting in the inner body pattern and water-damp collecting internally pattern pathoconditions that present with symptoms such as inhibited urination, water swelling (edema), vexation thirst with no desire to drink, and immediate vomiting of ingested fluids.

Dr. Lee commonly prescribes **Wu Ling San (Nephritis Formula)** for the treatment of post-acute and chronic water-damp collecting internally pattern pathoconditions that manifest in proteinuria, edema, uremia, and hypoalbuminemia (e.g., nephrotic syndrome, glomerulonephritis, chronic kidney failure); pulmonary edema (e.g., intrinsic lung disease, congestive heart failure, kidney failure); and increased intracranial pressure (ICP).

Wu Wei Yi Gong San (五味異功散/Five-Ingredient Special Achievement Powder)
Ren Shen, Bai Zhu, Fu Ling, Gan Cao, Chen Pi, Sheng Jiang, Da Zao

Wu Zhu Yu Tang (吳茱萸湯)
Wu Zhu Yu, Ren Shen, Sheng Jiang, Da Zao

Wu Zi Yan Zong Wan (五子衍宗丸/Five-Seed Progeny Pill)
Tu Si Zi, Wu Wei Zi, Gou Ji Zi, Fu Pen Zi, Che Qian Zi

Xi Ji – refer to **Antimicrobial Wash**

Xi Jiao Di Huang Tang (犀角地黃湯)
Xi Jiao (now use Shui Niu Jiao instead), Sheng Di Huang, Shao Yao, Mu Dan Pi

Xian Fang Huo Ming Yin (仙方活命飲/Immortal Formula Life-Giving Beverage/aka **Zhen Ren Huo Ming Yin)**

Chen Pi, Tian Hua, Jin Yin Hua, Ru Xiang	3 qian each
Mo Yao, Fang Feng, Zao Jiao Ci, Dang Gui	3 qian each
Niu Bang Zi, Chi Shao, Bai Zhi, Gan Cao	3 qian each
Cang Zhu	4 qian
Sheng Shi Gao	1 liang

The Yu Sheng version is virtually identical to the original formula except for the exclusion of Chuan Shan Jia, an endangered animal species that is now prohibited, and the use of Zhe Bei Mu (powder) instead of decocting pieces, which can be either added into the formula after decoction or taken separately. Plus, as a substitute for Chuan Shan Jia, Dr. Lee includes Niu Bang Zi, Cang Zhu, and Sheng Shi Gao.

Niu Bang Zi courses wind and dissipates heat, outthrusts macules and disinhibits the throat, resolves toxin and dissipates swelling; Sheng Shi Gao clears heat and drains fire and astringes and engenders flesh; and Cang Zhu dries dampness and fortifies the spleen and dispels wind-damp. These additions complement the blood-quickening and pus-expelling swelling-dispersing actions of Zao Jiao Ci, and provide an effective alternative for Chuan Shan Jia.

In TCM classical texts **Xian Fang Huo Ming Yin** is classified as a "sore sage formula" for its heat-clearing toxin-resolving, swelling-dispersing hardness-breaking, and blood-quickening pain-relieving actions. Traditionally, it is prescribed for the treatment of acute and post-acute stage swelling and toxin of sores and welling-abscesses (e.g., carbuncles, furuncles, boils), localized skin redness, heat, swelling, and pain, and generalized heat with mild aversion to cold (e.g., cellulitis, cinnabar toxin (erysipelas))

In addition to these types of external medicine pathoconditions, Dr. Lee may prescribe **Xian Fang Huo Ming Yin** for other pathoconditions such as innominate toxin swellings (both benign and malignant), cellulitis, appendicitis, postherpetic neuralgia (phantom pain), and pulmonary abscesses.

Xiang Sha Liu Jun Zi Tang (香砂六君子湯/Costus Root and Amomum Six Gentlemen Decoction)

Dan Shen, Cang Zhu, Fu Ling	3 qian each
Gan Cao, Mu Xiang, Sha Ren	3 qian each
Chen Pi, Ban Xia	4 qian each

The Yu Sheng version is virtually the same as the original formula except that Dan Shen replaces Ren Shen, Cang Zhu replaces Bai Zhu, and Sheng Jiang and Da Zao are subtracted.

Dan Shen quickens the blood and dispels stasis, cools the blood and disperses welling-abscesses, and relieves pain and quiets the spirit; and Cang Zhu dries dampness and fortifies the spleen, which is ideal for Taiwan's humid subtropical climate.

Depending on the presenting signs, symptoms, and pattern, Dr. Lee may also add the following medicinals into this formula: Ren Shen (powder) or Ren Shen/Chuan Qi Powder; Sheng Jiang, as in the original formula, for the treatment of morning sickness during the first trimester of pregnancy; and Gan Jiang for the treatment of interior cold pattern pathoconditions.

This formula's qi-boosting spleen-fortifying and qi-moving phlegm-transforming actions are traditionally administered for spleen and stomach qi vacuity and phlegm obstruction and qi stagnation pattern pathoconditions that present with symptoms such as spleen and stomach vacuity, dampness obstruction and qi stagnation, abdominal distention after food intake, acid reflux, and poor appetite.

Some specific pathoconditions Dr. Lee typically prescribes this formula for are gastrointestinal reflux disease (GERD), chronic gastritis, autoimmune diseases (e.g., SLE), ascites (e.g., hepatic disorders), renal disease (e.g., azotemia), and poor appetite and malnutrition during the late stages of cancer.

The qi-boosting spleen-fortifying and qi-moving phlegm-transforming actions of **Xiang Sha Liu Jun Zi Tang** form the foundation of the three formulas that treat the "allergic triad" manifestations of atopy—**Asthma Formula** treats the lung, **Atopic Dermatitis Formula** treats the skin, and **Tearing on Exposure to Wind Formula** treats the sinuses. These hyperallergic reactions may present as an inflammatory response in the upper respiratory tract (e.g., lungs, sinuses) or manifest on the skin.

In TCM theory, the spleen belongs to earth and engenders metal, governs the movement and transformation of the essence of grain and water and also governs the flesh. The lung belongs to metal and governs qi, skin and hair, opens at the nose, and has an upward and outward diffusing movement, which carries moisture and nourishment to the skin.

Xiao Ban Xia Jia Fu Ling Tang (小半夏加茯苓湯/Minor Pinellia Plus Poria Decoction)
Ban Xia, Sheng Jiang, Fu Ling

Xiao Ban Xia Tang (小半夏湯/Minor Pinellia Decoction)
Ban Xia, Sheng Jiang

Xiao Chai Hu Tang (小柴胡湯/Minor Bupleurum Decoction)

Huang Qin	3 qian
Dan Shen, Ban Xia, Gan Cao, Sheng Jiang	5 qian each
Chai Hu	6 qian
Da Zao	5 pieces

The Yu Sheng version is virtually identical to the original formula except for Dan Shen replacing Ren Shen. However, depending on the presenting signs, symptoms, and pattern, Ren Shen (powder) or Ren Shen/Chuan Qi Powder may also be included.

Traditionally, this is a commonly prescribed formula for the treatment of Shao Yang pattern pathoconditions (e.g., alternating heat and cold, fullness in the chest and rib-side, no desire for food and drink), general discomfort or pain in the hypochondriac region, heat entering the blood chamber, and pathoconditions of the liver, gallbladder, and spleen (e.g., hepatitis, cholecystitis, splenitis).

Dr. Lee's application of **Xiao Chai Hu Tang** can be classified into three broad categories: 1) Depressed heat (i.e., persistent low-grade fever) following external contraction (i.e., microbial infection), especially for pediatric patients and tuberculosis (TB) patients who *have* been administered antibiotic treatment; 2) Microbial infections, toxin (e.g., noxious chemicals), or autoimmune reactions leading to metabolic waste buildup that disrupts the autoregulation capacity of the nervous system (specifically, the coordinated interactions of the CNS, ANS, and PNS) to regulate bodily functions and maintain homeostasis, thus resulting in dyscrasias (e.g., leukemia, hemophilia, multiple myeloma); and 3) For complex pattern pathoconditions that are difficult to diagnose and/or pathoconditions that are in a transitional phase, which can be identified as half-interior half-exterior (mid-stage) pattern, this formula may be prescribed until a definitive diagnosis and/or pattern identification can be ascertained (e.g., whether a pathocondition is passing from the exterior into the interior or from the interior into the exterior).

Xiao Qing Long Tang (小青龍湯/Minor Green-Blue Dragon Decoction)
Ma Huang, Gui Zhi, Bai Shao, Gan Cao, Gan Jiang, Xi Xin, Ban Xia, Wu Wei Zi

Xiao Yao San (逍遙散/Free Wanderer Powder)
Chai Hu, Dang Gui, Bai Shao, Bai Zhu, Fu Ling, Gan Cao, Sheng Jiang, Bo He

Xie Xin Tang (寫心湯/Heart-Draining Decoction/aka **San Huang Xie Xin Tang)**
Da Huang, Huang Lian, Huang Qin

Xuan Fu Dai Zhe Tang (旋覆代赭湯)
Xuan Fu Hua, Sheng Jiang, Ren Shen, Da Zhe Shi, Gan Cao, Ban Xia, Da Zao

Xue Fu Zhu Yu Tang (血府逐瘀湯/House of Blood Stasis-Expelling Decoction)
Dang Gui, Sheng Di Huang, Tao Ren, Hong Hua, Zhi Ke, Chi Shao, Chai Hu, Gan Cao, Jie Geng, Chuan Xiong, Niu Xi

Xue Ku Fang – refer to **Blood Desiccation Formula**

Yang Dan Tang (陽但湯/Yang Dawn Decoction)

Rou Gui, Chi Shao, Sheng Cao, Sheng Jiang	5 qian each
Huang Qin	3 qian
Da Zao	5 pieces

This Yu Sheng version is virtually identical to the original formula, which is a derivative of **Gui Zhi Tang**—Gui Zhi, Bai Shao, Gan Cao, Sheng Jiang, Da Zao—except as is the case in many of Dr. Lee's other formulas, Chi Shao replaces Bai Shao and Rou Gui replaces Gui Zhi.

Huang Qin clears heat and dries dampness and drains fire and resolves toxin (antimicrobial and anti-inflammatory)) for the treatment of wind-heat and damp-heat in the upper burner; and **Gui Zhi Tang** resolves the flesh and dispels wind and harmonizes construction and defense for the treatment of external contraction wind-cold exterior vacuity. The addition of Huang Qin to **Gui Zhi Tang** broadens the scope of this classic formula's applications to encompass both exterior wind-cold and wind-heat pattern pathoconditions.

Traditionally, **Yang Dan Tang** is prescribed for the treatment of wind strike cold damage, floating pulse, alternating heat (fever) and aversion to cold, sweating and aversion to wind, stiff neck, noisy nose (鼻鳴 bí míng), and dry retching.

The basic composition of **Yang Dan Tang** forms the foundation of Dr. Lee's therapeutic approach for the treatment of exterior wind-cold and wind-heat pattern pathoconditions of the respiratory tract, eyes, and skin. Dr. Lee typically does *not* prescribe this formula in decocting pieces for decoction on its own, but *includes* these medicinals in other formula variants. However, if a patient presents with a relatively mild external contraction exterior wind-cold or wind-heat pattern pathocondition, he may prescribe this formula in the form of extract granules, possibly adding other medicinals as well.

Yao Xian – refer to **Yu Sheng Medicated Thread**

Yi Gan San (抑肝散/Liver-Repressing Powder)
Dang Gui, Bai Zhu, Fu Ling, Gou Teng, Chuan Xiong, Chai Hu, Gan Cao

Yi Qi Cong Ming Tang (益氣聰明湯/Qi-Boosting Sharp and Bright Decoction)
Huang Qi, Ren Shen, Ge Gen, Man Xing Zi, Bai Shao, Huang Bo, Sheng Ma, Gan Cao

Yi Wei Xing Pi Fu Yan Fang – refer to **Atopic Dermatitis Formula**

Yin Qiao San (銀翹散)

Jin Yin Hua, Lian Qiao, Jing Jie, Dan Dou Chi, Jie Geng, Bo He, Niu Bang Zi, Gan Cao, Zhu Ye, Wei Gen

Ying Feng Luo Lei Fang – refer to **Tearing on Exposure to Wind Formula**

You Gui Wan (右歸丸/Right-Restoring Pill)

Shu Di Huang, Shan Yao, Gou Qi Zi, Tu Si Zi, Du Zhong, Lu Jiao Jiao, Shan Zhu Yu, Dang Gui, Fu Zi, Rou Gui

You Gui Yin (右歸飲/Right-Restoring Beverage)

Dang Gui, Fu Ling	2 qian each
Gou Qi Zi, Huang Bo, Gan Jiang	3 qian each
Sheng Di Huang, Shan Zhu Yu, Shan Yao	4 qian each
Cang Zhu, Du Zhong, Tu Si Zi	4 qian each
Fu Zi, Niu Xi, Rou Gui	5 qian each

The Yu Sheng version combines medicinals from the original versions of **You Gui Yin** (Shan Yao, Gou Qi Zi, Shan Zhu Yu, Du Zhong, Fu Zi, and Rou Gui), **Shen Qi Wan** (Gan Di Huang and Fu Ling), and **You Gui Wan** (Tu Si Zi and Dang Gui). Plus, Huang Bo, Gan Jiang, Cang Zhu, and Niu Xi are added.

Niu Xi quickens the blood and frees the channels, supplements the liver and kidney, strengthens sinew and bone, disinhibits water and frees strangury, and conducts fire (blood) downward; and Du Zhong supplements the liver and kidney, strengthens sinew and bone, and quiets the fetus. Together, the medicinal pair Niu Xi and Du Zhong serves as a lumbus (spine) and lower limb conductor.

Huang Bo clears heat and dries dampness, drains lower burner fire, resolves toxin, serves as a foot Tai Yang channel conductor, and counteracts the heat of The Three Great Yang-Supplementers; and Cang Zhu dries dampness, fortifies the spleen, dispels wind-damp to counteract the potential of digestion impairment and loose stools that may result from large doses of blood-nourishing yin-enriching medicinals. Together, this medicinal pair clears heat and dries dampness, disperses swelling and relieves pain, and eliminates dampness for the treatment pain in the feet and knees, wilting pattern, and strangury-turbidity.

Dr. Lee commonly prescribes this formula for a wide range of yang vacuity and depletion pattern pathoconditions, including lumbar and back pain (e.g., radiculopathy (sciatica) from herniated intervertebral disc, spondylolisthesis, spinal stenosis), limp knees and weak legs (e.g., various post-acute articular cartilage, ligament, and tendon injuries), congenital development disorders, and atopy (especially in male patients) (e.g., chronic stage asthma, tearing on exposure to wind, atopic dermatitis).

Yu Ping Feng San (玉屏風散/Jade Wind-Barrier Powder)
Fang Feng, Huang Qi, Bai Zhu, Sheng Jiang, Da Zao

Yu Sheng Medicated Thread (育生藥線/Yu Sheng Yao Xian)

Da Huang	2 liang
Lu Gan Shi, Xiong Huang, Liu Huang	5 qian each
Tong Qing, Ru Xiang, Hua Shi Fen	5 qian each
Qing Fen, Bai Xin	3 qian each

This is a hybrid formula that contains a compilation of the most commonly prescribed external medicine essential medicinals in the Chinese medicine pharmacopoeia for drawing pus and eliminating putridity (提膿去腐 tí nóng qù fu) and eroding tissue and flattening excrescence (腐蝕平胬 fu shí píng nu).

It contains a litany of heavy metals (i.e., mercury, lead, arsenic, copper, zinc, and magnesium) along with sulfur to form a potent sore-eroding, putridity-eliminating, toxin-resolving, worm-killing, flesh-engendering, and sore-closing medicated thread. After thorough processing, these medicinals are ground into a fine powder and thoroughly blended together to form a homogenous mixture. Shan Yao (an excipient that moderates the toxicity of medicinals) is also ground into a fine powder and mixed in with the other medicinals, adding appropriate amounts of water to form a thick dough. This dough is pressed and rolled into threads about 1 mm in diameter and 15 cm in length, and then dried.

Bai Xin (White Arsenic/As2O3/arsenic trioxide) erodes sores and eliminates putridity; Qing Fen (Calomel/Hg_2Cl_2/mercury chloride) kills worms, eliminates putridity, and closes sores; Tong Qing (Verdigris/CuCO3/copper (II) carbonate) eliminates putridity, closes sores, and kills worms; Xiong Huang (Realgar/As_2S_2/arsenic sulfide) resolves toxin, kills worms, and dries dampness; Liu Huang (Sulfur/S) resolves toxin, kills worms, and relieves itch; Lu Gan Shi (Calamine/$ZnCO_3$/zinc carbonate) resolves toxin, engenders flesh, and closes sores; Hua Shi Fen (Talc/$Mg_3Si_4O_{10}(OH)_2$/magnesium silicate hydroxide) dispels dampness and closes sores; Da Huang (Rhubarb Root) clears heat and drains fire, resolves toxin and erodes pus, quickens the blood and dispels stasis, and removes the old and engenders flesh; and Ru Xiang (Frankincense) disperses swelling and engenders flesh, quickens the blood and moves qi, and relieves pain.

Yu Sheng Medicated Thread is effective for exterior damp-heat toxin, wind toxin, and fire-toxin pattern lesions such as scrofula (mycobacterial cervical lymphadenitis); all types of welling-abscesses, flat-abscesses, boils, and clove sores failing to heal and close; and other benign and malignant cutaneous tumors. It functions as an antimicrobial to resolve inflammation and infection, breaks down pus and pathogenic tissue, expedites the extrusion of pus and debridement of putrified tissue, and promotes the regeneration of healthy tissue.

Application involves breaking off a piece of the thread at an appropriate length, just long enough so that it can be inserted using the fingers or tweezers into the opening of the lesion. This may simply be one piece inserted into the "head" of a boil or it could be numerous pieces stuck into the diameter of a putrid tissue mass (e.g., tumor). Following insertion, the lesion is covered in sterile gauze and left inside anywhere from 1 to 3 days. At that time, the patient returns to assess whether the thread needs to be removed and/or changed.

In the case of pustular lesions (e.g., boils), if the pus is ready to be drawn (squeezed), then do so; and if not, then you can remove the thread and add more as needed. In the case of a tumor, the putrid tissue should be debrided along with the thread and more thread should be added as before. For tumors, this is an involved process that will require repeated insertion and debridement every 1 to 3 days, along with the administration of an appropriate formula that resolves toxin, engenders flesh, and if necessary, combats the cancer.

Yu Sheng Wan (育生丸/Yu Sheng Pill)

Jin Yin Hua	0.04 g/pill
Shan Yao	0.6 g/pill
Feng Mi (Honey)	

The sovereign medicinal in this original formula is Jin Yin Hua (*Datura metel* L./Flos Daturae/Datura Flower/aka Man Tuo Luo Hua), whose principal bioactive constituents are the anticholinergics scopolamine (hyoscine) and hyoscyamine (atropine).

Shan Yao and Feng Mi (Honey) serve the roles of assistant and envoy medicinals, respectively. Shan Yao boosts qi and nourishes yin, supplements the spleen, lung, and kidneys, secures essence, has a moderating effect on Jin Yin Hua, and functions as a bulking agent and diluent. Feng Mi (Honey) supplements the center, harmonizes the nature of Jin Yin Hua, and functions as a binder and preservative.

Feng Mi (Honey) is boiled slowly on low heat to reduce water content and increase its viscosity and then the pulverized powder of Jin Yin Hua and Shan Yao are thoroughly blended together in the honey to form a homogenous mixture. This mixture is made into pills and allowed to dry.

Yu Sheng Wan is a commonly prescribed pill that Dr. Lee includes in the therapeutic regimen for a broad spectrum of pathoconditions. Dr. Lee explains that the underlying pharmacodynamics of this pill is its capacity to stimulate cerebral collateral circulation and recalibrate the brain's self-regulating function (autoregulation). Cerebral circulation fluctuates in response to physical and mental activities and metabolic processes, and normally the brain is able to self-regulate in order to maintain homeostasis. However, certain pathoconditions, as well as the process of aging, may lead to microvascular changes, decreased vascular density, and pericyte degeneration. These changes cause the brain to *misinterpret* the internal environment it holds dominion over, functioning imperceptively in a compromised state of dyshomeostasis.

Dr. Lee utilizes the actions of these properties to supplement the brain, remedy insomnia and depression, eliminate anxiety and stress, slow the degenerative process of aging and disease (e.g., dementia, Alzheimer's disease (AD), Parkinson's disease (PD)), relieve all types of pain, check spasm, and stabilize panting (asthma). Its capacity to relax smooth muscle makes it effective for treating overactive bladder (females) and enlarged prostate (males) and for promoting the passage of urinary tract calculi and gallstones (i.e., using a large 1x dose of 4–6 pills for males and 4–8 pills for females accompanied by acupuncture). It is also prescribed as a part of Dr. Lee's cancer treatment protocol.

The efficacy of **Yu Sheng Wan** is very much dose-related, with large doses potentially causing side effects such as dry mouth, drowsiness, blurry vision, and confusion. Thus, it is essential to limit the standard dosage to 1–3 pills per day, unless certain cases warrant otherwise.

Yu Zhen San (玉真散/True Jade Powder)
Tian Nan Xing, Bai Zhi, Fang Feng, Qiang Huo, Tian Ma, Bai Fu Zi

Yue Bi Tang (越婢湯/Spleen-Effusing Decoction/aka **Maidservant From *Yue* Decoction)**
Ma Huang, Shi Gao, Sheng Jiang, Gan Cao, Da Zao

Yue Ju Wan (越鞠丸/Depression-Overcoming Pill)
Cang Zhu, Xiang Fu, Chuan Xiong, Shen Qu, Zhi Zi

Zao Fu Tang (棗附湯)
Fu Zi, Da Zao, Sheng Jiang

Zhen Wu Tang (真武湯/True Warrior Decoction)
Fu Ling, Shao Yao, Bai Zhu, Sheng Jiang, Fu Zi

Zhi Bo Di Huang Tang (知柏地黃湯)

Gan Cao, Huang Bo	3 qian
Zhi Mu, Shan Zhu Yu, Shan Yao, Fu Ling	4 qian each
Mu Dan Pi, Ze Xie, Niu Xi, Cang Zhu	4 qian each
Sheng Di Huang	8 qian

The Yu Sheng version is similar to the original formula except for Sheng Di Huang replacing Shu Di Huang and the addition of Niu Xi, Cang Zhu, and Gan Cao. These additions complement the overall yin-enriching fire-downbearing actions of the original formula and further provide blood-quickening channel-freeing, heat-clearing dampness-drying, and pain-relieving actions.

Niu Xi quickens the blood and frees the channels, supplements the liver and kidney, strengthens sinew and bone, disinhibits water and frees strangury, and conducts fire (blood) downward; Cang Zhu dries dampness, fortifies the spleen, and dispels wind-damp; and Gan Cao boosts qi and supplements the center, clears heat and resolves toxin, relaxes tension and relieves pain, and harmonizes the nature of medicinals.

The medicinal combination Huang Bo, Niu Xi, and Cang Zhu forms **San Miao Wan**, a commonly prescribed heat-clearing dampness-drying and medicinal downward-conducting formula for the treatment of pathoconditions that include damp-heat pouring downward pattern (e.g., strangury-turbidity, dribbling urinary block, vaginal discharge, damp-heat diarrhea), wilting pattern (e.g., myasthenia gravis), and arthritic ailments.

Traditionally, **Zhi Bo Di Huang Tang** is administered for effulgent yin vacuity fire pattern pathoconditions that present with symptoms such as steaming bone tidal heat, aching pain in the lumbar spine, seminal emission, and dry mouth.

Dr. Lee typically prescribes **Zhi Bo Di Huang Tang** for the treatment of steaming bone (e.g., osteomyelitis), pulling of the sinews and inhibited bending and stretching (e.g., sprains, strains, tears, osteoarthritis), bone fractures, heel pain syndrome, tuberculosis, yin vacuity cough (aka dryness cough), epilepsy, diabetes, genitourinary tract disorders, seminal emission, and symptoms of menopausal transition.

Due to its capacity for promoting self-repair and preventing the potential development of further degeneration (e.g., fibrosis, enthesopathy) that may arise from complications of aspiration, bleeding, or administration of anti-inflammatory agents, Dr. Lee considers **Zhi Bo Di Huang Tang** to be an essential formula for acute and sub-acute musculoskeletal injuries (e.g., arthritic, traumatic, autoimmune) that present with swelling and inflammation.

Zhi Zi Bo Pi Tang (梔子柏皮湯)

Shan Zhi Zi, Huang Bo, Gan Cao

Zi Jin Ding (紫金錠/Purple Gold Pill)

Quan Xie, Shan Dou Gen	1 liang each
Shan Ci Gu, Xiong Huang,	2 liang each
Zhu Sha, Qian Jin Zi	2 liang each
Wu Pei Zi, Da Xian	2.5 liang each
Da Huang	4 liang

Zi Yun Gao (紫雲膏/Purple Cloud Ointment/aka **Run Ji Gao)**

Zi Cao	120 g
Dang Gui	60 g
Ma You (Sesame Oil)	520 g
Mi La (Beeswax)	300 g

Dr. Lee purchases this ointment ready-prepared from a proprietary supplier. This formula is derived from the original composition presented in the *Orthodox Manual of External Medicine* (外科正宗 *Wai Ke Zheng Zong*).

Zi Cao enters the blood aspect of the liver channel, cools and quickens the blood, and resolves toxin and outthrusts papules; and Dang Gui quickens and supplements the blood, moistens dryness, disperses swelling and relieves pain, and engenders flesh. Ma You (Sesame Oil) functions both as an extractant, extracting the lipophilic active ingredients of the principal medicinals, and as a skin-conditioner and emollient (moisturizer). Mi La (Beeswax) functions as an excipient, both as an emulsifier, used to blend and stabilize liquids that are not mutually soluble and to improve the bioavailability of lipid-soluble compounds, and as a bulking agent.

Zi Yun Gao provides antibacterial and bactericidal actions for external injuries of the skin, promotes the growth of granulation tissue at the site of wounds, and enriches and moistens the skin. Dr. Lee commonly prescribes this medicinal ointment for topical application in the treatment of minor burns, eczematous dry fissured skin (e.g., pompholyx, cracked heels, atopic dermatitis), erosions (have reached the epidermis, but *not* for ulcerations, which have reached the dermis), chilblains, and hemorrhoids.

Zuo Gui Yin (左歸飲/Left-Restoring Beverage)

Dang Gui	2 qian

Gou Qi Zi, Fu Ling, Gan Cao	3 qian each
Sheng Di Huang, Shan Zhu Yu, Shan Yao	4 qian each
Tu Si Zi, Du Zhong, Cang Zhu	4 qian each
Niu Xi	5 qian

The Yu Sheng version is similar to the original formula except for Sheng Di Huang replacing Shu Di Huang and the addition of Niu Xi, Du Zhong, and Tu Si Zi. These additions enhance this formula's overall kidney yang-warming and -supplementing and essence-replenishing blood-supplementing actions and complement it with conductor medicinals that target the lumbus (spine) and lower limbs.

Niu Xi quickens the blood and frees the channels, supplements the liver and kidney, strengthens sinew and bone, and conducts fire (blood) downward; and Du Zhong supplements the liver and kidney, strengthens sinew and bone, and quiets the fetus. Together, the medicinal pair Niu Xi and Du Zhong serves as lumbus (spine) and lower limb conductor. And Tu Si Zi supplements the kidney and secures essence, nourishes the liver, and quiets the fetus.

In the early years of Dr. Lee's clinical practice, he would prescribe **Zuo Gui Yin** for insufficiency of kidney yin and yin vacuity with yang exuberance pattern pathoconditions, such as post-acute and chronic stage lumbar pain (e.g., degenerative disc disease) and limp knees and weak legs (e.g., articular cartilage, ligament, and tendon injuries of the lower limbs) presenting with pronounced heat (inflammation and swelling). Nowadays, Dr. Lee seldom prescribes this formula, often choosing to use **Zhi Bo Di Huang Tang** variants instead.

EPILOGUE

Our aim was to provide the reader with an insider's perspective on this subject matter through the compilation of these Q&A format case studies. We sincerely hope that TCM students, scholars, practitioners, physicians, and the interested layperson alike have gleaned valuable information on both the clinical application of TCM in primary and secondary care and as a first-line therapeutic option, as well as the integrative role TCM offers in neoadjuvant, adjuvant, complementary, and palliative therapy.

This fluid introduction of a broad spectrum of pathologies intends to inspire the reader to pursue further research and explore the vast potential for broader clinical applications.

We recognize that the development and expansion of TCM clinical applications is in part influenced by prevailing cultural factors and institutional barriers existing within each respective society and nation. Amidst these dynamics, TCM's increasingly manifest scientific basis and overwhelming efficacy continues propelling this 3,000 year-old medical system to the forefront of inquiry and discovery into its promising possibilities.

We hope that *Integrative Chinese Herbal Therapy Volume III Roots of Life* has piqued your interests for learning more and encourage you to read *Volume I Beyond the Being* and *Volume II Surfaces in Motion* of this series.

BIBLIOGRAPHY

Bensky, Dan, Steve Clavey, Erich Stoger. *Chinese Herbal Medicine: Materia Medica* (3rd Edition). Eastland Press, 2015.

Chang, Hsian-che; Tsai, Gui-hua. *Processing of Traditional Chinese Medicine Materia Medica* [Zhong Yao Pao Zhi Xue] Second Edition (Chinese). Taichung, Taiwan (R.O.C.): China Medical University, 2003.

Chen, John K.; Chen, Tina T. *Chinese Medical Herbology and Pharmacology.* USA: Art of Medicine Press, 2004.

Chen, Shi-gong. *Orthodox Manual of External Medicine* [Wai Ke Zheng Zong] (Chinese). China: Qing Dynasty (1617).

Cheng, Wu-ji. *The Clear Rationale of Cold Damage* [Shang Han Ming Li Lun] (Chinese). China: Jin Dynasty (1156).

Chinese Materia Medica [Zhong Hua Ben Cao] (Chinese). Shanghai, China: Shanghai Science Technology Publication, 1998.

Chinese Materia Medica Grand Dictionary [Xin Bian Zhong Yao Da Ci Dian] (Chinese). Taipei, Taiwan (R.O.C.): Xin Wen Feng Publishing Co., Ltd., 1982.

Clinical Applications of Traditional Chinese Medicinals [Zhong Yao Lin Chuang Ying Yong] (Chinese). Taipei, Taiwan (R.O.C.): Cheers Books Co., 1988.

Deng, Tie-tao. *Traditional Chinese Medicine Diagnostics* [Zhong Yi Zhen Duan Xue] (Chinese). Taipei, Taiwan (R.O.C.): Jyin Publishing Co., 2003.

Fundamentals of Chinese Medicine [Zhong Yi Ji Chu Xue] (Chinese). Taipei, Taiwan (R.O.C.): Cheers Books Co., 1994.

Harrison's Principles of Internal Medicine 19th Edition. McGraw-Hill, 2015.

Hong, Zhen-hui. *Dictionary of Chinese Medicine* [Zhong Guo Yi Xue Ci Dian] (Chinese). Taipei, Taiwan (R.O.C.): Li De Publishing Co., Ltd., 1983.

Huang, Wei-san. *Science of Acupuncture and Moxibustion* [Zhen Jiu Ke Xue] (Chinese). Taipei, Taiwan (R.O.C.): Zheng Zhong Publishing Co., Ltd., 1985.

Ke Qin. *Collected Writings on the Renewal of the 'Treatise on Cold Damage'* [Shang Han Lun Su Ji] (Chinese). China: Ming Dynasty (1674).

Keisetsu, □tsuka, *Thirty Years of Kampo Diagnosis and Treatment* [Han Fang Zhen Liao San Shi Nian] (Chinese). Tainan, Taiwan (R.O.C.): Zheng Yan Medical Publications, 1959.

Kou, Zong-yi. *Expanded Herbal Foundation* [Ben Cao Yan Yi] (Chinese). China: Song Dynasty (1116)

Lee, Chen-yu. *Neuropathy: Traditional Chinese Herbal Treatment in a Modern Medical Environment.* tr. Daniel L. Altschuler. Taipei, Taiwan (R.O.C.): Cheers Books Co., 2005.

Lee, Chen-yu. *Traditional Chinese Medicine Treatment of Common Liver Diseases* [Chang Jian Gan Bing Zhong Yi Liao Fa] (Chinese). Taipei, Taiwan (R.O.C.): Cheers Books Co., 2001.

Li, Dong-yuan. *Treatise on the Spleen and Stomach* [Pi Wei Lun] (Chinese). China: Jin Dynasty (1249).

Li, Nian-e. *Essential Knowledge of Internal Medicine* [Nei Jing Zhi Yao] (Chinese). China: Ming Dynasty (1642).

Li, Shi-zhen. *Herbal Foundation Compendium* [Ben Cao Gang Mu] (Chinese). China: Ming Dynasty (1590).

Li, Shi-zhen. *Supplement to the Herbal Foundation* [Ben Cao Gang Mu Shi Yi] (Chinese). China: Ming Dynasty (1590).

Ma, Jian Zhong. *Chinese Medicine Internal Medicine* [Zhong Yi Nei Ke Xue] (Chinese). Taipei, Taiwan (R.O.C.): Zheng Zhong Publishing Co., Ltd., 1986.

Neal, Anthony J., Peter J. Hoskin. *Clinical Oncology Basic Principles and Practice* (Third Edition). London, UK: Arnold, 2003.

Oswald, Cyril, Frank Delaigue. *Les Hommes de l'Art* (French). You-Feng (Librairie), 2013.

Taber's Cyclopedic Medical Dictionary (23rd Edition). Philadelphia, PA (U.S.A.): F.A. Davis Company, 2017.

Tang, Zong-zai. *Treatise on Blood Syndromes* [Xue Zheng Lun] (Chinese). China: Qing Dynasty (1884).

The Divine Husbandman's Herbal Foundation Canon [Shen Nong Ben Cao Jing] (Chinese). China: est. Qin or Han Dynasty.

The Yellow Emperor's Inner Cannon [Huang Di Nei Jing] (Chinese). China: Eastern Han Dynasty.

Wang, Ang. *Medical Formulas Gathered and Explained* [Yi Fang Ji Jie] (Chinese). China: Qing Dynasty (1682).

Wang, Ang. *The Essential Herbal Foundation* [Ben Cao Bei Yao] (Chinese). China: Qing Dynasty (1694).

Wang, Qing-ren. *Correction of Errors in Medical Classics* [Yi Lin Gai Cuo] (Chinese). China: Qing Dynasty (1830).

Wiseman, Nigel and Ye, Feng. *A Practical Dictionary of Chinese Medicine* (Second Edition). Brookline, Massachusetts: Paradigm Publications, 1998.

Wu, Qian. *Essential Teachings on Acupuncture and Moxibustion* [Ci Jiu Xin Fa Yao Jue] (Chinese). China: Qing Dynasty (1742).

Wu, Qian. *Essential Teachings on Miscellaneous Diseases* [Za Bing Xin Fa] (Chinese). China: Qing Dynasty (1742).

Wu, Qian. *The Golden Mirror of Medicin*e [Yi Zong Jin Jian] (Chinese). China: Qing Dynasty (1742).

Yakazu, D□ mei. *Kampo Prescriptions Explained* [Han Fang Chu Fang Jie Shuo] (Chinese). Tainan, Taiwan (R.O.C.): Zheng Yan Medical Publications, 1966.

Yang, Ji-zhou. *The Great Compendium of Acupuncture and Moxibustion* [Zhen Jiu Da Cheng] (Chinese). China: Ming Dynasty (1601).

Young, Wei-chieh. Annotated Explanations of The Yellow Emperor's Inner Classic: Basic Questions [Huang Di Nei Jing Su Wen Yi Jie] (Chinese). Taipei, Taiwan (R.O.C.): Chih-Yuan Publishing Co., Ltd., (1994).

Young, Wei-chieh. Annotated Explanations of The Yellow Emperor's Inner Classic: The Spiritual Pivot [Huang Di Nei Jing Ling Shu Yi Jie] (Chinese). Taipei, Taiwan (R.O.C.): Chih-Yuan Publishing Co., Ltd., (2006).

Young, Wei-chieh. *Practical Applications: Chinese Medicinal Formulas* [Shi Yong Zhong Yi Fang Ji Xue] (Chinese). Taipei, Taiwan (R.O.C.): Le Qun Cultural Publications, 1992.

Yun Tie-qiao, *Research on Treatise On Cold Damage* [Shang Han Lun Yan Jiu] (Chinese). China: 1923.

Zhang, Bo-yu. *Traditional Chinese Medicine Internal Medicine* [Zhong Yi Nei Ke Xue] (Chinese). Taipei, Taiwan (R.O.C.): Jyin Publishing Co., 1989.

Zhang, De-yu. *True Meaning of the Herbal Foundation* [Ben Cao Zheng Yi] (Chinese). China: Qing Dynasty (1828).

Zhang Ji [Zhong-jing]. *Treatise on Cold Damage and Miscellaneous Diseases* [Shang Han Za Bing Lun] (Chinese). China: Eastern Han Dynasty.

Zhang Xi-chun. *Records of Chinese Medicine with Reference to Western Medicine* [Yi Xue Zhong Zhong Can Xi Lu] (1918-1934) (Chinese). China: Chinese Medicine Classics Publications, 2016.

AMBOSS (Medical Knowledge Distilled)
https://www.amboss.com/us/

Cleveland Clinic
https://my.clevelandclinic.org/

DermNet NZ (All About the Skin)
https://www.dermnetnz.org/

Mayo Clinic
http://www.mayoclinic.org/

McMaster Pathophysiological Review
http://www.pathophys.org/

MSD (Merck) Manuals Professional Edition
http://www.merckmanuals.com/professional

Stat Pearls
https://www.ncbi.nlm.nih.gov/books/NBK430685/

UpToDate
https://www.uptodate.com/home

中醫世家 [Zhong Yi Shi Jia] (a Chinese language TCM databank)
http://www.zysj.com.cn/

醫砭 [Yi Bian] (a Chinese language TCM databank)
http://yibian.hopto.org/

ABOUT THE AUTHOR

Scott L. Herbster has spent the better part of the past 25 years in Taiwan and China immersed in Chinese culture and pursuing related studies in literature, philosophy, religion, music, martial arts, and traditional Chinese medicine (TCM).

From 1993 to 1996, he learned Mandarin at Normal Taiwan University Mandarin Training Center; from 2001 to 2007, he precepted under the tutelage of Dr. Lee Chen Yu at Yu Sheng Chinese Medicine Clinic; and from 2007 to 2012, he studied in the Postbaccalaureate Chinese Medicine program at China Medical University in Taichung, Taiwan, which included a Western medicine clerkship at Tri-Service General Hospital and TCM internships at Taipei Municipal Heping Hospital, Taipei City Hospital (Kunming TCM Branch), and Taipei City Hospital (Linsen TCM Branch).

Upon completion of his Chinese medicine degree in 2012 to the present, he has had the honor and privilege of returning to assist Dr. Lee in the clinical setting, as well as compiling and translating academic papers, case study presentations, and now this three-volume series of case studies.

ABOUT THE EDITOR

Marc Wasserman studied under Dr. Lee Chen-Yu from 2004 through 2014. During those years, he worked directly with patients in the clinic while also assisting Dr. Lee with research, translation, and publication projects. He and Dr. Lee often travelled together, making presentations at various international medical conferences.

Marc is a graduate of the doctoral program at Liaoning University of Traditional Chinese Medicine, a prestigious medical school in northeastern China. He is the first American of non-Asian heritage to complete the program. He holds a visiting professorship with Liaoning University of Traditional Chinese Medicine, and is an adjunct professor at Virginia University of Oriental Medicine.

Currently, Dr. Wasserman runs a small clinic in Hunt Valley, Maryland. For more information on his practice, please visit www.flowhealthclinic.com.

Made in United States
North Haven, CT
04 November 2026

21763950R00312